Alternative Pain Management:

Solutions for Avoiding Prescription Drug Overuse

Information Resources Management Association
USA

A volume in the Trending Topics
Book Series (TTBS) Book Series

IGI Global
DISSEMINATOR OF KNOWLEDGE

Published in the United States of America by
IGI Global
Medical Information Science Reference (an imprint of IGI Global)
701 E. Chocolate Avenue
Hershey PA, USA 17033
Tel: 717-533-8845
Fax: 717-533-8661
E-mail: cust@igi-global.com
Web site: http://www.igi-global.com

Library of Congress Cataloging-in-Publication Data

Names: Information Resources Management Association, editor.
Title: Alternative pain management : solutions for avoiding prescription drug overuse / Information Resources Management Association, editor.
Description: Hershey, PA : Medical Information Science Reference, [2020] | Includes bibliographical references and index. | Summary: "This book provides alternative solutions for managing and treating chronic pain, including through the use of mobile applications, online programs, self-management strategies, and virtual reality. It also promotes a further understanding of pain and how it is diagnosed and reviews pharmaceutical accountability when prescribing drugs for pain management"-- Provided by publisher.
Identifiers: LCCN 2019033337 (print) | LCCN 2019033338 (ebook) | ISBN 9781799816805 (hardcover) | ISBN 9781799816812 (ebook)
Subjects: MESH: Pain Management--methods | Complementary Therapies | Mobile Applications | Software | Prescription Drug Overuse--prevention & control
Classification: LCC RM143 (print) | LCC RM143 (ebook) | NLM WL 704.6 | DDC 615.1/4--dc23
LC record available at https://lccn.loc.gov/2019033337
LC ebook record available at https://lccn.loc.gov/2019033338

This book is published in the IGI Global book series Trending Topics (TTBS) (ISSN: pending; eISSN: pending)

British Cataloguing in Publication Data
A Cataloguing in Publication record for this book is available from the British Library.

Trending Topics Book Series (TTBS) Book Series

Mehdi Khosrow-Pour, D.B.A.
Information Resources Management Association, USA

ISSN:pending
EISSN:pending

MISSION

Every day all over the world, researchers are making groundbreaking discoveries that address current challenges and solve complex problems across a variety of fields. Due to advancements in technology, changes in demographics, adjustments to societal norms, the development of political and economic structures, and more, new theories, methods, strategies, techniques, and applications are constantly being established in response to both existing and evolving issues.

Based on the success of IGI Global's latest Trending Topics Campaign, which provides news snippets and trending research breakthroughs relevant to IGI Global content, IGI Global has launched this new book series, titled the **Trending Topics Book Series**, which offers small anthologies of reprinted IGI Global book chapters and journal articles hand-selected by IGI Global's Executive Editorial Board on topics currently trending and stirring up discussion and/or controversy.

Spanning across topics such as the multigenerational workforce, legislation for sustainability, emotional branding, privacy on mobile devices, robotics in healthcare, and bio-based product development, this book series aims to provide researchers, academicians, professionals, and students with the most up-to-date studies in order to advance knowledge across all industries.

COVERAGE

- Emotional Branding
- Privacy on Mobile Devices
- Bio-Based Product Development
- Library Budget Challenges
- Robotics in Healthcare
- Millennials
- Business Sustainability
- Aging Workforce
- Multi-Generational Workforce
- Environmental Legislation and Sustainability

IGI Global is currently accepting manuscripts for publication within this series. To submit a proposal for a volume in this series, please contact our Acquisition Editors at Acquisitions@igi-global.com or visit: http://www.igi-global.com/publish/.

The Trending Topics Book Series (TTBS) Book Series (ISSN pending) is published by IGI Global, 701 E. Chocolate Avenue, Hershey, PA 17033-1240, USA, www.igi-global.com. This series is composed of titles available for purchase individually; each title is edited to be contextually exclusive from any other title within the series. For pricing and ordering information please visit http://www.igi-global.com/book-series/trending-topics-book-series/228608. Postmaster: Send all address changes to above address.

Titles in this Series

For a list of additional titles in this series, please visit:
https://www.igi-global.com/book-series/trending-topics-book-series/228608

Five Generations and Only One Workforce How Successful Businesses Are Managing a Multigenerational Workforce
Information Resources Management Association (USA)
Business Science Reference • © 2020 • 364pp • H/C (ISBN: 9781799804376) • US $215.00 (our price)

Developing Eco-Cities Through Policy, Planning, and Innovation Can It Really Work?
Information Resources Management Association (USA)
Engineering Science Reference • © 2020 • 350pp • H/C (ISBN: 9781799804413) • US $195.00 (our price)

IGI Global
DISSEMINATOR OF KNOWLEDGE

701 East Chocolate Avenue, Hershey, PA 17033, USA
Tel: 717-533-8845 x100 • Fax: 717-533-8661
E-Mail: cust@igi-global.com • www.igi-global.com

Table of Contents

Preface

Countries all over the world and the United States in particular are currently facing an opioid crisis and prescription drug addiction problems. Doctors and medical professionals are providing care for chronic pain and other maladies, often by prescribing medicine with addictive properties, and when the prescription runs out, patients are finding themselves craving and needing more of the drug. Aside from the addictive properties in the medicine, the rising costs of pharmaceuticals cause patients to skip doses, reduce doses, or hoard medicine to make ends meet. These, along with other causes such as drug misuse, abuse, and theft by other household members, are driving medical professionals and patients to seek alternative approaches to alleviate chronic pain.

Drug misuse is a chronic issue across the globe in which the medicine is being taken in a manner not as it is prescribed, such as taking the wrong dosage or taking someone else's prescription. The most commonly misused medicines include opioids, depressants, and stimulants; these have all caused an increase in emergency room visits, overdose deaths, and prescription drug use disorders.

Chronic pain, most commonly noted in the neck, back, and knees, leave patients feeling uncomfortable and in a helpless position. With prescription medicine leaving the potential for harmful side effects and other potential problems, patients are seeking alternative pain management remedies and options. Popular alternative pain management approaches include acupuncture, chiropractic treatment, yoga, massage, herbal and holistic remedies, and hypnosis. Additionally, patients may seek out some less popular options such as aromatherapy, therapy, guided imagery, and mind-body therapy.

Acupuncture is one of the most common and sought-after pain management treatments. The practice uses disposable, stainless steel needles to stimulate the body's 14 major meridians—the energy-carrying channels—to correct the perceived imbalance causing the body's pain and/or illness. This centuries old treatment aims to decrease pain by increasing endorphin release near nerves that send a message to the central nervous system to block the pain. While acupuncture is one of the most common alternative pain management treatments, this and any other option is an important discussion between medical professionals and doctors as pain management is not a one-size-fits-all approach.

Alternative Pain Management: Solutions for Avoiding Prescription Drug Overuse is organized into five sections that provide readers with comprehensive coverage of important topics. The sections are:

1. Diagnosing and Understanding Pain
2. Drugs and Pharmaceutical Accountability
3. ICTs, Mobile Applications, and Online Programs
4. Self-Management and Therapy
5. Virtual Reality and Video Games

The following paragraphs provide a summary of what readers can expect from this invaluable reference work:

Section 1, "Diagnosing and Understanding Pain," opens this trending topic compilation by highlighting the latest trends in chronic pain symptoms and pain assessment. In the first chapter in this section, "Chronic Stress and Chronic Pain: Disability After Trauma and Global Trends," Prof. Branislav Starcevic from the Clinic for Orthopedic Surgery and Traumatology, Clinical Center of Serbia, Serbia explores the connections between chronic stress and chronic pain as well as their impact on the body. In the following chapter, "Pain Assessment Through Facial Expression," the authors, Prof. Sanjay Kumar Singh from the Indian Institute of Technology (BHU), India; Prof. V. Rastogi from the Institute of Medical Sciences (BHU), India; and Prof. S.K. Singh from the Indian Institute of Technology (BHU), India, review existing technology used in studying facial expressions as a form of pain assessment while highlighting the critical importance of them in young patients and nonverbal patients. In the final chapter of this section, "Stress Associated With Orthopedic Surgery and Feeling Pain," the authors, Prof. Kinga Sobieralska-Michalak of Ludwig Rydygier Collegium Medicum, Poland & Nicolaus Copernicus University in Toruń, Poland; Prof. Maciej Michalak of Kazimierz Wielki University in Bydgoszcz, Poland; Prof. Agnieszka Woźniewicz from Ludwig Rydygier Collegium Medicum in Bydgoszcz, Poland & Nicolaus Copernicus University in Toruń, Poland; and Prof. Aleksandra Pawlicka from The School of Language and Literature in Bydgoszcz, Poland, discuss the characteristics of pain in conditions that require surgical treatment, surgery-related stress reaction, psychological factors that influence how one feels pain, the consequences of pain in people's functioning, and postoperative pain and the assessment of pain level.

Section 2, "Drugs and Pharmaceutical Accountability," includes chapters on liability in the pharmaceutical industry and proper prescription practices. In the opening chapter, "Overview of Multicomponent Solid Forms," the authors, Prof. Rahul B. Chavan and Prof. Nalini R. Shastri from Solid State Pharmaceutical Research Group (SSPRG), National Institute of Pharmaceutical Education and Research (NIPER), Hyderabad, India, provide an overview of different multicomponent drugs that give the option of combining the drugs at a supramolecular level (nano-sized level). In the concluding chapter of this section, "OpTrak: Tracking Opioid Prescriptions via Distributed Ledger Technology," the authors, Prof. Peng Zhang, Prof. Breck Stodghill, Prof. Cory Pitt, Prof. Cavin Briody, Prof. Douglas C. Schmidt, and Prof. Jules White all from Vanderbilt University, USA; Prof. Alan Pitt of Barrow Neurological Institute, USA; and Prof. Kelly Aldrich from the Center of Medical Interoperability, USA, describe the structure and functionality of OpTrak, a decentralized app implemented using the Ethereum blockchain that targets the opioid epidemic currently plaguing the United States.

Section 3, "ICTs, Mobile Applications, and Online Programs," presents information on electronic and interactive approaches to pain management. In the first chapter, "An Innovative, Information and Communication Technology Supported Approach, Towards Effective Chronic Pain Management," the authors, Prof. Haridimos Kondylakis from Institute of Computer Science (ICS), Foundation for Research and Technology-Hellas (FORTH), Greece; Prof. Santiago Hors-Fraile from Salumedia Tecnologías, Spain; Prof. Lefteris Koumakis from Institute of Computer Science (ICS), Foundation for Research and Technology-Hellas (FORTH), Greece; Prof. Angelina Kouroubali from the Institute of Computer Science (ICS), Foundation for Research and Technology-Hellas (FORTH), Greece; Prof. George Notas from the University of Crete, Greece; Prof. Alejandro Rivero-Rodriguez from Salumedia Tecnologías, Spain; Prof. Prodromos Sidiropoulos from the University of Crete, Greece; Prof. Panagiotis Simos from the University of Crete, Greece; and Prof. Dimitrios G. Katehakis from the Institute of Computer Science (ICS), Foundation for Research and Technology-Hellas (FORTH), Greece, reports on the design of a novel technical infrastructure to support effectively and efficiently chronic pain management, based on an intelligent personal health record platform on top of already available ICT tools to improve patient data and effective communication channels. In the second chapter in this section, "Participant Perspectives on Benefits and Challenges of Engaging in an Online Pain Self-Management Program," Prof. Marian Wilson and Prof. Michele R. Shaw from Washington State University, USA evaluate participants' perspectives after engaging in an 8-week online pain self-management program in which the 47 participants were previously prescribed opioid medicines for chronic pain. In the following chapter, "Systematic Review and Evaluation of Pain-Related Mobile Applications," the authors, Prof. Anabela

G. Silva, Prof. Alexandra Queirós, Prof. Hilma Caravau, Prof. Alina Ferreira, and Prof. Nelson P. Rocha from the University of Aveiro, Portugal, explore the use of pain-related mobile applications to improve healthcare outcomes as well as hindrances to its potential among patients and medical professionals. In the final chapter, "Headache App: Usability Assessment and Criterion Validity," the authors, Prof. Tânia Dantas, Prof. Milton Rodrigues dos Santos, Prof. Alexandra Queirós, and Prof. Anabela G. Silva from the University of Aveiro, Portugal, aim to search for and characterize the mobile applications related to headache in terms of content, usability, and criterion validity.

Section 4, "Self-Management and Therapy," provides emerging information on therapies for pain management and strategies that allow patients to self-manage their symptoms. In the first chapter, "The Role of Self-Efficacy and Aging in Managing Disease," Prof. Debra N. Weiss-Randall of Florida Atlantic University, USA argues the efficacy of the Chronic Disease Self-Management Program (CDSMP), an evidence-based program that helps patients to boost their self-efficacy and improve their disease self-management when under the supervision of a physician. In the next chapter, "Research-Based Applied Psychophysiology: Yoga for Occupational Stress and Health," Prof. Ned Hartfiel and Prof. Rhiannon Tudor Edwards from Bangor University, UK explore the benefits yoga and yoga in the workplace can have on occupational stress and the body and decrease the amount of pain and sickness-related absences. In the concluding chapter of this section, "Whole-Body Cryotherapy as a Tool to Improving of Infrared Thermography Diagnostics," the authors, Prof. Armand Cholewka from the University of Silesia, Poland; Prof. Agata Stanek from the Medical University of Silesia, Poland; Prof. Karolina Sieroń-Stołtny from the Medical University of Silesia, Poland; and Prof. Joanna Kajewska from the University of Silesia, Poland, argue the benefits of cryotherapy on patients suffering from different diseases and its use as a rehabilitation tool.

Section 5, "Virtual Reality and Video Games," contains chapters with information on emerging uses of video games in pain reduction and rehabilitation. In the first chapter, "Uses of Virtual Reality (VR) for Chronic Pain," the authors, Prof. Bradley Chi from the Zucker School of Medicine at Hofstra/Northwell, USA; Prof. Brian Chau from Loma Linda University Health, USA; and Prof. Phillip Ta from Loma Linda University Health, USA, investigate the use of virtual reality as a therapeutic tool for chronic pain due to its impact on attention, emotion, and potentially central nervous system plasticity. In the following chapter, "Videogames as Therapy: An Updated Selective Review of the Medical and Psychological Literature," the authors, Prof. Mark D. Griffith and Prof. Daria J. Kuss from Nottingham Trent University, UK and Prof. Angelica B. Ortiz de Gortari from Nottingham Trent University, UK & the University of Liège, Belgium, examine video games as physiotherapy and occupational therapy, video games as distractors in the role of pain management, videogames and cognitive rehabilitation, video games and the development of social and communication skills among the learning disabled, video games and impulsivity/attention deficit disorders, video games and therapeutic benefits in the elderly, video games in psychotherapeutic settings, video games and healthcare, video games and anxiety disorders, and video games and psychological wellbeing. In the concluding chapter of this section and volume, "Look of Life: The Wonder Therapy," the authors, Prof. Vittoria Sichi, Prof. Giacomo Ercolani, Prof. Luca Franchini, Prof. Luca Golfari, Prof. Silvia Varani, Prof. Daniela Rizzoli, Prof. Raffaella Pannuti, and Prof. Daniele Roganti from the ANT Foundation, Italy, present a study of cancer patient usage of virtual reality in their treatments and the impact of it on their emotional wellbeing and pain symptoms.

Although the primary organization of the contents in this work is based on its five sections, offering a progression of coverage of the important concepts, methodologies, technologies, applications, social issues, and emerging trends, the reader can also identify specific contents by utilizing the extensive indexing system listed at the end.

Section 1

Diagnosing and Understanding Pain

Chapter 1
Chronic Stress and Chronic Pain:
Disability After Trauma and Global Trends

Branislav Starcevic
Clinic for Orthopaedic Surgery and Traumatology, Clinical Center of Serbia, Serbia

ABSTRACT

Pain and stress basically overlap in conceptual and physiological perceptions. Chronic stress and chronic pain share a common behavioral model of failure to extinguish negative memories as one of psychological and physiological mechanisms of defense. They also have discrepancies such that the final brain endophenotype of posttraumatic stress disorder (PTSD), depression, and chronic pain appears to be different among the three conditions, and the role of the hypothalamic-pituitary-adrenal axis remains unclear in the physiology of pain. Persistence of either stress or pain is maladaptive and could lead to compromised homeostasis. The effectiveness of interventions that may increase return to work and patient satisfaction in trauma victims should be a future directive of research.

INTRODUCTION

The concept of pain has remained a topic of long debate since its emergence in ancient times. It is considered that the initial ideas about pain as a new entity were defined before 1800. Since then, different theories of pain have emerged and become central topics of debate. The existing theories of pain may be appropriate for the

DOI: 10.4018/978-1-7998-1680-5.ch001

interpretation of some aspects of pain, but the history of pain problems is as long as that of human beings and the understanding of pain mechanisms is still far from very well defined and requires extensive research.

Modern theories sought a consensus definition for pain, and in 1975, the International Association for the Study of Pain defined the pain as "an unpleasant sensory and emotional experience associated with actual or potential tissue damage, or described in terms of such damage".(IASP,2011)

As a physical phenomenon, the emotional state of a person, as well as the context or situation associated with the pain also impacts the perception of the nociceptive or noxious event. For example, if a human experiences a painful event associated with any form of trauma a reoccurrence of similar physical pain will not only inflict physical trauma but also the emotional and mental trauma first associated with the painful event. That was a basic hypothesis primarily for defining the concept of posttraumatic stress disorder (PTSD). Research has shown that should a similar injury occur to two people, one person who associates large emotional consequence to the pain and the other person who does not, the person who associates a large consequence on the pain event will feel a more intense physical pain that the person who does not associate a large emotional consequence with the pain.

Acute pain with its unpleasant features plays an important role in protecting the body from potential injury and represents the characteristic evolutionarily created with the aim of survival. Painful sensation promotes a change in actions and behavior which could stop any further injury. On the other hand, chronic pain represents a pathologic condition which neither serves the defense of the organism nor is it harmless. By the International Association for the Study of Pain (IASP), the pain is considered to be chronic when it lasts or recurs for more than 3 to 6 months(Chadi,2017)

It is estimated that chronic pain affects about 20% of people worldwide3-6 and its treatment is considered to be a significant unmet therapeutic need.

The link between stress and chronic pain is a well known but this interaction still demands further investigation. It is possible that there are common central mechanisms that facilitate both stress and nociception. Investigation of this relationship that exist between stress and nociception could possibly lead us to the atypical approach in pain treatment (Ponsford,2008).

In this text the author aimed to give the overview of pain pathways and pain matrix, discuss the potential mechanisms that underlies transformation of pain from acute to chronic form and to point out the key site of action of the currently available medications. Special attention will be devoted to the reports of so far conducted investigations supporting and explaining potential synergistic mechanisms of stress and chronic pain, pointing out the direction for further investigations in search of more effective drugs or treatments for chronic pain.

Pain is a multidimensional sensation comprising sensory information, affective processing and a cognitive-evaluative component. Furthermore, pain leads to changes in autonomic body functions such as blood pressure, heart frequency. Pain perception can be substantially altered in different psychiatric disorders.

Experimental studies have described different mechanisms for altered pain perception and processing in several psychiatric disorders. Pain and stress basically overlap in conceptual and physiological perceptions. Chronic stress and chronic pain share a common behavioral model of failure to extinguish negative memories as one of psychological and physiological mechanisms of defense. They also have discrepancies such that the final brain endophenotype of posttraumatic stress disorder (PTSD), depression, and chronic pain appears to be different among the three conditions, and the role of the hypothalamic-pituitary-adrenal axis remains unclear in the physiology of pain. Persistence of either stress or pain is maladaptive and could lead to compromised homeostasis.(Chadi, 2017)

Neuroanatomical morphological supstrate assumed to be involved in pain processing and perception id dorsolateral prefrontal cortex(DLPFC). As previously mentioned, depression presents the final endophenotype of posttraumatic stress disorder. Depression is suppose to be overlapping in a majority of times when it is difficult to distinguish between PTSD and depression differentially in final diagnostic. Patients psychological characteristics induce the prevalence of PTSD morbidity as well as coping mechanisms. Neurophysiologically, in depression, reduced activity of the dorsolateral prefrontal cortex is found to be involved in psychomotoric slowdown and attention and memory deficit. Also a positive correlation is found to exist with the severity of trauma and pain perception.

The explanation of the reduced pain perception in depression lies in cognitive deficit of pain processing stimuli, and manages the visualisation of the hyperstimulation of this brain area.

Amygdala presents grey matter which activity is increased in depression, but decreased activity is shown in healthy patients when experiencing pain.

Stress is often described as a feeling of being overwhelmed. Stress can affect people of all ages, genders and circumstances and can lead to both physical and psychological health issues. Stress presents any uncomfortable emotional experience accompanied by predictable biochemical, physiological and behavioral changes. (Baum, 1990; Anderson, 2003)

Chronic stress can occur in response to everyday stressors that are ignored or poorly managed, as well as to exposure to traumatic events. The consequences of chronic stress could be very serious, particularly if it induces to anxiety and depression.

Chronic or ongoing pain includes several symptoms and conditions, including acute posttraumatic pain, depression, hostility, anxiety, sleep and rest disturbances (Castillo, 2006). In a study of Duivenvoorden et al., they found a high prevalence of anxiety and depressive symptoms in a population with end-stage hip and knee Osteoarthritis. After surgery a significant decrease of the prevalence of anxiety and depressive symptoms for both hip and knee patients was seen. In hip as well as knee patients, preoperative depressive symptoms predicted a lower Patient Reported Outcomes after surgery. Hip and knee patients with preoperative anxiety or depressive symptoms were less satisfied postoperatively. Because of the close relationship between psychological symptoms and pain and disability, the prevalence of psychological symptoms would be high in end-stage hip and knee Osteoarthritis patients. Preoperatively higher prevalence of depressive symptoms was found in hip than in knee Osteoarthritis patients. And that might be a result of the difference in ability to perform their activities of daily living preoperatively (Duivenvoorden,2103). Many trauma patients suffer from long term impairments, disabilities and handicaps, and at least half of all major trauma patients are left with one or more residual problems. Therefore, understanding the determinants of long-term functional consequences following trauma is important in order to improve the chances of a patient's recovery (Ponsord,2008). Trauma has been proposed as a causal factor or trigger of chronic or persistent pain.

Work disability due to chronic pain is estimated to be four times more than productivity lost due to lost workdays alone (Castillo, 2006). The results of the prevalence and early predictors of chronic pain of major lower extremity trauma patients, present that more than a quarter of the study group reported that their pain highly interfered with daily activities (Clay et al., 2010). Pain also has other consequences for its victims, including psychological regression (Clay et al, 2010). Those who suffer from chronic pain also use five times more health services than the general population (Castillo, 2006). As surgeons, we know that pain is an inevitable result of traumatic injury and the accompanying healing process. However, why do patients continue to endure pain long after they have been treated?

CONCLUSION

The biomedical model of health focuses on pain as the result of a physical injury (Clay et al., 2010). This makes it difficult to clinically explain the presence of disability after the pathology related to the injury has healed . Studies focusing on trauma populations suggest that factors during the course of recovery other than the injury are critical to the development of persistent pain and associated functional impairment. Such factors include high initial pain intensity, PTSD, worker's compensation status, education, low recovery expectations and depression (Clay et al., 2010). In the aforementioned study by Castillo et al. (Castillo, 2006), several early predictors of chronic pain were identified at baseline, including having less than a high school education, having less than a college education, low self efficacy for return to daily activities, and high levels of alcohol consumption. In addition, high reported acute pain intensity, sleep and rest dysfunction, depression and anxiety at 3 months post discharge were found to be predictors of chronic pain at 7 years (Castillo,2006).

Return to work is defined as a complete or almost complete return to pre-injury state. Return to work may represent the level of appropriate successful social reintegration after minor or major trauma and therefore coming back to work surrounding may indicate the level of personal fulfilment and sense of self-worth. The effectiveness of interventions that may increase return to work and patient satisfaction in trauma victims should be a future directive of research.

REFERENCES

Abdallah & Geha. (2017). Chronic Pain and Chronic Stress: Two Sides of the Same Coin? *Chronic Stress (Thousand Oaks)*, *1*. doi:10.1177/2470547017704763

Anderson, N. B., & Anderson, P. E. (2003). *Emotional Longevity: what really determines how long you live*. New York: Viking.

Baum, A. (1990). Stress, Intrusive Imagery, and Chronic Distress. *Health Psychology*, *6*(6), 653–675. doi:10.1037/0278-6133.9.6.653 PMID:2286178

Castillo, R. C., MacKenzie, E. J., Wegener, S. T., & Bosse, M. J. (2006). Prevalence of chronic pain seven years following limb threatening lower extremity trauma. *Pain*, *124*(3), 321–329. doi:10.1016/j.pain.2006.04.020 PMID:16781066

Clay, F. J., Newstead, S. V., Watson, W. L., Ozanne-Smith, J., Guy, J., & McClure, R. J. (2010). Bio-psychosocial determinants of persistent pain 6 months after non-life-threatening acute orthopaedic trauma. *The Journal of Pain*, *11*(5), 420–423. doi:10.1016/j.jpain.2009.12.002 PMID:20439055

Duivenvoorden, T. (2013). Anxiety and depressive symptoms before and after total hip and knee arthroplasty: a prospective multicentre study. *Osteoarthritis and Cartilage, 21*, 1834-1840.

International Association for the Study of Pain. (2011). *IASP Taxonomy*. International Association for the Study of Pain.

MacKenzie, E. J., Morris, J. A. Jr, Jurkovich, G. J., Yasui, Y., Cushing, B. M., Burgess, A. R., ... Swiontkowski, M. F. (1998). Return to work following injury: The role of economic, social, and job- related factors. *American Journal of Public Health*, *88*(11), 1630–1637. doi:10.2105/AJPH.88.11.1630 PMID:9807528

Ponsford, J., Hill, B., Karamitsios, M., & Bahar-Fuchs, A. (2008). Factors infl uencing outcome after orthopedic trauma. *The Journal of Trauma*, *64*(4), 1001–1009. doi:10.1097/TA.0b013e31809fec16 PMID:18404068

This research was previously published in Chronic Stress and Its Effect on Brain Structure and Connectivity edited by Ana Starcevic, pages 90-95, copyright year 2019 by Medical Information Science Reference (an imprint of IGI Global).

Chapter 2
Pain Assessment through Facial Expression

Sanjay Kumar Singh
Indian Institute of Technology (BHU), India

V. Rastogi
Institute of Medical Sciences (BHU), India

S. K. Singh
Indian Institute of Technology (BHU), India

ABSTRACT

Pain, assumed to be the fifth vital sign, is an important symptom that needs to be adequately assessed in heath care. The visual changes reflected on the face of a person in pain may be apparent for only a few seconds and occur instinctively. Tracking these changes is a difficult and time-consuming process in a clinical setting. This is why it is motivating researchers and experts from medical, psychology and computer fields to conduct inter-disciplinary research in capturing facial expressions. This chapter contains a comprehensive review of technologies in the study of facial expression along with its application in pain assessment. The facial expressions of pain in children's (0-2 years) and in non-communicative patients need to be recognized as they are of utmost importance for proper diagnosis. Well designed computerized methodologies would streamline the process of patient assessment, increasing its accessibility to physicians and improving quality of care.

DOI: 10.4018/978-1-7998-1680-5.ch002

INTRODUCTION

In a clinical setting, there is difficulty in reliably assessing and managing pain. Patient self-report is the most valid and widely used technique to measure pain due to convenience, does not demand advanced technology or specialized skills. It is typically checked and evaluated either through clinical interview, completing a questionnaire or by using a visual analogue scales (VAS). In the VAS, the intensity of pain is represented by marking a line on a horizontal scale, which is fixed at each end with words containing "no pain" and "worst pain". Though useful, these self-report procedures have significant limitations (Lewis, Allesandri & Sullivan, 1990), as they represent inconsistent metric properties across scale dimensions, they may facilitate efforts at impression management or deception, they may show reactivity to suggestion, and there may be differences between clinicians and sufferers' conceptualization of pain (Keefe, Williams, & Smith, 2001). Moreover, use of self-report cannot be used in significant populations, such as young children, patients who cannot communicate, the mentally retarded, and patients who have the need for assisted breathing. In these situations, an observer rating is required, and the Faces Pain Scale is commonly used where the observer chooses a face on the scale which best resembles the facial expression of the patient (Prkachin, 1986). This is highly impractical and inefficient if the observer is required for long periods of time which could be the case for a patient in an intensive care unit (ICU).

In addition to self-report and observer measures being highly subjective, these measures do not give a continuous output over time, as the only output measured coincides when the patient is at their emotional apex (e.g. highest pain intensity). They do not provide information on the patient's emotional state at times other than these peak periods. In an effort to address these shortcomings, many researchers have pursued the goal of obtaining a continuous objective measure of pain through analysis of tissue pathology, neurological "signatures", imaging procedures, testing of muscle strength and so on (Williams, 2002). These approaches are complex because they are often inconsistent with other evidence of pain, in addition to being highly invasive and constraining to the patient. Another aspect to this potential solution is to code pain using facial expressions.

Significant efforts have been made over a period longer than two decades, in identifying such facial expressions (Darwin, 1872; Hollander, 1939; Landis, 1929; Prkachin & Solomon, 1998). This measure of pain can be obtained by examining videotapes at each time step (video frame), and is the only such measure available. A limitation of this approach is that it needs to be performed offline, where manual observations are time-consuming and costly, which makes clinical use prohibitive. However, real-time automatic system can be used to train using such information which could provide significant advantage in cost reduction and patient care.

Faces in human species have evolved to express rich information for social interaction, including expressions of pain and emotions (Barlett, Littlewort, Frank & Kanglee, 2014). These expressions reflect behavioral sources of evidence about pain. Parents monitor their infant's facial expressions overtime, because they provide information about changes in their infants' affective states (Lewis, Allesandri & Sullivan, 1990; Rosenstein & Oster, 1988). Only the parent or carer can identify the source of distress, and they are the only ones who can take action to relive physical discomfort. At this age, the facial expression of the infant is one of the few behaviors an infant uses to change its world.

(Keefe, Bradley & Crisson, 1990) described pain behaviour as: People, who perceives pain, may vocalize their suffering by moaning, crying, complaining or may show signs of body postures or facial expressions related to pain. These are classified as verbal or nonverbal behaviors originating from pain behaviors, as they serve to communicate the information that pain is being experienced. Their description emphasizes that pain behaviours are informative and easily communicable. However, communication such as direct and indirect can be distinguished. Behaviours, for instance, facial expressions, appear to be exclusively adapted for social communication (Prkachin, 1986; Williams, 2002). Certain behaviours communicating pain serve primarily to modify it (e.g., rubbing an irritated part of the body). Pain expressions can be defined as salient behaviours, in any modality which accompany and are specific to pain, and appear to be adapted to function in interpersonal contexts. In principle, this definition includes other kinds of behaviour, such as vocalizations. The prime focus in this chapter is on the distinct features of facial expressions.

BACKGROUND

It is true that humans have perhaps always been sensitive to the facial expression of pain. Classic era artists were able to capture the sense of suffering by the representations of the face. An example is the sculpture Laocoön, depicting the death throes of a Trojan priest, which is notable for the facial expression representing agonizing pain. Pain assessment proves difficult when the patient suffers from brain damage, dementia or some other condition that compromises the patient's ability to engage in self-assessment and present a verbal report. In respect to the lack of pain assessment, clinicians may overlook new pathologies when they occur, resulting in failure to identify and alleviate the suffering of patients who actually experience pain that is not expressed verbally, and this may lead to higher costs of care (Chapman, 2008).

Charles Darwin characterized pain expression thus:

During the pain the mouth is compressed closely or the teeth are clenched, the lips are retracted, the eyes are wide spread as if in horrified astonishment (Darwin, pp. 173-182, 1955).

The study of pain expression on a scientific basis was the first major attempt proposed by Darwin. His views on emotions in general were steady with the approach to pain. He emphasized on expressive behaviors in order to understand the functions and origin of affective states and motivation. Nonverbal communication behaviors were acknowledged through the explicit role of functional adaptations. In a similar manner, he emphasized the concepts of inter-specific continuity and ontogeny. With higher priority given to the study of emotional communication, Darwin's contribution to the study of pain expression of which it was a part was largely forgotten for a century. One reason was the turn of behavioral science away from universalism and heading for cultural relativism that occurred at the cusp of the 20th century. Some early research (Landis, 1929) expressed the concern, questioning the notion was there anything universal and discrete to be found in facial expression. Despite the interest declining, there were occasional forays into the study of pain related facial expression. (Hollander, 1939) conducted an experiment on pain by placing a metal piece under a blood pressure cuff and inflating it, recording the pressure at which the subject 'winced.' Chapman and Jones (1944) used heat to evaluate the "pain-reaction". They noticed that: the initial contraction at the outer corner of the eyelids can thus represent the pain reaction end-points. There was no more appreciable alteration made by the participants, even when asked to keep from wincing.

These readings were interesting because they suggested that the region surrounding the eye carried important information about pain, and led to later interest in the ability to self-regulate displays of pain. In later work, Chapman (1944) noted that, pain reactions patients with 'neurosis' occurred at a lower threshold than in normal patients. After this work, studies of pain expression were intermittent and had little influence until the 1970s.

METHODOLOGICAL ADVANCES

Facial expressions, being complex in nature, are difficult to describe and quantify, as they evolves over time. Usually, they leave no record. These obstacles present a barrier to scientific analysis. Recent development in video technology which was affordable and accessible overcame this problem and stimulated growth of the field. However, technology does not, resolve the problem of quantification.

A major advance was the development of clearly described observational systems that addressed this problem, minimizing inference and maximizing 'objectivity'. (Some element of judgment was involved in the prevalent facial coding systems applied by humans, with the inherent subjectivity that entails due to which the word 'objectivity' is in quotation marks) Ekman and Friesen's (1978) Facial Action Coding System (FACS) has been the most significant. It provides facial expressions comprising of 44 'action units', representing distinctive changes produced by the muscle combinations or by individual facial muscles. Using FACS and obtaining autonomous datasets the system's performance is tested for ground truth. Through repeated review of video recordings, observers work from strict coding criteria to 'dissect' facial movements.

Gaining Interest in Pain Expression

Emerging interest in pain expression can be identified by four sources.

1. In the 1970s, psychologists working on the operant model came up with the concept of pain behavior. Based on these concepts it was proposed that almost all inferences about pain arise from behavioral observations (Fordyce, 1976) and focused attention on those behaviours.
2. Better methods for measuring pain were sought by researchers. Human studies have relied heavily on verbal reports, despite the concerns about their objectivity, susceptibility to bias and validity. As an observable behavior related to pain experience, it was considered that facial expression offered a means of evaluating pain that have avoided the issues of self-report and yielded a more 'objective' measure. Once the evidence of pain can be perceived by individuals in others then can render them assistance, or to take preventive measures to protect themselves against the threat shared with the person in pain. Thus, sensitivity to evidence of pain in others should be a universal human capacity. Early research showed that indexes of facial expression could be sensitive both to variables thought to influence pain and variations in pain (Prkachin, Craig, 1985).
3. Research on emotions by Ekman et al. (1969) and Izard (1971) supported the notion of a discrete set of universal, basic emotions which are identifiable in facial expressions.
4. The last and probably the, most important influence on the field were related to the advances in methodology.

The Structure of Pain Expression

The FACS was used to describe facial expressions in candid photographs of people in extreme pain. It was concluded that there was a characteristic pain expression, involving a lowered brow, skin drawn tightly around the eyes, and stretched open mouth horizontally with deepening of the nasolabial furrow.

Craig & Patrick (1985) performed experiments using FACS to describe the facial expressions of people's responses to the cold pressor test. They found significant pain-associated increases in at least six facial action categories: raising of cheek/lid-tightening, raising upper lip, lip-corner pulling, lips parting, eye closure/blinking and mouth opening.

Patrick, Craig & Prkachin (1986) studied reactions to pain on patients induced by electric shock, and found a significant increase in brow lowering apart from the aforementioned movements, to be associated with immense pain. The relative consistency of expressions associated with pain supported the concept of a characteristic 'pain expression'. Prkachin (1992) examined whether these expressions were consistent across painful stimuli using FACS to measure facial responses to four categories of nociceptive stimulation: pressure, cold, electric shock and ischemia.

The study demonstrated consistent increases in four actions – orbit tightening, brow lowering, eye closure and upper-lip raising/ nose wrinkling – across all four types of stimulation. In other similar studies, certain actions, (lip-corner pulling and eye blinking), were found to be only associated with some categories of pain. Thus, the conclusion reached from this evidence was that there is a basic pain signal involving four 'core' facial actions. A study of patients suffering from shoulder pain who were exposed to various potentially painful clinical range-of-motion tests (Prkachin & Solomon 2008) confirmed these findings.

Behavioral Pain Assessment Tools

Research by Li et al., (2008) identified six objective pain measures of psychometric properties that were developed to assess pain in non-communicative critically ill patients. Facial expressions are a common component of these behavioral pain tools. However, the descriptors vary across tools used to identify facial expression. The most common tools in use today, that include facial expression, are summarized below.

The component of these tools used for facial expression varies in their behavioral descriptors and scoring ranges. With a different intensity of pain score, each tool describes wincing, frowning and grimacing differently. The inclusion of the facial expression component in the majority of these tools was derived from previously described instruments (Mateo & Krenzischek, 1992; McGrath et al., 1985; Payen et al., 2001), chart review (Gelinas et al., 2004), and focus groups interviews (Gelinas et al., 2005). The Pain Assessment and Intervention Notation Algorithm (PAIN) (Puntillo et al., 1997) checklist of physiological and behavioral indicators of pain was derived from a review of available research and content validity was established by experts in critical care practice and pain.

The Pain Behaviour Assessment Tool (PBAT) (Puntillo et al., 2004) was then modified from the PAIN tool and the Children's Hospital Eastern Ontario Pain Scale (CHEOPS) (McGrath et al., 1985). Apart from, the PBAT was examined for reliability and validity of the facial expressions component of the tool, with much of the research centered on pediatrics studies. Both the PAIN and PBAT algorithm were developed not as a scoring instrument but as an observation tool to identify specific pain-related behaviours in patients who could respond to questions and were able to use a numeric rating scale of pain intensity.

The Post-Anaesthesia Care Unit Behavioural Pain Rating Scale (PACU BPRS) (Mateo and Krenzischek, 1992) along with the Non-Verbal Pain Scale (NVPS) (Odhner et al., 2003) was tested in a specialised population of the Post-Anaesthesia Care Unit. The PACU BPRS has four categories for assessing three types of pain (chronic, acute, and progressive pain) which were developed by (Chambers & Price, 1967). The four dimensions (restlessness, tense muscles, patient sounds and frowning or grimacing) range from none (0) to severe (2) with total pain score ranging from 0 to 10. The face and movement dimension of NVPS was based on the face, legs, cry, activity, consol-ability (FLACC) (Merkel, 1997) pain assessment tool. The FLACC was developed by clinicians in order to assure a simple, consistent method to identify, document, and evaluate pain in the pediatric population. One of the major drawbacks of the FLACC tool is that the cry and consol-ability dimensions are not appropriate for the critically ill or incubated adults. Thus, NVPS used only the movement and face dimensions of FLACC tool.

To assess pain in mechanically ventilated patients the Behavioural Pain Scale (BPS) (Payen, 2001) was developed. The BPS focuses on three dimensions (facial expressions, compliance with ventilation and upper limbs movement) ranging from 1 to 4 points with total pain score ranging from 3 to 12. Facial expression scoring from 1 (no response) to 4 (full response) was based on the hypothesis that these behaviours reflect increases in pain intensity in critically ill patients. The facial expressions were derived from the study of facial muscle actions related to pain states (Prkachin, 1992). The Facial Action Coding System (Ekman and Friesen, 1978) was used to measure facial actions during painful and non-pain periods in healthy adult volunteers. Prkachin categorized facial expressions of pain into four groups through graded pain intensity: tightening and closing of the eyelids, brow lowering, nose wrinkling and upper lip is rising. This classification was modified to a large extent by Payen et al., (2001) in the BPS to make it easier for evaluators to rate.

The Critical Care Pain Observation Tool (CPOT), a more recently developed tool, (Gelinas et al., 2006) comprises components of facial expressions that were derived from previous established tools, such as the PACU, BPRS, PAIN and BPS. The CPOT also consists of four components with ratings of 0 to 2 for each behaviour: facial expression, muscle tension, body movements and compliance with the ventilator for incubated patients and vocalization for extubated patients.

Although facial expressions have been included in these tools, they have not been rigorously tested. Since facial expressions are an important component of pain evaluation tools, the scoring should be based on objective data extracted from facial expression during pain in the critically ill. Recently developed tools, which are in use, include a wide range of facial expression descriptors, such as relaxed, no facial response, smile, wince, frown, and grimacing. It has been suggested that more research is required to identify facial indicators that are involved in pain-related distress. Systematic and accurate identification of facial expression during pain is, therefore, crucial.

Insight into Facial Expressions

The face reveals a wealth of information about emotions and human behaviour. The pain behaviour most commonly used in pain evaluation scales for people who cannot verbally communicate is, facial expression (Ambuel, 1992; Jonghe, 2003; Gelinas, 2006; Merkel, 1997; Payen, 2001; Puntillo, 2002; Salmore, 2002). Facial expression has long been studied, dating back to Charles Darwin's ''The Expression of Emotions in Man and Animals'' (Darwin, 1898) reporting observations and detailed explanations of why particular facial expressions occur with particular emotions (Black, 2002).

Ekman and Friesen, experts in facial expressions studies, performed extensive cross-cultural studies to determine if facial expressions are universal or specific to each culture (Ekman et al., 1969, 1971, 1987, 1972, 1993, 1999). They found that observers judgments of fear, anger, disgust, surprise, sadness and happiness made by preliterate people as isolated as New Guineans (Ekman & Friesen, 1971) were similar to the judgments made by college students. They arrived at the conclusion that regardless of gender, age, and race/ethnicity, facial expressions are real evidence of universal expressions across cultures with variation due to the expression itself, and in what the expression conveys to the person showing the expression and to others (Ekman, 1999).

Their studies contributed to the development of the Facial Action Coding System (FACS) (Ekman & Friesen, 1978), which distinctly identifies facial muscle movements during an emotional response. These facial muscle movements are typically identified by use of slow action video and stop-frame feedback. There are

44 action units (AUs) identified in FACS. Each Action Unit (AU) represents the movement of a single facial muscle or an association of muscles, which move as a unit. The 44 AUs can be reliably recognized by trained FACS coders and can also be upgraded on a five-point scale for intensity (degree of muscle excursion). Once the pain expressions are known, the relevant data on the number of expressions per minute during the course of each condition can be derived (Ekman & Friesen, 1978). The FACS has proved to be highly reliable in many studies and represents a distinct pattern of facial actions that are characteristic of pain (Ambuel, 1992; Craig, 1991, 1994, 2001). Facial Action Coding takes a long time if processed manually but advances in automated face analysis with the use of computer vision are being developed (Cohn et al., 1999). A high concurrent validity is reported with automated face analysis by feature point tracking and manual FACS in the eye, brow, and mouth regions.

Pain Related Facial Expression

Facial expression specifically related to pain has been studied using the Facial Action Coding System (FACS) (Craig et al., 1991, 2001;Craig & Patrick, 1985; Prkachin & Craig, 1985; Patrick et al., 1986; Prkachin & Mercer, 1989; Poole and Craig, 1992; Prkachin, 1992). Several facial actions correlated with pain that have been identified includes raised cheeks, lowered brows, closed eyes, tightened eyelids and a raised upper lip or opened mouth (Craig et al., 1991, 2001).

Expressions of acute pain-related facial activity have been identified in the general population, i.e. brow lowering, narrowing of the eye aperture from below, raising the upper lip, and blinking (Craig & Patrick, 1985; Patrick et al., 1986). Using FACS, facial activity associated with exposure to the painful stimulus in healthy adults was recorded and six action units (AU) categories that occurred more usually during exposure to the stimulus than during a baseline experience were identified.

Prkachin, (1992) concentrated on pain behaviour of healthy adults (n=41), focusing on facial expression during four different types of pain stimulus (cold, electric shock, pressure, and muscle ischemia). Using the FACS, he identified four actions during pain, increasing in intensity or duration amongst all modalities: brow lowering (AU4), closing and tightening of the eyelids (AU6/AU7), and nose wrinkling/upper lip raising (AU9/AU10). Hadjistavropoulos (2000) examined the validity of non-verbal measures to detect pain amongst adults who were experiencing movement related exacerbations of musculoskeletal pain and recorded the utility of behavioral coding of pain related body/limb movements (e.g., guarding and bracing). The results clearly showed that the FACS not only differentiated between pain and absence of pain but could also provide relevant information about the variability of the pain experience (Hadjistavropoulos, 2003).

Another study was performed Kunz et al., (2006) to evaluate gender differences in facial expressiveness to pain, using the FACS and focusing on 4 AUs: eye closure (AU 43), brow lowering (AU4), tightening of the orbital muscles surrounding the eye (AUs 6/7) and nose wrinkling/upper lip raising (AUs 9/10). They concluded that in young and pain-free individuals (male n=20, female n=20) both men and women were equally facially expressive while given tonic heat stimulation at painful and non-painful intensities. These observations were similar to previous findings of lack of gender differences in the facial expressiveness of pain (Craig, 1991; Prkachin, 1992).

In summary, it has been shown that the FACS provides an objective assessment of facial reactions that are the most reflexive and automatic non-verbal indices of pain related. Even when facial expressions have been reliably identified in children, infants, adults and the elderly using FACS, there is much less evidence of its utility in critically ill patients and more research is required.

Facial Expression of Pain in Children

The facial expressions of pain in children's (0-2 years) and non-communicative patients need to be recognized as they are of utmost importance for proper diagnosis. Researchers interested in the study of facial expressions of children must appreciate that, due to differences in skin texture, the absence of wrinkles and creases, and immaturity of neuromuscular systems, the expressions on face of children differ from those of adults. Grunau & Craig (1987) developed a measure of potential pain-related actions in newborns: the Neonatal Facial Coding System (NFCS). Nine specific facial movements are identified by the NFCS: eye squeeze, brow bulge, deepening of the nasolabial furrow, vertical mouth stretch, open lips, horizontal mouth stretch, taut tongue, lip purse, and chin quiver. Measurements of facial activity were taken during lancing of the heel to draw blood samples. Heel lancing was directly related to eye squeezing, brow bulging, nasolabial furrow deepening, taut tongue and lip parting. A hybrid technique, the Child Facial Coding System (CFCS) (Chambers, Cassidy & McGrath, 1987) was developed in order to evaluate facial expressions in preschool children.

The CFCS comprises codes for 13 facial behaviours. Gilbert et al. (1999) applied the CFCS on children who were of 13 to 74-month-old, recovering from surgery. Principal components analysis indicated loading at 0.60 or higher for the following actions: brow lowering, cheek raising, vertical mouth stretch, nasolabial furrow, flared nostril, nose wrinkle, horizontal mouth stretch, eye squeeze and lip corner pulling. Among children undergoing immunizations similar findings have been reported (Breau, McGrath, Craig, Cassidy & Reid, 2001). The findings suggested that there are similarities between the actions that have been directly associated with pain in children, neonates and adults, indicating continuity from the earliest days of life to adulthood. In a study of responses of young (21 to 38 years of age) and elderly (65 to 84 years of age) persons to mechanical and electric stimulation, both types of pain were directly associated with increase in orbit tightening (Kunz, Mylius, & Lautenbacher, 2008). Mechanical pain, too, led to an increase in brow lowering.

In brief, there is strong evidence that there is a similar facial response to different types of pain extending across the life span (Table 1). Prkachin, (1992) findings imply that the majority of the information about pain contained in facial expression comes from a limited set of facial actions, notably those produced by orbicularis oculi, corrugator, and levator muscles. There may be other actions recruited, but their occurrence is less reliable. Fundamentally, this suggests that researchers interested in assessing pain expression can safely limit their attention to these actions without missing information of key importance.

Changing Scenario

To find out relevant facial behaviours and to prove their validity is an important aspect, but it is limited as a goal in itself. It would add value if new dimensions or new interpretations were provided. This has begun to be realized in a number of areas, only a sample of which can be given here.

A question, commonly asked about the value of facial measurement is why it should be used if alternative methods are available and adequate. Indeed, it is commonly argued that the best and most effective method, of collecting data is the

Table 1. Homology of pain expression across the various stages of human life

Muscular Basis	Adult(FACS)	Neonate(NFCS)	Child(CFCS)	Elderly (FACS)
Corrugator	Brow lower (AU 4	Brow bulge	Brow lower	
Orbicularis oculi	Lids tighten, cheek raise (AU6, AU7)	Eye Squeeze	Eye Squeeze, squint, cheek raiser	Lids tighten, cheek raise AU6, AU7)
Levator	Nose wrinkle,upper lip raiser (AU9, AU10)	Nasolabial furrow, vertical mouth stretch	Nose wrinkle, Nasolabial furrow, upper lip raiser	Nose wrinkle, lip raiser (AU9, AU10)
Zygomatic	Lip corner pull (AU 12)	Lip corner puller		Lip corner pull (AU 12)
Risorius	Horizontal mouth stretch		Horizontal mouth stretch	
Plerygoid			Vertical mouth stretch	
Nasalis			Flared nostril	

Descriptors are from the system used to code expressions. AU Facial Action Coding System (FACS) action unit; CFCS Child facial coding system; NFCS Neonatal facial coding system. (Pain, 51, pp. 297-306)

verbal report, which is the 'gold standard' for assessing pain, although this has been criticized (Hadjistavropoulos & Craig, 2004). Of course, facial expression may prove to be useful in those significant instances in which verbal report is unavailable, as is the case with infants, neonates, and young children, or people with non verbal communication (Craig, Prkachin & Grunau, 1993).

Both the verbal report and the assessment of pain using facial expression brings added value. For instance, in a study by Kunz, Scharmann, Hemmeter, Schepelmann & Lautenbacher (2007), responses to five levels of mechanical pain were studied in patients with dementia. Participants were asked to rate the pain verbally and their facial expressions were measured using the FACS. Verbal ratings of pain usually supported the experience of patients and controls; however, facial responses to pressure stimulation were significantly enhanced in demented patients compared to healthy. This finding suggests a novel phenomenon – enhanced pain reactivity among those with dementia, the existence of which might not have been known had the researchers relied only on verbal report.

Developmentally, pain expression reflects the relationship between complex experiential, constitutional and environmental factors. These factors could be properly described and understood if investigations that incorporate assessment of pain expression were explored. Rocha et al. (2003) measured the intensity of pain expression among five-year-old children undergoing immunization.

Individual differences in pain reactivity were directly related to parent's reports of their children's somatization. While extending the study further a follow-up of this sample, at five years of age pain reactivity was associated with the children's own self-reports of somatic symptoms at 10 to 11 years of age (Rocha et al., 2003). These findings conclude that the intensity of pain expression in childhood (4-5 years) may serve as a marker of resilience.

Applications in Special Populations

Facial behaviour opens a new paradigm into the pain experience of populations who find difficult to express or communicate about pain in any language, including preverbal children. Many assessment instruments have been developed that make use of behavioral observations of facial expression.

For example, the Non- Communicating Children's Pain Checklist (Breau, McGrath, Camfield, Finley, 2002) was designed to assess pain in children with verbal communication impairments, and incorporate the five categories of facial expression: wrinkled brow, changing of look around the eyes, turning down of mouth, grinding teeth and tongue activity and clenching.

In one study (Grunau, 2002) the NFCS was used to study the influence of past pain experiences on pain reactivity among newborns with low birth weights undergoing heel lancing at 31 to 33 weeks post conceptional age. Infants who had undergone a greater number of painful procedures, judged to have more severe illnesses and who had been administered higher doses of steroids, showed diminished reactivity with respect to the test stimulus.

Stevens, McGrath & Gibbins (2007) studied neonates who were admitted to neonatal intensive care units. Three cohorts were described according to their risk of neurological impairment: pulmonary hypertension, respiratory distress (low risk) and meningitis or necrotizing enterocolitis (intermediate risk), and perinatal asphyxia (high risk). Facial actions with respect to heel lancing for blood sampling were measured with the NFCS. All the three cohorts displayed an increase in pain expression following exposure to the heel lance procedure. The cohorts with intermediate and high risk of neurological impairment displayed diminished facial responsiveness, suggesting either that the cohorts differed in their pain experience or the risk of neurological impairment is associated with diminished ability to express pain.

CLINICAL APPLICATION

Measurement of pain expression is mostly limited to research investigations due to its resource intensive nature. Moreover, investigators have worked toward the designing of systems for making routine observations of facial behaviour during pain which would be of great use in clinical settings. Observers have been provided ample training to perform real-time measurement of pain expression through physical examinations of low-back pain patients (Prkachin, Hughes, Schultz, & Hunt, 2002).

In children, the NFCS has been fruitful in real-time assessment of 32 to 33 week post-conceptional age infants who were undergoing heel lance (Oberlander, Grunau, Holsti & Whitfield, 1998). It was observed that the reliability of observations was high, especially with four movements (eye squeeze, brow lower, nasolabial furrow deepen and open mouth) showing clear discrimination amongst painful and nonpainful phases of the procedure.

In preterm infants, there are difficulties for assessment because there is evidence that facial pain expression is absent (Grunau, Oberlander, Whitfield & Fitzgerald, 2001). Holsti and Grunau (2007) developed the Behavioural Indicators of Infant Pain scale, an instrument for assessing pain behaviours in preterm infants. It combines pain-related facial actions from the NFCS with hand movements and sleep/wake indicators. The Behavioral Indicators of Infant Pain was applied in preterm infants using real-time video recordings as they underwent heel lancing. The scale was applied reliably by both experienced and inexperienced raters. It effectively distinguished between painful and non-painful phases of the procedure. It was concluded that in the ready availability of video recording equipment and evidence of the consistency of the procedures, these studies convey that clinical and real-time applications are possible and feasible.

SOLUTIONS AND RECOMMENDATIONS

Limitations of Facial Measurement, Alternatives and New Perspectives

Despite evidence of their value and reliability in a variety of people, facial measures have been of interest only to a small group of scientists and clinicians (Prkachin, 2009).

- The main reason is that assessment of pain by facial expression is burdensome. If the measurement is concentrated on the FACS, there is a considerable amount of time (approximately 100 h) which is involved in training. Observation is directly dependent on access to hardware and software for performing frame-by-frame analysis of any video sequence.
- A significant issue is the time required for observation. If one uses the full FACS procedure, a reasonable approximation is that for every unit of real time, coding requires 100 units. Based on all these observations and what have been learned, it is feasible to restrict attention to a smaller number of facial actions. However, in this approach coding still needs a significant amount of time.
- Facial coding techniques have other limitations too. Although characterized as 'objective', they are based, in the final analysis, on human judgments. There is always some element of subjectivity in deciding an action has occurred or when minimum requirements for coding are met.

In addition, the human observer may be biased or has inherent limitations in their capacity to make precise discriminations at the margins. Alternatives exist or are being developed. As the FACS has limitations in describing pain related expressions, it becomes necessary to adopt some other means of assessment. The next step towards application must involve computer technology that can recognize human AUs and, identifying and scoring pain dynamically. Both research and application will greatly advance the development of automated coding technology.

Judgment Studies

A relatively simple solution to this is the judgment study (Rosenthal, 1993). In a judgment study, untrained judges often rate some underlying dimension of behaviour. For example, samples of children's facial responses to an extreme painful event may be edited from the video recordings and presented to experts/judges to rate on a scale of pain intensity. The judgments of observers are of utmost importance in such studies as they are highly reliable (Prkachin, Berzins & Mercer, 1994) and can be summed into overall scores that signify the intensity of the reaction.

If such studies are properly designed, they have the advantage of providing additional insight into the social component related to the pain-expression nexus. Such methods have been valuable in shedding light on commonly observed underestimation bias in pain judgments: the fact that observers, including health care providers, generally underestimate others pain, when the criterion is of the pain reports of others. For example, it has been shown that the experience of observing higher levels of pain in others makes observers not so willing to judge others as being in pain, and they may not be able to differentiate between pain of different intensities. Prkachin, Mass and Mercer (2004) investigated the effects of exposure on perception of pain expression. Using similar methodology, studies show that children below five years of age are already sensitive to pain in others and they are capable of making quantitative distinctions (Deyo, Prkachin & Mercer, 2004).

FUTURE RESEARCH DIRECTIONS

Active investigations of facial expressions of pain began in the 1970s. Research involving processes such as direct measurement methods has come up with characteristic changes that appear to be homologous throughout the lifespan. Studies based on use of direct measurement have established novel insights into pain in children and adults, while studies, which have been centered on dimensional judgments, have also increased our understanding of how pain behavior is actually processed and acted on by others. Facial assessment however has historically been resource-intensive, recent developments in computer-vision assisted automated assessment and real-time assessment protocols promise to advance understanding of pain in clinical and research settings.

It is clear that facial expression of pain needs to be extracted effectively and efficiently for better results. A machine assessment system for expressions of pain needs to be developed to assist clinicians in diagnosing pain. However, little work has been done, and this will be discussed in brief. For this, an automated system for monitoring facial expressions could increase the sensitivity, reliability and precision of the research with respect to the relationship between facial signs and experiences of pain, and further it could lead to new insights and diagnostic methods. This commentary examines whether the procedures defined through research on facial expression of pain as reported by Williams (2002), provides a platform for machine understanding of pain-associated facial expressions.

This review may contribute towards the development of a computer-assisted system using machine learning techniques to be used as a tool for reliable, uncomplicated and effective clinical decision-making for pain assessment. This Intelligent Computing System is also intended to assist nurses to perceive the intensity of patient's pain successfully and to manage it effectively. Facial expression is an important channel for human communication. Current approaches to facial expression recognition (FER) in static images do not provide sufficient data regarding facial elements, muscle movements, geometric and appearance characteristics of facial expressions. Salient distance features using patches and their matching have been shown to give a good result (Zhang, 2011).

Intelligent Computing Systems (ICS) involving the details of the patient's symptoms and analgesia have significantly contributed to a drastic change in the old traditional concept of pain assessment making it more reliable and fast in clinical decision making. However this too has limitations with respect to the system's accuracy, reduced integration with mobile devices, web-based interfaces and above all, a scarcity of pain related databases. On searching the literature it was observed that the current state of the art focuses on the real-time aspects of pain assessment through facial expressions, demanding the design of ICS to incorporate these issues for higher accuracy. The configuration of facial actions revealing pain reduces the problem to that of pattern recognition. Advances in information technology approaches hold considerable promise to progress in this area. Substantial progress has been made toward the development of automated analysis of computer-based facial expression (Deyo, Prkachin & Mercer, 2004).

The advancements in related fields, especially image processing, machine learning and human cognition has helped to take a further step in detecting such facial expressions automatically. Zhang (2011) suggested improving the performance of facial expression recognition (FER) by automatically capturing facial movement features in static images based on distance features. The performance of such systems to detect pain -related facial actions has been examined among a sample of patients undergoing range of motion testing for assessing shoulder pain (Tian, Cohn, Kanade, 2005). Digital videos containing pain expressions were processed using Active Appearance Model (Ashraf, Lucey & Cohn, 2007).

Lucey et al. (2006) introduced a technique that allows variations in the geometric shape and appearance of the face to be separated. Machine learning algorithms were used to train a system for depicting predictions of pain versus no pain. The study displayed a hit rate of 83%, with a false alarm rate of 30% which was obtained with the best performing predictive model. A significant advantage of this technique is its ability to represent the dynamic changes in pain-related actions that can provide insight into motor control processes associated with regulating pain expression. Schiavenato et al. (2008) suggested an alternative approach, the point-pair method. Individual video frames of neonates before and after heel lancing were used. Landmarks relating to NFCS actions were selected, and standardized distances between pairs of points were compared. Results were very consistent with behavioral studies representing major pain associated differences like brow lowering, mouth opening, and tightening of orbit. Systems based on information technology are currently not so prevalent, but it is clear that their use in assessing pain expression is feasible and they will add value with further research.

Active Appearance Model (AAM) is a computer vision system which can automatically detect pain based on facial expressions coded using FACS. The shoulder pain archive contains images of patients with rotator-cuff injuries, with spontaneous facial expressions associated with pain which are not posed or feigned. These facial actions vary in duration and intensity and often coincide with abrupt changes in head position. The AAM approach specifies that both shape (i.e. contour) and appearance (i.e. texture) are both vital for gaining accurate detection performance (Ashraf et. al., 2009).

When the head is in motion there are difficulties associated with detecting spontaneous data, for example with pain, where there is a lot of head motion. This is a particular problem for systems that use similarity normalized appearance features (i.e. normalized for rotation, translation, and scale), as some portions of the face may not be visible, prohibiting accurate detection. On fusing all the dimensions of AAM representations (i.e. appearance, similarity normalized shape and canonical normalized appearance which are synthesized) using linear logistical regression (LLR), improves the efficiency of both pain detection performance and AU.

In the literature there are several existing classes of methods that are proposed regarding facial expression analysis, such as those based on the measurements of the geometrical shapes of facial features and their spatial arrangements, analysis of facial motion, spatial pattern analysis using techniques based on Principal Component Analysis (PCA), pattern analysis at gray level using local spatial filters and so forth. In the literature, there is no predominant methodology therefore choosing the right method is highly relevant to objectives of a system. Depending on the applications for instance, if high performance in speed is desired then PCA algorithm is the optimum, although it has around 75% success. For a higher success rate the Gabor wavelet algorithm is the best with nearly 95% success.

Two important related issues, to tackle in automatic pain recognition, are how to take into account the bidirectional influence and the contextual information between the person in pain and others. Audio-visual indicators of pain need to be merged with contextual and social information related to pain to create a context-sensitive multimodal and interpersonal system for an objective measurement of pain and its intensity, which is again a difficult job.

One of the biggest obstacles to date for the automatic measurement of pain has been the lack of appropriate and accessible audio-video archives of patients or participants in a clinical context. To learn relevant features and train classifiers, well-labeled unscripted behavior related to the experience of different kinds and severity of pain is necessary. Interdisciplinary efforts to address this need have begun.

Another weakness of this facial expression-driven pain assessment is the lack of a database, as we know that pain is spontaneous and thus expressions on the face appear only for few second, so tracking this is a difficult task. Coding of Action Units in FACS involves great expertise and above all it is very time consuming.

CONCLUSION

This paper has proposed that an intelligent computing system will help patient assessment and research to overcome the existing barriers to quality pain assessment and facilitate patient-physician communications in real time.

Pain assessment is a significant challenge in noncommunicative seriously ill adults, as they are unable to communicate the intensity of their pain level. In critical care, many factors alter verbal communication with patients including reduced level of consciousness, tracheal intubation, sedation and administration of paralyzing drugs.

Therefore, accurate assessment is of utmost importance in non-verbal pain behaviours such as facial expression, generally in the critically ill. Emotions, cognitive processes and social interactions (Ekman, 1999) are represented by facial expressions providing a critical behavioral measure. Facial expressions, in particular, are recommended by experts as a standard in pain assessment (Craig, 1998) because they represent the most specific and frequent indicators of pain.

A thorough understanding of facial expressions may assist in the development of strategies to enhance pain assessment tools. Tools which have been recently in use to assess pain in the non-communicative critically ill patient have not been universally accepted although they provide a broad range of descriptors of facial expressions. It is quite interesting that most of the facial descriptors that are identified in the pain assessment tools are concerned with the upper face (eyes and brow). Using the Facial Action Coding System (FACS) to study facial expressions in this region may be feasible since other facial areas (mouth, nose) are generally distorted by the presence of a nasogastric or endotracheal tubes. Liossi et al., (2014) showed that eye tracking is one of the most promising methodologies for future research on pain disorders and is being combined with previously used tools and techniques for pain assessment. Specifically, data on facial action coding may provide empirical evidence to validate the use of facial expressions accurately in assessment tools that are reliable, practical, appropriate and valid across patient groups.

REFERENCES

Ambuel, B., Hamlett, K. W., Marx, C. M., & Blumer, J. L. (1992). Assessing distress in pediatric intensive care environments: The COMFORT scale. *Journal of Pediatric Psychology, 17*(1), 95–109. doi:10.1093/jpepsy/17.1.95 PMID:1545324

Ashraf, A. B. L., Simon, C. F., Chen, T., & Ambadar. (2009). The painful face – Pain expression recognition using active appearance models. *ACM Journal Image and Vision Computing, 27*(12), 1788-1796.

Ashraf, A. B., Lucey, S., & Cohn, J. F. (2007). The painful face: Pain expression assessment of pain behavior during clinical assessment of low-back pain patients. back pain: identification of pain behavior subgroups. *Pain, 40*, 153–160.

Barlett, M. S., Littlewort, G. C., & Frank, M. G. (2014). Automatic decoding of facial movements reveals deceptive pain expressions. *Current Biology, 24*(7), 738–743. doi:10.1016/j.cub.2014.02.009 PMID:24656830

Black, J. (2002). Darwin in the world of emotions. *Journal of the Royal Society of Medicine, 95*(6), 311–313. doi:10.1258/jrsm.95.6.311 PMID:12042386

Brahnam, S., Chuang, C.F., Sexton, R.S., & Shih, F.Y. (2007). Machine assessment of neonatal facial expressions of acute pain. *ACM Journal on Decision Support Systems, 43*(4), 1242- 1254.

Breau, L. M., McGrath, P. J., Camfield, C. S., & Finley, G. A. (2002). Psychometric properties of the non- communicating children's pain check list revised. *Pain, 99*(1), 349–357. doi:10.1016/S0304-3959(02)00179-3 PMID:12237214

Breau, L. M., McGrath, P. J., Craig, K. D., Santor, D., Cassidy, K. L., & Reid, G. (2001). Facial expression of children receiving immunizations: A principal components analysis of the Child Facial Coding System. *The Clinical Journal of Pain, 17*(2), 178–186. doi:10.1097/00002508-200106000-00011 PMID:11444720

Chambers, C. T., Cassidy, K. L., & McGrath, P. J. (1996). *Child Facial Coding System: A Manual Nova Scotia and Vancouver*. Dalhousie University and University of British Columbia.

Chambers, W., & Price, G. (1967). Influence of nurse upon effects of analgesics administered. *Nursing Research, 967*(16), 228–233.

Chapman, C. R. (2008). Progress in Pain Assessment: The Cognitively Compromised Patient. *Current Opinion in Anaesthesiology, 21*(5), 610–615. doi:10.1097/ACO.0b013e32830a4bfd PMID:18784487

Chapman, W. P. (1944). Measurements of pain sensitivity in normal control subjects and in psychoneurotic patients. *J. Psychosom. Med., 6*(3), 252–257. doi:10.1097/00006842-194407000-00008

Chapman, W. P., & Jones, C. M. (1944). *Variations in cutaneous and visceral pain sensitivity in normal subjects*. Clin. Invest.

Craig, K. D., Hadjistavropoulos, H. D., Grunau, R. V., & Whitfield, M. F. (1994). A comparison of two measures of facial activity during pain in the newborn child. *Journal of Pediatric Psychology, 19*(3), 305–318. doi:10.1093/jpepsy/19.3.305 PMID:8071797

Craig, K. D., Hyde, S. A., & Patrick, C. J. (1991). Genuine, suppressed and faked facial behavior during exacerbation of chronic low back pain. *Pain, 46*(2), 161–171. doi:10.1016/0304-3959(91)90071-5 PMID:1836259

Craig, K. D., & Patrick, C. J. (1985). Facial expression during induced pain. *Journal of Personality and Social Psychology, 48*(4), 1080–1091. doi:10.1037/0022-3514.48.4.1089 PMID:3989673

Craig, K. D., Prkachin, K. M., & Grunau, R. V. E. (1993). *The facial expression of pain. Handbook of pain assessment*. New York: Guilford.

Darwin, C. (1872). *The expression of emotion in man and animals*. New York: Philosophical Library.

DeJonghe, B., Cook, D., Griffith, L., Appere-de-Vecchi, C., Guyatt, G., Théron, V., ... Outin, H. (2003). Adaptation to the Intensive Care Environment (ATICE): Development and validation of a new sedation assessment instrument. *Critical Care Medicine, 31*(9), 2344–2354. doi:10.1097/01.CCM.0000084850.16444.94 PMID:14501966

Deyo, K., Prkachin, K. M., & Mercer, S. R. (2004). Development of sensitivity to facial expressions of pain. *Pain, 107*(1), 16–21. doi:10.1016/S0304-3959(03)00263-X PMID:14715384

Ekman, P. (1999). *Handbook of cognition and emotion.* New York: Wiley.

Ekman, P., & Cole, J. (1972). *Universals and cultural differences in facial expressions of emotion.* Lincoln, NE: University of Nebraska Press.

Ekman, P., & Friesen, W. V. (1971). Constants across cultures in the face and emotion. *Journal of Personality and Social Psychology, 17*(2), 124–129. doi:10.1037/h0030377 PMID:5542557

Ekman, P., & Friesen, W. V. (1978). *Investigator's guide to the Facial Action Coding System.* Palo Alto, CA: Consulting Psychologists Press.

Ekman, P., Friesen, W. V., O'Sullivan, M., Chan, A., & et al. (1987). Universals and cultural differences in the judgments of facial expressions of emotion. *Journal of Personality and Social Psychology, 53*(4), 712–717. doi:10.1037/0022-3514.53.4.712 PMID:3681648

Ekman, P., Sorenson, E. R., & Friesen, W. V. (1969). Pain cultural elements in facial displays of emotions. *Science, 164*(3875), 86–88. doi:10.1126cience.164.3875.86 PMID:5773719

Fordyce, W.E., & Louis, S. (1976). *Behavioral Methods for Chronic Pain and Illness.* Academic Press.

Gelinas, C., Harel, F., Fillion, L., Puntillo, K. A., & Johnston, C. C. (2008). Sensitivity and specificity of the critical care pain observation tool for the detection of pain in intubated adults after cardiac surgery. *Journal of Pain and Symptom Management.* PMID:18599262

Gilbert, C. A., Lilley, C. M., Craig, K. D., McGrath, P. J., Court, C. A., Bennett, S. M., & Montgomery, C. J. (1999). Postoperative pain expression in preschool childen: Validation of the Child Facial Coding System. *The Clinical Journal of Pain, 15*(3), 192–200. doi:10.1097/00002508-199909000-00006 PMID:10524472

Grunau, R. E., Oberlander, T., Holsti, L., & Whitfield, M. F. (1998). Bedside application of the Neonatal Facial Coding System in Pain assessment of premature neonates. *Pain, 76*(3), 277–286. doi:10.1016/S0304-3959(98)00046-3 PMID:9718246

Grunau, R. E., Oberlander, T. F., Whitfield, M. F., Fitzgerald, C., & Lee, S. K. (2001). Demographic and therapeutic determinants of pain reactivity in very low birth weight neonates at 32 weeks postconceptional age. *Pediatrics*, *107*(1), 105–112. doi:10.1542/peds.107.1.105 PMID:11134442

Grunau, R. V., & Craig, K. D. (1987). Pain expression in neonates: Facial action and cry. *Pain*, *28*(3), 395–410. doi:10.1016/0304-3959(87)90073-X PMID:3574966

Hadjistavropoulos, T., Chapelle, D. L., MacLeod, F. K., Snider, B., & Craig, K. D. (2000). Measuring movement- exacerbated pain in cognitively impaired frail elders. *The Clinical Journal of Pain*, *16*(1), 54–59. doi:10.1097/00002508-200003000-00009 PMID:10741819

Hadjistavropoulos, T., & Craig, K. D. (2004). *Pain: Psychological Perspectives*. New York: Erlbaum.

Hadjistavropoulos, T., LaChapelle, D. L., Hadjistavropoulos, H. D., & Green, S. (2002). Using facial expressions to assess musculoskele-tal pain in older persons. *European Journal of Pain (London, England)*, *6*(3), 179–187. doi:10.1053/eujp.2001.0327 PMID:12036305

Hollander, E. (1939). A clinical gauge for sensitivity to pain. *The Journal of Laboratory and Clinical Medicine*, 524–537.

Holsti, L., & Grunau, R. E. (2007). Initial validation of the Behavioral Indicators of Infant Pain (BIIP). *Pain*, *132*(3), 264–272. doi:10.1016/j.pain.2007.01.033 PMID:17382473

Izard, C. E. (1971). *The Face of Emotion*. New York: Appleton-Century-Crofts.

Keefe, F. J., Bradley, L. A., & Crisson, J. E. (1990). Behavioral assessment of low back pain: Identification of pain behavior subgroups. *Pain*, *40*(2), 153–160. doi:10.1016/0304-3959(90)90066-M PMID:2137905

Keefe, F. J., Williams, D. A., & Smith, S. J. (2001). Assessment of pain behaviors. In D. C. Turk & R. Melzack (Eds.), *Handbook of Pain Assessment* (2nd ed.; pp. 170–187). New York: Guilford.

Kunz, M., Mylius, V., Schepelmann, K., & Lautenbacher, S. (2008). Impact of age on the facial expression of pain. *Journal of Psychosomatic Research*, *64*(3), 311–318. doi:10.1016/j.jpsychores.2007.09.010 PMID:18291247

Kunz, M., Scharmann, S., Hemmeter, U., Schepelmann, K., & Lautenbacher, S. (2009). The facial expression of pain in patients with dementia. *Pain*, *133*(1), 221–228. doi:10.1016/j.pain.2007.09.007 PMID:17949906

Landis, C. (1929). The interpretation of facial expression in emotion. *The Journal of General Psychology*, *2*(1), 59–72. doi:10.1080/00221309.1929.9918042

LeResche, L. (1982). Facial expression in pain: A survey of candid photographs. *Journal of Nonverbal Behavior*, *7*(1), 45–56. doi:10.1007/BF01001777

Lewis, M. J., Allesandri, S. M., & Sullivan, M. W. (1990). Violation of expectancy, loss of control and anger expressions in young infants. *Developmental Psychology*, *26*(5), 745–751. doi:10.1037/0012-1649.26.5.745

Li, D., Puntillo, K., & Miaskowski, C. (2008). A review of objective pain measures for use with critical care adult patients unable to self-report. *The Journal of Pain*, *9*(1), 2–10. doi:10.1016/j.jpain.2007.08.009 PMID:17981512

Liossi, C., Schoth, D. E., Godwin, H., & Liversedge, S. P. (2014). Using eye movements to investigate selective attention in chronic daily headache. *Pain*, *155*(3), 503–510. doi:10.1016/j.pain.2013.11.014 PMID:24287436

Lucey, S., Matthews, I., Hu, C., Ambadar, Z., & Cohn, J. F. (2006). AAM derived face representations for robust facial action recognition. In *Proceedings of Seventh IEEE International Conference on Automatic Face and Gesture Recognition* (pp. 155-60). IEEE. 10.1109/FGR.2006.17

Mateo, O. M., & Krenzischek, D. A. (1992). A pilot study to assess the relationship between behavioral manifestations and self-report of pain in post anesthesia care unit patients. *Journal of Post Anesthesia Nursing*, *7*, 15–21. PMID:1531235

McGrath, P. J., & Johnson, G. (1985). CHEOPS: A behavioral scale for rating postoperative pain in children. *Adv. Pain Res.*, *9*, 395–402.

Merkel, S. I., Lewis, T., Shayevitz, J. R., & Malviya, S. (1997). The FLACC: A behavioral scale for scoring post operative pain in young children. *Pediatric Nursing*, *23*, 293–297. PMID:9220806

Patrick, C. J., Craig, K. D., & Prkachin, K. M. (1986). Observer judgments of acute pain: Facial action determinants. *Journal of Personality and Social Psychology*, *50*(6), 1291–1298. doi:10.1037/0022-3514.50.6.1291 PMID:3723341

Payen, J. F., Bru, O., Bosson, J. L., Lagrasta, A., Novel, E., Deschaux, I., ... Jacquot, C. (2001). Assessing pain in critically ill sedated patients by using a behavioral pain scale. *Critical Care Medicine*, *29*(12), 2258–2263. doi:10.1097/00003246-200112000-00004 PMID:11801819

Prkachin, K. M. (1986). Pain behaviour is not unitary. *Behavioral and Brain Sciences*, *9*(04), 754–757. doi:10.1017/S0140525X00052316

Prkachin, K. M. (1992). The consistency of facial expressions of pain: A comparison across modalities. *Pain, 51*(3), 297–306. doi:10.1016/0304-3959(92)90213-U PMID:1491857

Prkachin, K. M. (2007). The coming of age of pain expression. *Pain, 133*(1), 3–4. doi:10.1016/j.pain.2007.10.015 PMID:17959311

Prkachin, K. M., Berzins, S., & Mercer, S. R. (1994). Berzins S, Mercer SR. Encoding and decoding of pain expressions: A judgement study. *Pain, 58*(2), 253–259. doi:10.1016/0304-3959(94)90206-2 PMID:7816493

Prkachin, K. M., & Craig, K. D. (1985). Influencing nonverbal expressions of pain:Signal detection analyses. *Pain, 21*(4), 399–409. doi:10.1016/0304-3959(85)90168-X PMID:4000689

Prkachin, K. M., Hughes, E. A., Schultz, I., Joy, P., & Hunt, D. (2002). Real-time assessment of pain behavior during clinical assessment of low-back pain patients. *Pain, 95*(1), 23–30. doi:10.1016/S0304-3959(01)00369-4 PMID:11790464

Prkachin, K. M., Mass, H., & Mercer, S. R. (2004). Effects of exposure on perception of pain expression. *Pain, 111*(1), 8–12. doi:10.1016/j.pain.2004.03.027 PMID:15327803

Prkachin, K. M., & Solomon, P. E. (2008). The structure, reliability and validity of pain expression: Evidence from patients with shoulder pain. *Pain, 139*(2), 267–274. doi:10.1016/j.pain.2008.04.010 PMID:18502049

Puntillo, K. A. (1990). Pain experiences of intensive care unit patients. *Pain, 19*, 526–533. PMID:2211161

Puntillo, K. A. (1997). Stitch, creating an effective pain management program for critically ill patients. *Journal of Critical Care, 6*, 259–260. PMID:9215421

Puntillo, K. A., Miaskowski, C., Kehrle, K., Stannard, D., Gleeson, S., & Nye, P. (1997). Relationship between behavioral and physiological indicators of pain, critical care patients' self-reports of pain, and opioid administration. *Critical Care Medicine, 25*(7), 1159–1166. doi:10.1097/00003246-199707000-00017 PMID:9233742

Puntillo, K. A., Morris, A. B., Thompson, C. L., Stanik-Hutt, J., White, C. A., & Wild, L. R. (2004). Wild LR. Pain behaviors observed during six common procedures: Results from Thunder Project II. *Critical Care Medicine, 32*(2), 421–427. doi:10.1097/01.CCM.0000108875.35298.D2 PMID:14758158

Puntillo, K. A., Neighbour, M., O'Neil, N., & Nixon, R. (2003). Accuracy of emergency nurses in assessment of patients' pain. *Pain Management Nursing, 4*(4), 171–175. doi:10.1016/S1524-9042(03)00033-X PMID:14663795

Puntillo, K. A., Pasero, C., & Li, D. (2009). Evaluation of pain in ICU patients. *Chest, 135*(4), 1069–1074. doi:10.1378/chest.08-2369 PMID:19349402

Puntillo, K. A., Stannard, D., Miaskowski, C., Kehrle, K., & Gleeson, S. (2002). Use of a pain assessment and intervention notation (PAIN) tool in critical care nursing practice: Nurses' evaluations. *Heart & Lung, 31*(4), 303–314. doi:10.1067/mhl.2002.125652 PMID:12122394

Puntillo, K. A., White, C., & Morris, A. B. (2001). Patients' perceptions and responses to procedural pain: Results from Thunder Project II. *American Journal of Critical Care, 10*, 238–251. PMID:11432212

Rocha, E., & Prkachin, K. M. (2007). Temperament and pain reactivity predict health behavior seven years later. *Journal of Pediatric Psychology, 32*(4), 393–399. doi:10.1093/jpepsy/jsl036 PMID:17038414

Rocha, E., Prkachin, K. M., Beaumont, S. L., Hardy, C., & Zumbo, B. D. (2003). Pain reactivity and illness behavior in kindergarten-aged children. *Journal of Pediatric Psychology, 28*(1), 47–57. doi:10.1093/jpepsy/28.1.47 PMID:12490631

Rosenthal, R. (1993). *Judgment Studies: Design, Analysis and Meta-analysis*. Cambridge, UK: Cambridge University Press.

Salmore, R. (2002). Development of a new pain scale: Colorado Behavioral Numerical Pain Scale for sedated adult patients undergoing gastro intestinal procedures. *Gastroenterology Nursing, 25*(6), 257–262. doi:10.1097/00001610-200211000-00007 PMID:12488689

Schiavenato, M., Byers, J. F., & Scovaner, P. (2008). Neonatal pain facial expression: Evaluating the primal face of pain. *Pain, 138*(2), 460–471. doi:10.1016/j.pain.2008.07.009 PMID:18692963

Stevens, B., McGrath, P., & Gibbins, S. (2007). Determining behavioural and physiological responses to pain in infants at risk for neurological impairment. *Pain, 127*, 94–102. doi:10.1016/j.pain.2006.08.012 PMID:16997468

Tian, Y., Cohn, J. F., & Kanade, T. (2005). Facial expression analysis. In Handbook of Face Recognition. New York: Springer. doi:10.1007/0-387-27257-7_12

Williams, A. C. (2002). Facial expression of pain: An evolutionary account. *Behavioral and Brain Sciences*, 439–488. PMID:12879700

Zhang, L., & Tjondronegoro, D. (2011). Facial expression Recognition using facial movement features. *IEEE Trans. On Affective Computing, 2*(4), 219–229. doi:10.1109/T-AFFC.2011.13

ADDITIONAL READING

Black, J. (2002, June). Darwin in the world of emotions. *Journal of the Royal Society of Medicine*, *95*(6), 311–313. doi:10.1258/jrsm.95.6.311 PMID:12042386

Boerner, K. E., Chambers, C. T., Craig, K. D., Pillai, R. R. R., & Parker, J. A. (2013). Caregiver accuracy in detecting deception in facial expressions of pain in children. *Pain*, *154*(4), 525–533. doi:10.1016/j.pain.2012.12.015 PMID:23375511

Butler, D. S., & Moseley, G. L. (2003). *Explain pain*. Adelaide City West, South Australia: Nolgroup Publications.

Chambers, C. T., Hardial, J., Craig, K. D., Court, C., & Montgomery, C. (2005). Faces scales for the measurement of postoperative pain in children. *The Clinical Journal of Pain*, *21*, 277–285. doi:10.1097/00002508-200505000-00011 PMID:15818080

Craig, K. D. (2009). The social communication model of pain. *Canadian Psychology*, *50*(1), 22–32. doi:10.1037/a0014772

Craig, K. D., & Hadjistavropoulos, T. (2004). Psychological perspectives on pain: Controversies. In T. Hadjistavropoulos & K. D. Craig (Eds.), *Pain: Psychological Perspectives* (pp. 303–326). New York, NY: Lawrence Erlbaum.

Craig, K. D., & Korol, C. T. (2008). Developmental issues in understanding, assessing, and managing pediatric pain. In G. Walco & K. Goldschnieder (Eds.), *Pediatric Pain Management in Primary Care: A Practical Guide* (pp. 9–20). Totowa, NJ: The Humana Press Inc. doi:10.1007/978-1-59745-476-6_2

Craig, K. D., Prkachin, K. M., & Grunau, R. V. E. (2011). The facial expression of pain. In D. C. Turk & R. Melzack (Eds.), *Handbook of pain assessment* (3rd ed., pp. 117–133). New York: Guilford.

Craig, K. D., & Versloot, J. (2011). Psychosocial perspectives on chronic pain. In M. E. Lynch, K. D. Craig, & P. Peng (Eds.), *Clinical Pain Management: A Practical Guide* (pp. 24–31). Oxford, UK: Wiley- Blackwell Press.

Dobson, K. S., & Craig, K. D. (Eds.). (1996). *Advances in cognitive-behavioral therapy*. Thousand Oaks, CA: Sage Publications.

Ekman, P. (Ed.). (2003). *Emotions Inside Out: 130 Years after Darwin's The Expression of the Emotions in Man and Animals* (1st ed.). New York: New York Academy of Sciences.

FitzgibbonB. M.GiummarraM. J.Georgiou-KaristianisN.EnticottP. G.BradshawJ. L. (2010).

Goubert, L., Craig, K. D., & Buysse, A. (2009). Perceiving others in pain: Experimental and clinical evidence on the role of empathy. In W. Ickes & J. Decety (Eds.), *The Social Neuroscience of Empathy* (pp. 153–166). MIT Press. doi:10.7551/mitpress/9780262012973.003.0013

Hadjistavropoulos, H. D., & Williams, A. C. deC. & Craig, K.D. (2011). Psychological interventions: Cognitive behavioral and stress management approaches. In Lynch, ME., Craig, K.D., & Peng, P. (Eds.). Clinical Pain Management: A Practical Guide. pp. 200-206. Oxford, UK: Wiley-Blackwell Press.

Hill, M. L., & Craig, K. D. (2004). Detecting deception in facial expressions of pain: Accuracy and training. *The Clinical Journal of Pain*, *20*(6), 415–422. doi:10.1097/00002508-200411000-00006 PMID:15502685

Jamison, R. N., & Craig, K. D. (2011). Psychological assessment of persons with chronic pain. In M. E. Lynch, K. D. Craig, & P. Peng (Eds.), *Clinical Pain Management: A Practical Guide. Oxford* (pp. 81–90). UK: Wiley-Blackwell Press.

Langford, D. J., Bailey, A. L., Chanda, M. L., Clarke, S. E., Drummond, T. E., Echols, S., ... Mogil, J. S. (2010). Coding of facial expressions of pain in the laboratory mouse. *Nature Methods*, *7*(6), 447–449. doi:10.1038/nmeth.1455 PMID:20453868

Larochette, A. C., Chambers, C. T., & Craig, K. D. (2006). Genuine, suppressed and faked facial expressions of pain in children. *Pain*, *126*(1), 64–71. doi:10.1016/j.pain.2006.06.013 PMID:16860478

Lynch, M. E., Craig, K. D., & Peng, P. (Eds.). (2011). *Clinical Pain Management: A Practical Guide*. Oxford, UK: Wiley-Blackwell Press.

McCrystal, K. N., Craig, K. D., Versloot, J., Fashler, S. R., & Jones, D. N. (2011). Perceiving pain in others: Validation of a dual processing model. *Pain*, *152*(5), 1083–1089. doi:10.1016/j.pain.2011.01.025 PMID:21388739

Messmer, R. L., Nader, R., & Craig, K. D. (2008). Judging pain intensity in children with autism undergoing venepuncture: The influence of facial activity. *Journal of Autism and Developmental Disorders*, *38*(7), 1391–1394. doi:10.100710803-007-0511-0 PMID:18161016

Moon, E. C., Chambers, C. T., Larochette, A. C., Hayton, K., Craig, K. D., & McGrath, P. J. (2008). Sex differences in parent and child pain ratings during an experimental child pain task. *Pain Research & Management*, *13*, 225–230. PMID:18592059

Nader, R., Job, E. A., Badali, M., & Craig, K. D. (2004). Infant crying in context. Commentary for Solsti, J. The signal functions of early infant Cry. *Behavioral and Brain Sciences*, *27*(4), 469.

Pillai Riddell, R. R., & Craig, K. D. (2007). Judgments of infant pain: The impact of caregiver identity and infant age. *Journal of Pediatric Psychology*, *32*(5), 501–511. doi:10.1093/jpepsy/jsl049 PMID:17182668

Schiavenato, M., & Craig, K. D. (2010). Pain assessment as a social transaction: Beyond the "Gold Standard". *The Clinical Journal of Pain*, *26*, 667–676. PMID:20664341

Sellam, G., Cignacco, E., Craig, K. D., & Engberg, S. (2011). Contextual factors influencing pain response to heel stick procedures in preterm infants: What do we know? A systematic review. *European Journal of Pain (London, England)*, *15*(7), e1–661.e15. PMID:21330173

Shankland & Dr. Wesley E. (2001). *Face the Pain - The Challenge of Facial Pain*, Pain in the elderly: Validity of facial expression components of observational measures. *The Clinical Journal of Pain*, *27*(7), 593–601.

Simon, D., Craig, K. D., Gosselin, F., Belin, P., & Rainville, P. (2008). Recognition and discrimination of prototypical dynamic expressions of pain and emotions. *Pain*, *135*(1), 55–64. doi:10.1016/j.pain.2007.05.008 PMID:17583430

Williams, A. C de C., & Craig, K. D. (2006). A science of pain expression? *Pain*, *125*(3), 202–203. doi:10.1016/j.pain.2006.08.004 PMID:16962239

KEY TERMS AND DEFINITIONS

Active Appearance Model: A computer vision algorithm for matching a statistical model of object shape and appearance to a new image. They are built during a training phase. A set of images, together with coordinates of landmarks that appear in all of the images, is provided to the training supervisor.

Acute Pain: Pain of less than 6 months duration for which an underlying pathology can be identified by their appearance on the face.

Facial Action Coding System (FACS): Is a system to taxonomize human facial movements by their appearance on the face.

Intelligent Computing System: Is a computer system that aims to provide immediate and customized instruction or feedback to learners, usually without intervention from a human teacher. These are used in the medical planning, diagnosis and treatment.

Pain Scale: Measures a patient's pain intensity or other features. Pain scales are based on self-report, observational (behavioral), or physiological data.

Pain: An unpleasant sensory and emotional experience associated with actual or threatened tissue damage.

Self-Reports: Self-report is the primary measure of pain intensity in non communicative patients.

This research was previously published in Improving Health Management through Clinical Decision Support Systems edited by Jane D. Moon and Mary P. Galea, pages 59-80, copyright year 2016 by Medical Information Science Reference (an imprint of IGI Global).

Chapter 3
Stress Associated with Orthopedic Surgery and Feeling Pain

Kinga Sobieralska-Michalak
Ludwig Rydygier Collegium Medicum, Poland & Nicolaus Copernicus University in Toruń, Poland

Maciej Michalak
Kazimierz Wielki University in Bydgoszcz, Poland

Agnieszka Woźniewicz
Ludwig Rydygier Collegium Medicum in Bydgoszcz, Poland & Nicolaus Copernicus University in Toruń, Poland

Aleksandra Pawlicka
The School of Language and Literature in Bydgoszcz, Poland

ABSTRACT

Injuries and degenerative disease of the skeletal and articular systems are the most common reasons for undergoing orthopaedic surgery. Those diseases are often associated with pain, which is experienced by the patient long before the surgical procedure. Strong stress reaction is the main source of adjustment disorders of patients undergoing surgical treatment. Orthopaedic surgery, like any other surgery, upsets body's homeostasis. The results of the surgery are not completely predictable, but are always closely related to life and health. Patients' strong stress reaction is also connected with anaesthesia (emergence from anaesthesia), being worried of complications caused by central neuraxial anaesthesia – the fear of paresis or death. The factor which influences worse adaptation process is the patients' post-surgery mood. Right after the surgery, patients feel worse than before it, they are weak, move less freely, they are anxious about their consciousness being dimmed due to medicine

DOI: 10.4018/978-1-7998-1680-5.ch003

intake and pain. The expectations concerning the ways of controlling the dynamics of the pain one experiences are crucial. According to the researchers, in the central nervous system there exist neural circuits that may cause physiological reactions according to one's expectations, and due to this fact the pain one experiences may become stronger or alleviated depending on one's expectations. The lack of positive pain-reducing experience may lead to the learned helplessness or no sense of one's control over pain, both of which make the pain stronger. The pain-influencing factors include cognitive processes and emotions. The role of attention processes, one's cognitive appraisal and one's attitude towards pain has been emphasised, as well as the pain-modelling influence of emotions, all of which emphasise the complexity of one's pain experience. Patients, when asked to point out the factors that hinder effective pain therapy, indicate frustration caused by the lack of information, numerous worries concerning the treatment and the stereotypical image of pain. Relieving tension influences the patient's mood positively, whilst stress influences it in a negative way. The stress one experiences and one's emotions lower one's pain threshold, which leads to greater pain experience and thus makes the healing process last longer. The quality of pre- and post-operational care is thus crucial, as it influences the level of the experienced stress. The pain components influence one another, there occur interactions of biological, psychological and situational factors, which makes it advisable to personalise one's pain treatment. The need of an interdisciplinary approach towards a person, especially to their health, has been recently emphasised. Pain is a biopsychosocial occurrence, which makes pain therapy an interdisciplinary problem. This chapter discusses the following issues: 1) The characteristics of pain in conditions that require surgical treatment,2) Surgery-related stress reaction, 3) Psychological factors which influence how one feels pain, 4) The consequences of pain in people's functioning, and 5) Postoperative pain, the assessment of pain level and its relieving.

INTRODUCTION

The Characteristics of Pain in Ailments Which Require Surgical Treatment

In the neurophysiologic sense experiencing pain is connected with the nociceptive tract, owing to which the stimuli are transmitted from the peripheral to the central nervous system. The nociceptive tract consists of specialized free nerve endings which respond to harmful stimuli and nerve fibres which transmit the information from peripheral cells to the spinal cord and then to the brain structures. It is a complicated and dynamic system, in which, besides the pain transmitting tracts, there also exist regulation mechanisms, which can modify the degree of pain and how long it lasts. The process which results in a subjective experience of pain in an individual is called nociception and is divided into four stages:

- **Transduction:** The change of the harmful stimuli's action potential into an electrical impulse,
- **Transmission:** Transmission of the impulse to the dorsal horn and to the central nervous system, through two types of nerve fibres – fast, myelinated A delta fibres and slow unmyelinated C fibres,
- **Modulation:** Stimulating, inhibiting, and accumulating the stimuli.
- **Perception:** The conscious experience of pain, its assessment and affective reactions (Suchocka, 2008).

In the medical sense there exist various classifications of pain, some of them being:

1. Classification due to the pain mechanisms:
    - **Nociceptive Pain:** The result of mechanical, thermal, chemical stimulation of pain receptors. There exist two kids of nociceptive pain:
        - **Somatic Pain:** Divided into bone pain and pain resulting from deep tissue damage: skin, subcutaneous tissue or muscles. It is well-localized and easy to describe.
        - **Visceral Pain:** Diffused pain which is difficult to localise, originates from the internal organs; abdominal cavity, pelvis minor, coronary.
    - **Non-Nociceptive Pain:** A chronic pain caused by dysfunction of either peripheral or central nervous system:
        - **Neuropathic Pain:** Is characterized by sudden, seizure-like pain which lasts from a few seconds up to several minutes, either intermittent or constant, along with the sensations of burning, twisting, tearing, crushing - at first in the damaged area, then in a wider area, with lower intensity – tingling or stabbing paraesthesia, the feeling of heaviness and numbness
        - **Psychogenic Pain:** The second kind of non-nociceptive pain, appears despite no tissue damage, but is reported by the patients in the same ways as pain caused by tissue damage. It is caused by mental, emotional or personal (hysterical/hypochondriac) factors; related to depression; delusional, phantom pain
2. Classification due to the kind of pain-causing nociceptive stimuli:
    - **Physiological Pain:** With the nociceptors being activated (no tissue damage involved),

- **Clinical Pain:** The consequence of damage to the tissues, it is characteristic for the post- surgery and post-injury pain.

3. Classification due to time the pain lasts:
    - **Acute Pain:** Arising quickly and suddenly, usually of high intensity, it is usually possible to find the causal and temporal connection between the onset of pain and injury or disease.
    - **Chronic Pain:** Lasting longer than 3 months, persistent or recurrent, of various aetiology, needs constant pain-managing treatment, it lasts despite the tissues having healed. It does not have a clear cause; long-lasting pain loses its meaning as a warning against damage, it becomes an independent syndrome. Pain seems to turn into an illness itself (Filipczak – Brynierska, Brynierski, Woroń & Wodliczek, 2010; Korzeniowska & Szałek, 2010).

One of the condition that need surgical treatment is in the degenerative disease; the following is the characteristics of pain in this disease. Degenerative disease is an ailment in which the clinical symptoms arise quite slowly and deceitfully. It usually affects the hip joint or knee. One of the most significant symptoms of the degenerative disease of the hip is pain located in one's groin, buttock and in the hip area, radiating towards knee. The pain intensifies during long-lasting physical activity; sometimes it arises spontaneously, waking the patient up from their sleep. When the pathological changes progress the pain arises even in small physical activity, there occurs joint rigidity, especially after a period of a longer immobility, there increase joint deformation and joint dysfunction. The patients who are offered fitting joint prosthesis are mainly those, who suffer from extensive degenerative lesions or lesions which are the result of previous bone fractures, e.g. femoral neck fracture, or other various ailments one had previously suffered from, usually undiagnosed hip dysplasia or dysplasia the treatment of which was delayed too late. A significant number of patients are those who suffer from rheumatoid joint inflammation. Nowadays, the standard treatment of degeneratively changed hip joints is based on total hip arthroplasty, which is replacing the degenerated joint with a prosthetic one. The surgery consists in removing the cartilaginous and fibrous layers along with the under-cartilaginous part of the hip acetabulum and removing the head and neck of the femur. The removed parts are replaced with a head fitted to the acetabulum and a prosthetic acetabulum (Kiwerski, 2006; Marciniak & Szulc, 2004).

Gonarthrosis of the knee joint usually results from previously existing deformations, such as: valgus or varus deformity of knees or a fracture within the knee joint. The dominating symptom is pain localized in the front or medial part of the knee, as well as in the top-medial part of the shin. There appear: pain which intensifies when applying load, the feeling of the knee joint being tense, limited mobility, exudates and contractures. The pain that arises after the patient starts walking is typical; the patient says they have to walk for some time before the pain subsides. The occurrence of the following symptoms indicated the need for surgical treatment: permanent pain, which is resistant to preventive therapy, progressive deformity and instability of the knee joint or its significant rigidity. During the surgery the knee joint is replaced by a prosthetic knee made from metal and plastics. After cutting through the skin on the front part of the knee, the further part of the femur and closer part of the shinbone are cut off and replaced with prosthesis, the part fitted to the femur being made of metal and the one fitted to the shinbone – made of metal and plastics (Kramer, 1997).

Another way of treatment, especially in the early stages of degenerative disease, is arthroscopy – a modern and minimally invasive surgical procedure on a joint. In this method, a small fiberoptic camera, also called an arthroscope, is inserted into the joint through a small incision; surgeons view the joint area on a video monitor. This surgical procedure is used to perform an examination, and owing to its high sensitivity it allows to assess the joint, the stage of progression and range of lesions; the procedure is also used to treat other orthopaedic conditions, such as torn cartilage, loose bone fragment in the joint or joint destabilisation or dislocation of patella. It is also helpful in certain stages of the full orthopaedic surgery, e.g. the reconstruction of cruciate ligament (Widuchowski, Widuchowski & Paściak, 2005).

The degenerative disease of the glenohumeral joint also causes strong, chronic pain and significant limitations in fulfilling everyday duties, as the arms are used in to perform thousands of tasks. The degenerated joint hurts both when moving and resting. The patients find it difficult to make the simplest movements, e.g. grasping one's neck, rotating one's arm. In this joint, arthroscopy is also used as a therapeutic method. This method is used in diagnosing and treatment of the ankle joint, too; the ankle joint is the most heavily loaded joint of the body, and at the same time vulnerable to injuries and lesions caused by excessive loading. The patients experience oversensitivity, pain, swelling, limited joint mobility, rigidity, walking with a limp (Kobus, Wójcicki, Dydymski, Węgrzyn & Hamlawi, 2007; Piontek, Ciemniewska-Gorzela, Szulc, Naczk & Słomczykowski, 2012). Tunnel syndromes are medical conditions which occur due to compression of the peripheral nerves in their physiological localisation. They cause stabbing, shooting, burning, penetrating and electric-like pains, as well as paresthesia and neuropathic sensory disorders in the area supplied by the nerve. In the syndrome, the damage to the fibres lead to the occurrence of accompanying symptoms, such as redness or paleness of skin, lividity, swelling, excessive or insufficient transpiration and trophic skin changes. The most common form of is the carpal tunnel syndrome, the symptoms of which being: pain and numbness of the middle and index finger, in the further stages atrophy and palsy of the thenar eminence muscles. In the treatment, there are two ways of applying successful pain-relieving analgesia; pharmacological analgesia, that is using analgesics; and non-pharmacological analgesia, i.e. physiotherapy and exercise. Invasive treatment: peripheral nerve blocks and surgical treatment – releasing compressed nerves. It is a group of patients which is difficult to treat, which should be taken care of in the pain management centres (Kübler, 2008).

SURGERY: RELATED STRESS REACTION

Stress is a very important part of life. It serves an adaptive function, thanks to which it is possible to regain balance by eliminating disturbances from the external or internal environment. When a person falls ill, there arises the feeling of threat to health and life. It is the situation that is one of the main stress-inducing factors. For most people, illness and experiences related to it are a serious burden, as the possibility of achieving one's previously set goals becomes disturbed, there emerge physical ailments, usually followed by negative emotions. According to the T.H. Holmes & partners' scale, which assesses the level of stress, measured with Life Change Units (LCU), it turns out that illness is the fifth most stressful event (out of 40 considered). There emerge strong emotions, most of all anxiety which increases even more if the treatment requires surgical intervention. Strong stress that patients experience is connected with the possibility of experiencing pain, of suffering, but also anaesthetics (emergence from it), worrying about complications of neuraxial anaesthesia, the possibility of serious consequences, i.e. paresis or death. Being hospitalized is a specific, stress-inducing experience (ZięSbicka & Gajdosz, 2006). Stress reaction is caused by limitation of serving one's social roles: in family, professional life. The patient feels rather incapacitated, feels the lack of being fully independent in deciding about oneself and one's affairs, the decrease in the level of activity and self-reliance and being dependent on other people. Hospital is perceived as a strange and unfriendly place, where patients feel anonymous, helpless, dependent on doctors' and nurses' decisions. The patient faces the challenge of dealing with the loss of autonomy and support, which induces stress, leading to decrease in immunity (Bishop, 2000.)

There appears the prospect of losing health or health hazard, a threat to physical safety as well as psychological and economic safety; the prospect also causes the feeling of losing one's self-esteem (Motyka & Załuski, 2010).

The patient is sensitive to what the medical staff says about them and their condition, observes the behaviour of doctors and nurses, tries to deduce the actual opinion the doctors have on their state, based on the heard words, ambiguities and gestures. The patient who does not understand what is being spoken about or does not understand what is said to him, feels more stressed, which makes it more difficult to positively approach the treatment. Depending on their own observation and other people's opinions, the patient can be either happy with or regret their decision. Each person experiences the necessity of being hospitalized and undergoing surgery in their own, unique way (Lesińska - Sawicka, Grygorowicz E

& Jałtuszewska 2007). The patients experience the feelings of anxiety and stress related to illness before being admitted to the hospital ward. There exist three stages of stress caused by hospitalization: 1) the period from being admitted to hospital to decision on surgical treatment, 2) anaesthesia and surgery, 3) the postoperative period. In connection with this, one can distinguish the three stages of operational stress, which correspond with the preoperative period, the surgery and the postoperative period.

During each stage the patient's body is under the influence of different factors, which are able to significantly change the physiological response to injury. The most important factors include:

- **Preoperative:** Age, gender, nutritional status, anxiety, fear;
- **Surgical:** Anaesthetics, surgical stimulation, the level of tissue damage, hypothermia;
- **Postoperative:** Pain, infections, oxygen deficiency, immobilization.

In that period patients may also experience anger, pain and suffering, may be oversensitive or even hostile towards the hospital environment, although these reactions occur less often than anxiety states. The emotional reaction is independent on the physiological reaction. (Salmon, 2002). Surgical treatment is a significant emotional burden to patients and the risk of serious, dangerous consequences leads to their anxiety (Ziębicka & Gajdosz, 2006).

The patient who requires surgical intervention due to orthopaedic condition usually has problems moving on their own, needs other person's support, uses a walking stick, crutches or a wheelchair. Because of it, they expect some form of help, some assistance in moving within the hospital area. The first contact with the medical staff usually takes place in the admission room; the patient hopes for kind and quick taking care of the formalities. It is usually the moment when the tension and stress begin to rise as the result of the long wait for the admission. Additionally, being among unfamiliar people who are asking questions, giving orders, making decisions concerning the patient's health, who are often younger than the patient, which may contribute to the feeling of reluctance and the patient reacting by mounting resistance.

After filling in the documentation the patient is admitted to the hospital ward. The nurse in the ward takes the medical history, shows the patient round the ward, informs about the customs, daily ward routine, privileges and duties, the hospital's regulations. The accumulation of information may be the factor causing anxiety and the feeling of threat, the patient is unsure if they managed to remember everything correctly. The patient also acquires information about the upcoming surgery. The whole procedure of admission, medical examination and consultation are tiring and stressful for the patient, mostly because the situation is new and unknown, the patient loses the sense of control and predictability, which is crucial for the feeling of balance and safety.

Health is the basic constituent of human capital, thus the fear of losing it causes strong emotions, such as anxiety, fear, sadness, helplessness and fright. In the period preceding and following the surgery the social status of patient changes entirely and they do not always have the ability to deal with this fact. Due to this the patient's behaviour may be characterised by mistrust and suspiciousness, an aversion to talk or even anger and aggression (Chodkiewicz, 2004).

The patient, when becoming a member of the hospital society, ceases to serve their previous roles in favour of taking up actions, the effect of which should be regaining one's health. The actions taken up by the patient, especially at the initial stage of hospitalization, are called learning the patient's role. One of the first important tasks is making a conscious, deliberate decision about treatment and surgery, followed by one's written consent. This document is the written confirmation of the fact that the patient understands the nature of their condition, the kind of treatment, prognosis, consequences and the risk of treatment, as well as the consequences of not undergoing the treatment. It is important for the patient to have enough time to carefully consider everything and make their decision, however, it is not always possible, especially if surgery should be performed urgently. It is easier to deal with difficult situation – hospitalization - if one has enough time (arranging everything at home and at work). Expressing one's anxiety, fear, uncertainty, the possibility of consultation with other specialists, has a crucial influence over dealing with a difficult situation and convalescence (Kurowska & Czepek, 2009).

Providing information concerning diagnosis and the causes of the condition, the next steps of treatment, possible undesirable consequences of the applied medical procedures as well as practical tips about taking actions in the post-operative period (concentrated on the actions one should avoid) are a common, easily accessible form of preparing the patient to their surgery.

Patients' reactions are various, due to individual features and also to using different types and techniques of adapting to certain conditions.

Patients can be divided into two groups:

- People who tend to avoid difficult situations, who improve their mood (they are confined to defence – by avoiding information); these patients, when being given information about possible threat experience worse functioning. Despite the fact it causes their emotional state become worse, the patients must receive this basic, essential information.

- People dealing with stress in an active way (by undertaking stress-relieving actions, searching for information) profit from better post-operative functioning, even in uncontrollable situations (Włodarczyk & Skuza, 2007).

The patients' expectations about nurses concern both physical and mental preparations to the upcoming surgery. Above all, they expect to be informed about the procedures that they are going to undergo, what their purpose is, until when they are allowed to eat and drink, how long the surgery is going to last, if they will be transported back to their room immediately after the surgery, what is going to happen right after the surgery, how long they are going to be forced to stay in bed, and if the patient requires applying plaster cast – how long they will have to wear it. The expectations also concern taking into consideration one's cultural diversity, applying hygienic procedures or performing their religious practices. The patients also expect the nurse to inform their family about the details of the nursing process.

Most patients are afraid of the surgery itself, but there also exist other factors, which may intensify stress. According to the research, the time of the day (morning, night) is one of them. In the morning patients wait for the doctor's consultation, various medical procedures and their outcome. At night patients, being in an unknown place, experience sleeplessness, the sounds of the ward increase anxiety, the ailments and pain seem to be stronger. The awareness of lower number of medical staff also increases stress (Lesińska - Sawicka, Grygorowicz E & Jałtuszewska 2007).

In the period right after the surgery, when one's independence is limited, patients feel unsure, they keep thinking about questions such as: if they will be able to expect manual work to be done skilfully, if they will experience kindness, friendliness, thoughtfulness, willingness to help, if they can expect their dignity and intimacy to be respected whilst undergoing all the medical procedures (Kapała, Chudziński & Hyrcza, 2008).

Anxiety is the basic source of the adaptive problems of patients undergoing surgical treatment.

Orthopaedic surgery, like any other surgery, upsets the patient's homeostasis. The effects of the surgery are not fully predictable, but they are always connected with patient's health and life. Patients' anxiety is connected with anaesthesia (emerging from anaesthesia), the fear of complications of the neuraxial anaesthesia – being afraid of paresis or death. The patient's mood after surgery is one of the factors which negatively affect the adaptive process. Patients after surgery feel worse than before it, they feel weak, move less freely, they are anxious about their consciousness being dimmed as the result of taking medicines, they experience pain. Patient's behaviour can also be caused by the way their perceive their own illness. It is the patient's „diagnosis", as the patient collects the information about their state from various sources, which are often non-professional sources, the information is seldom gained from a doctor. Due to this fact, the patient's picture of their own illness is often incomplete, may not reflect the actual state of health and may be resistant to being changed (Jakubowska - Winecka & Włodarczyk 2007; Hasiak 2012).

The reason for the patient feeling anxious about being discharged from hospital is that they are unsure how to deal with the surgical wound – its care, not knowing how long the wound needs to be covered with a dressing, the way the wound is going to heal, the fear of not noticing alarming symptoms which should be consulted by a doctor as well as the rehabilitation process.

The Psychological Factors Affecting How One Feels Pain

Pain is an important factor in medical care, it is one of the five vital signs along body temperature, respiratory rate, heart rate and blood pressure. (Dobrogowski & Wordliczek, 2004). According to the definition introduced by the International Association for the Study of Pain it is „an unpleasant sensory and emotional experience associated with actual or potential tissue damage, or described in terms of such damage" (Saint-Maurice, Muller & Meynadier, 1998). Pain is a psychosomatic occurrence, which the definition of J. Wordliczek also takes into account: „Pain is a sensory experience associated with both the influence of damaging pain (nociceptive) stimuli or a factor the influence of which may cause this kind of damage, but is also the perception which is caused by psychical interpretation of the occurrences modified by previous experience and psychosomatic causation" (Dobrogowski & Wordliczek, 2004). The pain a person experiences is not only determined by the stimuli that caused it. Apparently, the level and quality of the pain one feels is dependent not only on the sensory experience, but also on many various psychological factors. In 1968 Sternbach suggested that the way one experiences pain is dependent on:

- Their perceptual style and behavioural pattern, mostly on their way of reacting to fear,
- Learnt, fixed associations of certain physical stimuli and pain, which are associated with social situations,
- Interpreting, cognitive appraisal.

How a person experiences pain is a very individual question, it is subjective and associated with different aspects of human functioning. Pain is a very complex and dynamic process, which covers the following aspects: sensory-discriminative, cognitive-motivational and affective-motivational, which are processed simultaneously. In such an approach the pain model which is the most universal has been described by Wade and Price and consists of four stages:

Stage 1. Sensory: Discriminative experience.
Stage 2. Pain Unpleasantness: Is related to affective response, involves limited cognitive processing
Stage 3. Suffering
Stage 4. Behavioural reaction to pain.

At the first stage the information concerning pain experiencing is transmitted from the peripheral nervous system to the central levels of the nervous system. It concerns the way one feels pain (the sensory experience, e.g. piercing, ripping), where it is localised (in a particular body part or widespread). The level of intensity and strength of pain influences the feeling of unpleasantness in the second stage, i.e. how unbearable and unpleasant it is. Both in the first and the second stage the intensity of the experienced pain is measured using tools like the visual analogue scale (VAS). How strong is the pain one experiences in the third stage is dependent on many factors, that is individualistic features, previous experience, one's approach to pain or the ability of coping with stress. The fourth stage is the behavioural expression to pain, which is reflected in everyday functioning, one's mobility, it is related to behaviours leading to eliminating or decreasing pain. This stage depends on the source of pain, pathomechanics of its origin as well as individualistic features. People who are more emotionally expressive tend to show their pain in a more expressive way than people who are emotionally reserved.

When considering the pain perception from the psychological point of view, one can identify the threshold of pain and the pain tolerance. The pain threshold is the point of perception of a stimulus at which pains begins to be felt. This value is relatively constant and not much dependent on individual features (lower pain threshold is usually observed in females and older people). Pain tolerance is the maximum level of pain that a person is able to tolerate. This value is variable and depends on many various factors. The pain threshold depends mostly on the somatic factors, whilst pain tolerance depends on psychological factors [de Walden-Gałuszko, 2001). One of the most important factors which influence how a person feels pain is their emotional state, which depends on the cognitive appraisal, which consists of the idea about the cause and consequences of pain. The beliefs concerning one's condition and pain cause the feeling of helplessness and the emotional reactions of anxiety and bad mood. Thus, the kind and intensity of the patient's emotions, be it strong fear, anger or misery, is closely related to their dominating way of thinking. Strong negative emotions lower one's pain tolerance, which leads to feeling stronger pain. The fact that pain is an unpleasant experience often causes worsening one's mood, it is true especially for the patients suffering from chronic pain. People who experience pain are twice as prone to depression as the rest of the society. One must remember that there exists the risk of depression without its characteristic, distinct features, the so called masked depression. The emotional reaction resulting from the pain one feels is also dependent on how concentrated on their pain experiences the person is. Focusing one's attention and constant self-observation makes the person's experience of pain much more intense (de Walden-Gałuszko, 2001; Golec, 2000).

The patient's experience also provides a lasting memory in the emotional context. When pain stimuli appear similar to ones previously experienced, there is a possibility that similar reactions will occur according to the interpretation one gives them. Life experiences, especially those fixed in ones childhood, are taken as a norm, which can become the basis of thinking and behaving. The meaning the person in pain gives their experiences, illness and situation in which they are in, may significantly create the pain experience, which is a very individual feature of a person (Golec, 2000). Another, equally significant factor determining the feeling of pain is the subjectivity and the locus of one's sense of control over health. It is very important to have the inner sense of having the ability to decide upon and influence one's destiny. It is the sense of being able to influence one's health and improving its state (the so called internal locus of health control) or perceiving one's situation as a result of luck, coincidence, fate or as a result of other people's actions (the so called external locus of control). People with an external locus of control subject to pressure and external influences, they feel they are helpless and have no control over their situation. An external locus of control correlates with the sense of low level of control over one's pain. The patients with an internal locus of control believe in their abilities, they feel they can control their destiny, which leads to the ability of dealing with one's pain as well. It has a great meaning for the patient; interpreting pain as a threat may be the reason for mobilising patient's powers to relieve the pain. If patients awaiting surgery are informed about pain they may experience and how they should deal with it, they may find it easier to ease the pain. The study results show that personal, individualistic features are significant to the image of experiencing post-operative pain. Patients whose personalities allow them to deal with life difficulties, usually apply available strategies of coping when being exposed to threat, in this case – a surgery. People who expect complications, feel stronger and more intense pain. A person lives in a society, is shaped in it, cultural values play a big role in perceiving pain and reacting to it. Ethnic differences influence the attitude towards suffering and the ways of expressing it.

Giving support is a normal and desired thing in some cultures. Expressing pain can mean both the lack of support and be a form of searching for help. However, when the culture praises „being strong", the members of the group will not tend to show their ailments. The same applies to teaching behaviours within a family – a child mimics their parents and their attitudes. Spirituality and religiousness may also be a pain modifying factor. Emotional and spiritual development is another factor that may be the basis of accepting pain and oneself as a person who is suffering, it can make the suffering meaningful. Experiencing pain becomes easier, when it is embedded within the structure of one's religious life; the same is true for the non-believers who are highly soulful (Melzack & Wall, 2006).

Pain is an experience which causes suffering and discomfort, which along with the coexisting symptoms result in the feeling of lack of self-sufficiency, being dependent on others and low self-esteem (Rolka et al., 2009). When considering the particular significance of psychological factors of feeling pain, when taking actions in raising the threshold of pain the following factors are of significance: giving the patient psychical comfort by enabling them to communicate their needs – equipping with a nurse call button, providing them with peace and rest, not allowing the patient to focus their attention on negative emotions. It is crucial to give the patient social support; even being and talking with them positively affects the patient's emotional security.

The Consequences of Pain for the Person's Functioning

Experiencing pain is a complex and subjective matter, which consists of the physiological process of transmitting nerve impulses as well as of emotions, suffering, attitude and expressing one's pain. Prolonged, untreated pain worsens the quality of one's life. The idea of quality of life can be considered in two ways, as the quality of life independent on the health state and the quality of life dependent on health state. The factors that influence the quality of life dependent on the health state can be divided into:

Subjective factors (the sense of quality of life), which are (Chwałczyńska et al., 2004):

- Physical state;
- Mental state;
- Social situation;
- Human relations

Objective:

- **Health State:** The results of laboratory examination,
- Clinical picture of the illness,
- Social - economic state,
- Social contacts.

Suffering can thus have influence over the various levels of quality of life at the same time: at the somatic experience level, physical state and one's mobility.

The pain can lead to: tiredness, dizziness, pollakiuria, tachycardia, perspiration, muscle tremor. Furthermore, it can cause restlessness, disorders of attention and memory, irritability, insomnia. There exist different possibilities of relieving pain, depending on if it is acute or chronic. In acute pain, owing to the current knowledge and available resources, patients receive help which satisfies them; in chronic pain helping the patients may be problematic – 80% of doctor's appointments concern pain and the ways of relieving it, one may thus treat pain as a separate condition. It is important to remember that human functions as a psycho-physical unity, according to the holistic approach. That is why every disturbance in how the organism functions is reflected in the affective sphere and one's behaviour (Czubalski, 1995). When a person functions in pain, the proper interaction with their environment is disturbed and the relations between the person and their closest environment are unbalanced as well. Due to the experiencing of pain, the patient avoids various activities that cause pain but at the same time they lower the level of or cease other activities, which results in leading sedentary lifestyle. As a result, the patient burns less fat, which leads to them becoming overweight, that results in problems with circulatory system. The lack of activity causes weakening of muscles and joints and thus extending one's disabilities. Another effect is weakening one's immune system and being more prone to illnesses. Limiting one's physical activity causes specific problems to appear in the everyday life of the patient. Pain is the reason for various limitations in life. One's illness as well as the pain that accompanies it are both a biological and psychosocial threat, which disturbs or disables fulfilling one's life needs, makes realising one's life goals more difficult, and contributes to losing one's precious values. The ailments the patient experiences cause emotional, cognitive and motivational disturbances, they contribute to decreasing one's interest and life activity level (Heszen & Sęk, 2007; Hilgier, 2002).

Strong and chronic pain, experienced for a prolonged time, makes it more difficult to function in a normal way, to do one's chores and performing one's previous social roles. It leads to gradual eliminating of showing social activity, as the patient concentrates their thoughts on their pain and continuous searching for its causes, which results in lowering the quality and efficiency in one's work. It can also cause conflicts in the family or among friends, becoming excessively dependent on one's relatives and caretakers. Unreasonable fear of pain is connected with significant financial costs, being absent at work leads to losing one's source of income; the family, as well as the patient's employer, become financially burdened. All these factors result then in misusing and abusing the health care system, medical services and medicines; it is also connected with bearing costs of damages and compensations, disability pension and sickness benefit (Stachowiak et al., 2005).

The patient in pain may experience depression, increased feelings of sadness, annoyance, being trapped, outbursts of anger, fear, anxiety, bitterness, frustration, depression. There exists a significant relationship between depression and chronic pain. Stronger physical pain makes the physical state worsen (one's depression and anxiety intensify) and vice versa – the worse the mental state is, the stronger one experiences pain. Chronic pain may contribute to one's mental isolation and crawling into one's shell. The patient feels their own world has significantly narrowed down. Pain also influences one's suicidal thoughts – the more intense it becomes, the more often and more intensively one thinks about death (Hilgier, 2002; Wasilewski et al., 2010)

The actual consequences the experiencing pain has for the patient's functioning depend on the person's approach to illness. According to what Lipowski suggested, the patient's approach to illness and emotional and behavioural reactions connected to it are mainly dependent on the person's cognitive appraisal of the situation connected with illness. In other words, what is one's assessment or interpretation of the situation one is in. The assessment's result may be positive, negative or neutral, which relates to having a certain approach. Lipowski (as cited in Steuden, 2002) distinguishes several approaches to one's illness, classified according to the way the patient interprets their condition as the result of secondary cognitive appraisal (the assessment of one's possibilities of coping with a difficult situation) and behaviours related to those interpretations. One of the possible ways is assessing one's illness as an obstacle, a situation which disables realizing important life goals, this kind of appraisal leads to mobilising one's efforts in order to face the illness and defeat it. Another way of interpreting causes one to perceive illness as a loss; it makes the patient concentrate on limitations and deficiencies resulting from their illness, and finds them impossible to cope with. The results of this approach are: depression, sadness, self-destructive tendencies, as well as feelings of emptiness and grieving over the loss of certain mobility or function of the body. The illness can also be perceived as a kind of relief, not having to carry out one's duties, being free from the assignments one has to perform and from the resulting responsibility. A characteristic feature of this approach is aiming at getting acceptance from others, or justifying some certain behaviours. The fourth approach distinguished by Lipowski is the one where the patient perceives their illness as a kind of profit. As a consequence of this approach, the patient is able to have their needs fulfilled by receiving care from one's closest environment. Having this kind of approach may also be caused by the patient willing to profit financially, by receiving sick benefit or damages. Interpreting illness as a value usually occurs in its further stages and results from the patient accepting their illness and the resultant disabilities and limitations. Choosing this approach is connected with reflexions over one's life, with a positive experience, it also positively influences the process of growing as a person as well as creating relations with other people (as cited in Steuden, 2002). The approach of perceiving one's illness as a value that Lipowski has distinguished corresponds with Frankl's concept; he perceived illness as a chance of making the values of approach true and realizing one's personal existence (Frankl, 1998).

It can be assumed that the process of giving the meaning to a certain situation is the basis of creating emotional reactions and influences the choice of the strategy of coping with pain, which is going to have consequences in one's everyday functioning.

Obviously, the quality of how the patient functions is going to depend on the progression of the chronic illness, the dynamics of its clinical picture, the severity of illness, the results of treatment and prognosis, as well as life dynamics and personal and social resources of the patient.

POSTOPERATIVE PAIN, THE ASSESSMENT OF PAIN INTENSITY, PAIN MANAGEMENT

Postoperative pain is an unpleasant sensory and emotional experience, and the basic cause of patient's discomfort. It results from the surgical wound of the tissues and arises when the anaesthesia wears off. It is classified as a kind of acute pain. The source of postoperative pain are damaged cutaneous and subcutaneous tissues, as well as the damage to the deeper structures (such as muscles, fascias, ligaments, periosteum) and foreign bodies, like sutures and drains. Postoperative pain is the most intense on the first day after the surgery and gradually decreases on consecutive days. It is dependent on the kind of surgery, how long it lasted, how extensive it was and how much the tissues were traumatized. One of the kinds of the postoperative pain is the pain caused by wrong placement of a patient as well as by the applied dressing. Postoperative complications may also be the reason for a high analgesic requirement. Good communication and pain documenting lead to diagnosing pain in the early stage of the postoperative period. It is crucial to differentiate between the kinds of pain, e.g. chest pain may be the symptom of myocardial infarction, pulmonary embolism, pneumonia. Experiencing pain in certain patients, even whilst undergoing similar surgical procedures, may significantly vary in intensity, duration and analgesics requirement. In the postoperative pain management it is important for the patient to be made aware of the cause of pain, and to take an attitude towards it. Patients often exaggerate previous ailments, e.g. back pain caused by a prolonged lying position or headache being the result of ceasing to take medicines they had been previously prescribed. The proper method of treatment is chosen dependening on different components of one's pain (Kübler, 2008; Wodliczek & Dobrogowski, 2011)

Pain has always been an inseparable element of every surgical procedure. The breakthrough of treating postsurgical pain took place in 1809, when opium was used to alleviate pain during the surgery for the first time. Since that moment the development of pharmacotherapy has made it possible to relieve pain both during the surgery and afterwards, and various techniques and analgesics has allowed to successfully relieve pain.

Managing clinical pain, postoperative pain included, is based on scales and questionnaires that are used to assess the intensity of the ailments one experiences.

The most commonly used scales are:

- **Verbal Rating Scale (VRS):** A descriptive scale; the patient describes their pain using the following expressions: no pain, mild pain, moderate pain, severe pain, worst pain. The scale is mostly used with patients who have vision problems, children up to the fifth year of age and elderly people. According to the research, the patients who use the verbal scale seldom choose the most extremepossible answers and thus it is not quite clear if the pain they experience is properly interpreted.
- **Numeric Rating Scale (NRS):** The assessment of pain using the numeric scale from 0 to 10. According to this scale 0 means no pain, whilst 10 symbolises the worst pain the patient can imagine, an unbearable pain.
- **VAS Visual Analogue Scale (VAS):** It is a numeric scale with a 10-centimetre long graphic element, on which the patient is supposed to mark the level of pain they are experiencing. At the ends of the graphic element there are two extremes of pain assessment: the „0" point represents no pain, whilst the „10" point stands for the maximum pain. Along the graphic line there may be present verbal descriptions of the pain level (mild, moderate, severe).
- **Picture scale:** The pain level is represented by pictures of various face expressions. It is used mostly with children and elderly patients, with slight and moderate cognitive impairments, dyslexic patients, or the patients who do not know the language. All the scales assess the somatic dimension of pain, thus not covering the whole experience of patients. In order to gain the most complex assessment, one may use various additional questionnaires, for example:
- Melzack's questionnaire allows to assess the qualities of the patient's pain as well as its level of intensity, it also includes the socio-psychological factors which influence how one experiences pain. The questionnaire allows doctors to gain important information. The questionnaire is composed of a long list of adjectives. Owing to the list, a doctor may help the patient precisely verbalise the experience which is unpleasant and needs immediate reaction. Patients are given the questionnaire and told to choose only those words which describe their experience at that moment, e.g. the pain one experiences may be:
    1. Tearing
    2. Piercing
    3. Prickling
    4. Sharp
    5. Cramping

6. Gnawing
7. Hot/burning
8. Nagging
9. Heavy
10. Arising when touching the affected area
11. Splitting
12. Tiring/exhausting
13. Nauseating
14. Dreadful
15. Vivious/cruel

- The questionnaire concerning beliefs about managing pain is used to assess the strength of one's individual beliefs related to pain management.
- The questionnaire of pain management strategies, used to assess the pain management strategies one uses and the effectiveness of those strategies (Juszczak, 2009; Korzeniowska & Szałek, 2010; Ulatowska, Bączyk & Lewandowska, 2012).

Nowadays, relieving the postoperative pain successfully is a part of modern surgery treatment and should have a multidimensional character.

The basis of the pain management therapy is its measurement, based on the following principles:

- The assessment of the pain intensity at rest as well as when moving, which allows to evaluate the patient's functional status,
- Pain management therapy is applied or modified, when, according to the numerical scale, the pain is scored 3 points or more when at rest and 4 points or more when moving.
- Documenting the reactions to the applied therapies, including undesirable symptoms.

The collected data concerning the level of pain intensity is one of the elements influencing the choice of proper analgesics and their form. Other elements that must be taken into consideration are: the expected duration of the treatment, the kind and the possible risk of using a certain kind of analgesic, as well as the type of the surgical procedure and its range, the level of patient's awareness concerning the pain they are going to experience after the surgery. The choice of method should be made depending on the category of surgery. There are four categories of surgical procedures:

- Surgical procedures which involve small tissue damage - Category I – it includes small orthopaedic procedures, pain being scored <4 points on a scale, lasting one day,
- Surgical procedures which involve average tissue damage – Category II, pain < 4 points on a scale, lasting shorter than 3 days (procedures exclude pelvis' area operations)
- Surgical procedures which involve significant tissue damage – Category III, pain >4 on the scale, lasting from 3 to 7 days (pelvis' area operations),
- Surgical procedures which include severe tissue damage – Category IV, pain > 6, lasting longer than seven days (reconstructive surgery).

The way of giving the patient medications is significant. In the postoperative period, hypothermia and lower filling of blood vessels (blood loss, the loss of plasma or extracellular fluid) influence the medicament absorption from the subcutaneous and muscular tissues, which results in poor effectiveness of treatment, despite proper dosage of medicaments. Thus, analgesics after an extensive surgery should be applied intravenously in the postoperative period. The management of postoperative pain should begin before the pain stimuli caused by the surgery arises. Based on the research, there was developed a strategy, the aim of which was to prevent hypersensitivity from progressing; this kind of procedure is called „analgesia in advance" (giving analgesics in a calculated way).

Relieving postoperative pain is based on three therapeutic principles: the first one is applying analgesics according to the three-stage analgesic ladder (I stage – non-opioid and nonsteroidal anti-inflammatory drugs; II stage – weak opioids, the medicaments from the I stage; III stage – strong opioids, the medicaments from the I stage and coanalgesics); the second principle is using the regional anaesthesia techniques, which stop the pain transmitting (constant epidural and subarachnoid anaesthesia, blocking peripheral nerves, infiltration anaesthesia) and the multimodal analgesia technique, that is mixing medicaments of different mechanisms, in order to achieve better and more efficient pain relieving, with lower level of undesirable symptoms. In addition to those, the medicaments should be given according to the patient's weight and applied at fixed hours (Dobrogowski et al., 2008; Kübler, 2008, Paszkiewicz – Mes, 2011; Wodliczek & Dobrogowski, 2011).

During the development of medical sciences, the postoperative pain was defined as a crucial medical problem concerning both the patient and the medical staff. The nursing care of the patient suffering from the postoperative pain is multifaceted, comprising the following elements:

Teaching Patients

Nurses take care of the patient in a holistic way, according to the nursing process, which consists of preparing the patient to the surgery by teaching them about the possibility of experiencing pain, about the available methods of relieving it, they also ask questions concerning the previous pain experiences of the patient and their pain-managing preferences.

Observation

An observation is made to get to know the cause of pain and the factors which intensify it. The level of the postoperative pain is checked with the scales several times during the day and documented. The patient becomes a subject of observation themselves, their reactions which may show they are experiencing pain are being observed:

- Their face expression: grimace or clenching their teeth, sharp facial features, clenching one's eyelids, widely opened mouth;
- Sounds: crying, moaning, sighing;
- The patient's body movements: general restlessness, akinesis, limited physical activity, the body posture whilst walking;
- Controlling the vital signs: quicker or shallow respiration, increased pulse rate, perspiration, raised arterial blood pressure;
- Patient's state of mind: anxiety, hostility, regret, helplessness, fear.

Therapeutic Actions

The medicaments are given by the pain-managing therapy standards: according to the patient's age, weight, condition, regularly. Analgesics may cause different undesirable symptoms, such as nausea and vomiting, hypoventilation (respiratory depression), itching skin, constipation, all of which influences the patient in a negative way; that is why this occurrence is fought against according to the rule: maximum comfort, minimum undesirable symptoms. The nurse who makes a careful observation of a patient may help choosing the effective analgesic and the best way of applying it.

Nursing Procedures

All the nursing procedures are performed after giving the patient analgesics, in order to minimize the unpleasant experience. An important aspect of pain management is changing the patient's position, supervised by the nurse, who uses all the available facilities, such as rollers, props, wedges. If it is necessary, the nurse applies immobilization. To alleviate of relieve the pain, the nurse applies warm or cold compresses or other procedures in cooperation with physiotherapists. The nurse also takes actions in order to increase the patient's pain threshold: takes care of the patient's psychological comfort by enabling them to communicate their needs – by the nurse call system, provides the patient with peace and rest, makes the patient not focus on their negative emotions by conversation, by being with them, by raising the patient's sense of safety. The nurse has to cooperate closely with the multispecialty staff in coordinating the pain-managing process (Paszkiewicz – Mes, 2011, Niechwiadowicz - Czapka, 2009).

General Recommendation for the Patients Leaving the Hospital

The patient is discharged from hospital being rehabilitated to the point where they are able to sit, walk, perform simple tasks.

- When coming back home they should not drive, the advised position for the patients undergoing a leg surgery – at the back seat, with the extended leg resting on the seat; if the way home takes long time the patient is advised to take breaks and take a few steps.
- If the patient underwent a knee surgery, they should not put anything, like a blanket or a pillow under the leg, they also should keep their leg extended – it helps to prevent flexion contractures.
- In the postoperative period there may occur swelling and pain in the area affected by the surgical procedure. The non-pharmacological ways of pain management: keep the leg raised, apply cold compress to the area affected by the surgery for 20 minutes, up to 3-5 times a day (in order to avoid frost-caused injury the ice should be insulated with thin fabric and a plastic bag), take breaks during everyday activities (time for rest). When the swelling and pain begin to subside, the patient is advised to increase the level and frequency of activity.
- Using relaxation techniques as a non-pharmacological way of pain management: The relaxation should begin with taking several deep and calm diaphragmatic breaths (diaphragmatic/ abdominal respiration), then the patient should begin muscle relaxation by repeating „I'm relaxing my...." and naming the part of the body which is concerned; another exercise is alternate stretching tight and relaxing certain muscle groups.

- If there is need for immobilizing the body part (stabilizer, plaster cast), the immobilisation should be kept until the tissues have completely healed. The rehabilitation should be applied gradually. Applying any load should be consulted with the physician.
- The patient must not undertake activities which cause pain, not apply too much pressure to joints by avoiding lifting heavy objects, walking on uneven surfaces, prolonged standing or kneeling position. The housework activities which affect the therapeutic effects negatively are: washing the dishes whilst applying full load to the operated limb – the leg should be raised, with the knee slightly bent, supported with a footstool; the patient is forbidden to clean the floors until the intensive part of the therapy has finished, too.
- The rules concerning walking up the stairs – the uninjured leg goes first, then goes the injured one and then go the crutches; walking down the stairs – crutches, then the injured leg, and then the uninjured one.
- The instruction of safe falling and getting up after falling down: throwing crutches to the side, so that they would not cause any additional injury, supporting oneself with arms.
- Self-care and self-control: the patient should avoid making the wound wet, they should take showers instead of baths, after securing the wound with plastic foil or a special protective pad.
- Control visit in the orthopaedic outpatient clinic on a fixed date; in case of redness, oozing, fever, more intense pain or swelling the patient should contact the doctor immediately.
- If there is any need to continue the anticoagulant treatment at home, the patient must be reminded of the procedures of doing hypodermic injections, which they should have learnt when being hospitalized (supplying the patient with an instruction containing the description of the procedure and the places of applying the injections). Before discharging the patient from hospital, the medical staff should check if the patient can inject anticoagulants by themselves.
- Preparing the home environment for the safe functioning of the convalescent (removing obstacles – home appliances that are not necessary, but take up the room, carpets, installing daily living aids – grab bars, raised toilet seats, non-slip mats).
- If the patient is overweight, they should be advised to lose weight (dietician – obesity management clinic).
- Informing the patient about the possibility of getting help from the community/ public health nurse at the regional outpatient clinic.
- Buying the prescribed medicament.

It is difficult to foresee how the patient is going to react to pain and manage it, both in the physiological, psychological and the social aspects, due to the complex, multifaceted character of pain experiencing. (Juczyński, 2001, 2002) The way one experiences pain is closely dependent on one's cognitive appraisal. The meaning of pain is determined based on one's personal experience, beliefs concerning one's health and illness, as well as on information one gains from one's environment. Often this kind of situation is accompanied by anxiety, one experiences stress, which leads to the increase in the inner tension, which leads to pain intensifying, physical and mental exhaustion. The physical state of the patient, the quality of their lives and their closest ones are dependent on the patient's pain-related behaviours, i.e. frequent lying in bed, grumbling and complaining about their ailments, taking analgesics, seeking specialists' help. (James, 1992).

Mental aspects play a crucial role both in experiencing pain and in managing it. The cognitive appraisal concerning one's focus of attention, the assessment of one's possibilities, the effectiveness of coping, has a great meaning as well. (Kostarczyk, 2003). The empirical research shows that pain managing, the sense of locus of control and the cognitive appraisal of pain influence the intensity and character of the experienced pain. The sense of control is connected with the sense of being in power and with the ability of having influence over one's life and environment. People who do not have the sense of control suffer from bad mood, their general feeling worsens. This kind of approach influences effective pain management in a negative way and thus raises the level of the mental discomfort one experiences. On the other hand, people who have the sense of control show higher pain tolerance, manage pain better, which also comprises to better cooperation with the medical staff. (Suchocka, 2008). The sense of control and predictability are the factors owing to which patients manage pain better and need to be given analgesics less often. In Chapman's research in 1989 the patients who had the chance of giving themselves analgesics after the surgery (the drip infusion containing analgesic was connected during the whole time) managed their pain better, took the analgesics less frequently and in smaller doses than the patients who did not have this opportunity. Those effects are connected with the sense of having control over the situation and the sense of predictability. It turns out that people who choose active forms of coping, who have a high sense of pain control, who present a high self-esteem and think in a rational way, experience lower levels of pain and stress. (Golec, 2004, Keefe et al., 2005) The patients who learnt to apply active pain- and stress-management techniques, e.g. used relaxation techniques, visualisation, experienced less severe postoperative pain than the patients who had not been taught those techniques. (Golec, 2002).

The patient's illness and hospitalization causes changes in all the aspects of their life. The most common reaction to illness is anxiety, which is experienced especially if undergoing the surgical procedure turns out to be necessary. Surgical treatment is connected with experiencing pain, which is usually seen as one of the most serious life obstacles, which alienates the patient form their environment. The sole consciousness of the possible pain experience may affect a person's behaviour and burden their mental regulation mechanisms. In many cases stress and pain are like a vicious circle, seemingly with no escape. That is why it is necessary to teach patients techniques and methods other than pharmacological ones, especially if analgesics do not give desired results or if they significantly worsen the patient's functioning. These methods are psychological methods, such as relaxation, visualisation, biofeedback or the cognitive-behavioural therapy.

The social support the patient receives also plays a vital role in their pain management. Support is a form of interaction, between the patient and one or many participants in a problematic, difficult, stressful or critical situation; experiencing pain can be regarded as one of them as well. Depending on what is the supporting contents of the social exchange, one can distinguish different kinds of support:

- Emotional support, which consist of sending supporting and comforting emotions during the interaction, which express care about and positive approach towards the person who receives support. Additionally, creating the sense of affinity, care, raising one's self-esteem. People who are suffering or having a crisis, thanks to this kind of supportive interaction, release their own tension and negative feelings, they may express their concerns and sadness. Proper behaviour of the person giving support give other hope. This kind of support is most expected.
- Informative support is exchanging, during the interaction, this kind of information which helps to understand the situation, circumstances and the problem better.
- Instrumental support is giving instructions and information about the certain, specific ways of behaviour. It can also be a form of modelling effective remedial behaviours, it also consists of offering help in performing the everyday tasks, such as housework.
- Material support, which is material, objective and financial help, as well as direct physical help to those who need it. It can consist of giving someone resources they need to live, feeding, sheltering someone or buying them medicaments. (Sęk & Cieślak, 2004). The patient in pain needs special support and help coping with somatic, emotional and spiritual ailments, from the people who are important for them, usually their family and friends.

CONCLUSION

For some patients, the onset of pain may be a crucial turning point in their lives, which might inspire them to revalue and change their lives. The stress which is induced by one's illness and one's situation may be an opportunity to get to know oneself better and to prove oneself, to check one's mental strength and resilience. It may become the time of seeking and building new ways of controlling and influencing one's life, changes in thinking about the symptoms, body reactions and pain experience. A person might learn to perceive loss as one of the natural things. The situation also helps to create new, more adaptive ways of thinking, verify the previous ones and reject the ineffective ones (Motyka & Załuski, 2010). However, there exists a chance that illness may become a „recipe for life". Being ill may be the way of forcing other people to take an interest in them. The person wants to be in the limelight and „gains" from it. As a result of the actions taken by the patients is a certain way of adapting, which is influenced by the individual biological and mental features of every person. This is the reason for the existence of various pain and stress-management strategies and there is no universal way of coping with them (Kurowska & Czepek, 2009).

REFERENCES

Bishop, G. D. (2000). *The Psychology of Health*. Wrocław, Poland: Astrum.

Chodkiewicz, J. (2004). *The Psychology of Health – chosen issues*. Łódź, Poland: Akademia Humanistyczno – Ekonomiczna.

Chwałczyńska, A., Woźniewski, M., Rożek-Mróz, K., & Malicka, I. (2004). The quality of life of women undergoing mastectomy. *Medical News*, *57*, 5–6.

Czubalski, K. (1995). Indirect influence of illness over a person's functioning. In Chosen issues of psychosomatic medicine and the psychology of a somatic patient. Warsaw, Poland: Dział Wydawnictw Akademii Medycznej w Warszawie.

de Walden-Gałuszko, K. (2001). Psychological aspects of pain. *Przewodnik Lekarza*, *4*(4), 58–59.

Dobrogowski, J., & Wordliczek, J. (2004). *The medicine of pain*. Warsaw, Poland: Wydawnictwo Lekarskie PZWL.

Filipczak-Brynierska, I., Brynierski, K., Woroń, J., & Wodliczek, J. (2010). Pain-transmitting mechanisms. The role of immune system in regulating the way one experiences pain. *Anestezja i Ratownictwo*, *4*, 500–509.

Golec, A. (2000). The basic psychology of pain. *Nowa Klinika*, *7*(9), 933–938.

Golec, A. (2002). Acute pain – psychological aspects. In Ból Ostry. Kraków, Poland: Wydawnictwo Uniwersytetu Jagielońskiego.

Golec, A. (2004). Psychological aspects of pain. In J. Dobrogowski & J. Wordliczek (Eds.), *Medycyna Bólu*. Warsaw, Poland: Wydawnictwo Lekarskie PZWL.

Hasiak, J. (2012). Pre-and post-operative pain. Part I. Genesis. *Przegląd Urologiczny*, *13*(72), 19-24.

Heszen, I., & Sęk, H. (2007). *The psychology of Health*. Poland: Wydawnictwo Naukowe Naukowe PWN.

Heszen-Niejodek, I. (1990). Psychological problems and the tasks of a psychologist in surgery. In The role of psychologist in diagnosing and treating somatic diseases. Warszawa, Poland: Wydawnictwo Lekarskie PZWL.

Hilgier, M. (2002). Chronic pain – a medical and social problem. *Przewodnik Lekarza*, *5*(1/2), 6–11.

James, P. T. (1992). Psychological dimension of chronic pain. Cambridge: Butterworth – Heinemann. doi:10.1016/B978-0-7506-0573-1.50008-1

Juczyński, Z. (2001). *Measurement tools in promoting of health and psychology of health*. Warszawa, Poland: Pracownia Testów Psychologicznych Polskiego Towarzystwa Psychologicznego.

Juczyński, Z. (2002). Coping with chronic pain. In Theoretic and clinical ways of coping with stress. Poznań, Poland: Stowarzyszenie Psychologia i Architektura.

Juszczak, K. (2009). The role of nurse in relieving postoperative pain. *Pielęgniarstwo Chirurgiczne i Angiologiczne*, *4*, 131–134.

Kapała, W., Chudziński, S., & Hyrcza, S. (2008). *The expectations of hospitalized patients towards the nursing staff*. Pielęgniarstwo.

Keefe, F. J., Abernethy, A. P., & Campbell, L. C. (2005). Psychological approaches to understanding treating disease – related pain. *Annual Review of Psychology*, *56*, 601–630. doi:10.1146/annurev.psych.56.091103.070302 PMID:15709948

Kiwerski, J. (2006). Medical rehabilitation. Warsaw, Poland: Wydawnictwo Lekarskie PZWL.

Kobus, K., Wójcicki, P., Dydymski, T., Węgrzyn, M., & Hamlawi, F. (2007). The evaluation of the results of treatment of patients suffering from Dupuytren contraction, based on analysis of the authors' own materials. *Ortopedia, Traumatologia, Rehabilitacja, 9*, 134–140. PMID:17538519

Korzeniowska, K., & Szałek, E. (2010). Pain. *Contemporary Pharmacy, 3*, 9–14. PMID:20467575

Kostarczyk, E. (2003). *Neuropsychology of pain*. Poznań, Poland: Państwowe Towarzystwo Przyjaciół Nauki.

Kramer, J. (1997). Orthopaedics. Warsaw, Poland: Springer PWN.

Kübler, A. (2008). *Anaesthesiology*. Wrocław, Poland: Elsevier Urban & Partner.

Kurowska, K., Czepek, K. (2009). The feeling of coherence and the preferred styles of coping with illness in cholelithiasis patients. *Nowiny Lekarskie, 78*(5–6), 3–306.

Lesińska-Sawicka, M., Grygorowicz, E., & Jałtuszewska, S. (2007). Chosen elements of the quality of the medical care in relation to hospital patients' stress level. *Pielęgniarstwo XXI wieku, 3-4*(20-21), 51 – 56.

Marciniak, W., & Szulc, A. (Eds.). (2004). Orthopaedics and Rehabilitation by Wiktor Dega. Warsaw, Poland: Wydawnictwo Lekarskie PZWL.

Melzack, R., & Wall, P. (2006). *The secret of Pain*. Kraków, Poland: Wydawnictwo WAM.

Motyka, M., & Załuski, M. (2010). Illness as a crisis and developmental changes. *Pielęgniarstwo XXI wieku, 3-4*(32-33), 99-103.

Niechwiadowicz-Czapka, T. (2009). Coping with postoperative pain. *Magazyn Pielęgniarki i Położnej, 1*.

Paszkiewicz-Mes, E. (2011). The role of nurse in relieving postoperative pain. *Pielęgniarstwo XXI wieku, 4*, 37-41.

Piontek, T., Ciemniewska-Gorzela, K., Szulc, A., Naczk, J., & Słomczykowski, M. (2012). All-arthroscopic AMIC procedure for repair of cartilage defects of the knee. *Knee Surgery, Sports Traumatology, Arthroscopy, 20*(5), 922–925. doi:10.100700167-011-1657-z PMID:21910000

Rolka, H., Krajewska-Kułak, E., Kułak, W., Drozdowski, W., Gołębiewska, A., & Kondzior, D. (2009). Accepting one's illness and the pain-coping strategies as important components of life quality evaluation, depending on the state of migraine patients. Initial report. *Problemy Pielęgniarstwa, 17*(3), 178–183.

Saint-Maurice, C., Muller, A., & Meynadier, J. (1998). *Pain: diagnosing, treatment and preventing*. Warsaw, Poland: Wydawnictwo Gebethner i S-ka.

Salmon, P. (2002). *Psychology in medicine supports copperation with patient and the treatment*. Gdańsk, Poland: Gdańskie Wydawnictwo Psychologiczne.

Sęk, H., & Cieślak, R. (Eds.). (2004). Social support, stress and health. Warsaw, Poland: Wydawnictwo Naukowe Naukowe PWN.

Stachowiak-Andrysiak, M., & Mikstacki, A. (2005). The influence of chronic pain over the functioning of patients and their families. *Nowiny Lekarskie*, *74*(2), 255–258.

Steuden, S. (2002). Psychological issues concerning health and illness. In P. Oleś, S. Steuden, & J. Tuczołowicz (Eds.), *How I see less of the world: Vision problems and life quality*. Lublin, Poland: Towarzystwo Naukowe KUL.

Suchocka, L. (2008). Pain psychology. Warsaw, Poland: Wydawnictwo Delfin.

Ulatowska, A., Bączyk, G., & Lewandowska, H. (2012). The review of literature concerning postoperative pain and the quality of nursing care. *Surgical and Angiological Nursing*, *1*, 7–12.

Wasilewski, D., Wojnar, M., & Chatizow, J. (2010). Depression and pain: National epidemiological research. *Psychiatria Polska*, *44*, 435–445. PMID:20672522

Widuchowski, J., Widuchowski, W., & Paściak, M. (2005). Knee arthroscopy – past and present. *Wiadomości Lekarskie*, *58*(1–2), 111–115. PMID:15991563

Włodarczyk, D., & Skuza, B. (2007). The meaning of the patient – medical staff relation within the treatment. In Psychology in medical practicej. Warsaw, Poland: Wydawnictwo Lekarskie PZWL.

Wodliczek, J. (2011). *Dobrogowski J.: Pain treatment*. Wydawnictwo Lekarskie PZWL.

Ziębicka, J., & Gajdosz, R. (2006). Chosen aspects of anxiety of patients awaiting surgical procedure. *Anestezjologia Intensywna Terapia*, *1*, 41–44.

This research was previously published in Organizational Culture and Ethics in Modern Medicine edited by Anna Rosiek and Krzysztof Leksowski, pages 372-392, copyright year 2016 by Medical Information Science Reference (an imprint of IGI Global).

Section 2

Drugs and Pharmaceutical Accountability

Chapter 4
Overview of Multicomponent Solid Forms

Rahul B Chavan
National Institute of Pharmaceutical Education and Research (NIPER), India

Nalini R Shastri
National Institute of Pharmaceutical Education and Research (NIPER), India

ABSTRACT

Multi-drug therapy involves the simultaneous or sequential administration of two or more drugs with similar or different mechanisms of action and is efficient in combating various ailments such as cancer, diabetes, and rheumatoid arthritis. It has emerged advantageous due to larger therapeutic benefits, an increase in patient compliance, lower administrative costs, and reduced number of prescriptions. In the recent past, the clinical success of the Novartis product Entresto (sacubitril, disodium valsartan and water) and Esteve product E-58425 (tramadol and celecoxib) has boosted the development of multi-drug . The present article is hence designed to provide an overview of different multicomponent addicts which provide option of combining the drugs at a supramolecular level (nano-sized level). Key features of multi-drug cocrystal, co-amorphous system and eutectics are described with major emphasis on screening tools, preparation methods, characterization techniques, biopharmaceutical aspects and scale up.

DOI: 10.4018/978-1-7998-1680-5.ch004

INTRODUCTION

Concurrent administration of two or more therapeutic agents which have similar or different mechanisms of action are termed as multi drug therapy and can be used to combat various ailments (Shin et al., 2009). In comparison to single drug therapy, this approach helps in targeting different key signal transduction pathways which can be more efficacious in management of diseases, since they can evade cellular resistance mechanisms. The advantages offered by multi-drug therapy are schematically depicted in Figure 1. To date, this approach has been successfully implemented for management of diseases such as HIV/AIDS, cancer, multiple sclerosis, malaria, infectious diseases, cardiovascular and metabolic diseases, hypertension, auto immune disorders and many psychiatric maladies (Conway et al., 2010; Thipparaboina et al., 2015). Multi-drug therapy when administered in fixed dose combinations (FDC) are cost-effective which help in reducing pill load without any additional risk of adverse events or drug resistance and hence improve the patient compliance. FDC also facilitate the reduction of managerial and manufacturing costs by reducing the outflow related to packaging and drug prescriptions. FDC products contain simple drug–drug combinations or drug–device combinations, such as drug-eluting stents or drug-biological products for use in cancer therapy. The benefits offered by FDC are often overshadowed because of its severe disadvantages such as stability issues, and solubility differences and incompatibility between the parent drugs (Thipparaboina et al., 2015). Hence, there is a need to develop alternative approach which will facilitate the development of therapeutic hybrids to counter such problems. Multicomponent solids such as cocrystals, co amorphous system (CAM) and eutectics may provide solution required for delivering the drug-drug combinations with improved benefits in terms of stability, improved solubility and dissolution when compared to FDC.

Clinical success of Novartis product Entresto a multi drug cocrystal which was approved in 2015 for effective management of chronic heart pain, is comprised of monosodium sacubitril, disodium valsartan and water, and has given a boost to pharmaceutical industry to improve the pharmaceutical attributes using multi component systems. However, developments of such multi component solid system need careful attention as it requires supportive evidence on its pharmacological action and safety such as synergistic or additive effect of two drugs in addition to stability and formulation related attributes. This review article aims to provide a brief overview on multi component solid forms (cocrystals, CAM and eutectics) and furnish information ranging from preparation, characterization, scale up and regulatory concerns related to these systems.

Figure 1. Advantages offered by multi drug therapy: MDR multi-drug resistance

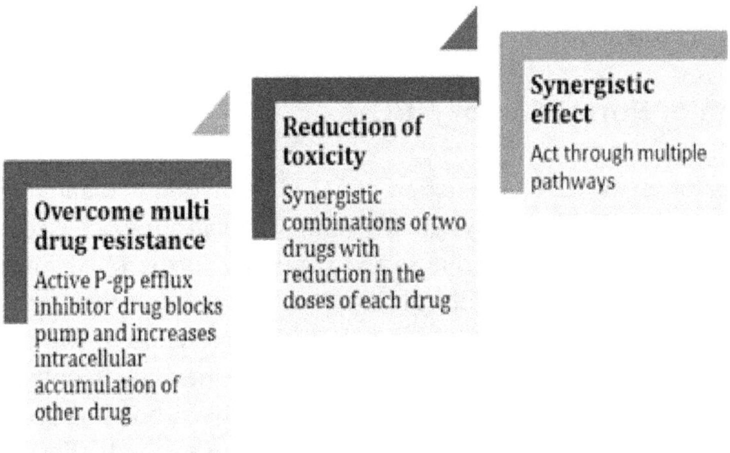

MULTI-DRUG COCRYSTALS

Multi drug cocrystals (MDC) are a subset of pharmaceutical cocrystals wherein the conformer is a bioactive molecule which possess independent drug activity instead of being an inert coformer. As per FDA, co-crystals are dissociable multicomponent solid crystalline supramolecular complexes which contain two or more components within the same crystal lattice where in the components are in neutral state and interact via nonionic interactions' (Aitipamula et al., 2012). MDC offer numerous advantages from enhanced bioavailability to reduction of multidrug resistance, synergistic and/or additive effects, enhanced solubility and dissolution of at least one component, possible stabilization of unstable components through intermolecular interactions, lifecycle management of existing products, and finally combination therapies (Thipparaboina et al., 2016). Our research group was the first one to propose the definition of co-crystals to MDC systems, and defined it as 'dissociable solid crystalline supramolecular complexes comprising two or more therapeutically effective components in a stoichiometric ratio within the same crystal lattice, wherein the components may predominantly interact via nonionic interactions and rarely through hybrid interactions (a combination of ionic and nonionic interactions involving partial proton transfer and hydrogen bonding) with or without the presence of solvate molecules' (Thipparaboina et al., 2016). Approval of Entresto a MDC appeared just after the EMA reflection paper and US-FDA guidance stimulated the interest of the pharmaceutical industry in MDCs as materials for drug products. Interestingly, the first MDC was reported by Nakao et al., way back in 1977 who developed theophylline: phenobarbital MDC (Nakao et al., 1977). A partial list of some of the reported MDC along with their preparation methods and applications are depicted in Table 1.

Prediction of Formation of MDC

Before preparation of MDC, prediction of MDC formation is found to be crucial. To date, there are no confirmed systematic computational approaches for prediction the MDC formation. However, due to the similarity in the bond formation, the well-developed prediction models of co-crystal formation between drugs and coformers can be successfully extrapolated for the prediction of MDC formation. These approaches may be based on knowledge or experimental screening (Figure 2). pKa based models, use of molecular descriptors, hydrogen-bonding propensity and synthonic engineering are promising knowledge based methods (Duggirala et al., 2016). These methods can be successfully applied to any two molecule systems and, thus, can be used for drug–drug systems. Synthon based approach is most widely used strategies to understand molecular interactions. Structural units of supramolecular system are identified that can be assembled to form intermolecular interactions. Use of this synthon-based retrosynthetic strategy for the development of lamivudine and zidovudine MDC was reported by Prashant et al (Bhatt et al., 2008). This approach can predict with reasonable degree of success using simple molecules, but become complex in molecules with multiple hydrogen-bond donors and acceptors. Numerous attempts have been made to develop new prediction model for coformer selection. Delori et al., implemented hydrogen bonding propensity calculations for predicting the formation of an MDC of pyrimethamine with theophylline and carbamazepine (Delori et al., 2013). Etter et al., developed a set of empirical rules to determine the tendency for hydrogen bonding of various donor/acceptor combinations. These rules are based on the fact that the best proton donors will form a hydrogen bond with the best proton acceptor (Etter et al., 1990). Apart from these approaches, Childs et al., proposed ΔpKa based method which involves pKa values of drug and coformers. In their work on theophylline–acid complexes, they categorized a $0 < \triangle pKa < 2.5$ region as a salt/co-crystal continuum zone (Childs et al., 2007). Cruz Cabeza et al., after studying the 6465 crystalline complexes in the CSD, and validating and quantifying the △pKa rule, stated that △pKa would be one of the most prominent and simplest methods to use in predicting co-crystal formation. They concluded that $\triangle pKa < -1$ would exclusively result in a non-ionized complex; $\triangle pKa < 4$ would result in an ionized complex; and between $1 \leq \triangle pKa \leq 4$, a 1 △pKa difference would increase the probability of proton transfer by 17% from 10% at $\triangle pKa = -1$ to 95% at $\triangle pKa = 4$ (Cruz-Cabeza, 2012). Use of Hansen solubility parameters

(Mohammad et al., 2011), lattice energy calculations (Issa et al., 2008) and many other knowledge based methods are also available for prediction of cocrystal preparation which can be extrapolated to MDC (Duggirala et al., 2016).

Similar to these knowledge-based prediction methods, literature also lacks in experimental screening methods for MDC formation. However, methods such as Ternary phase diagrams based on solubility and melting, liquid-phase excess enthalpy predictions, pulsed gradient spin-echo nuclear magnetic resonance (PGSE NMR), and intermolecular site pairing energy which were investigated for cocrystals can be extrapolated for MDC preparation but require proper validation before developing robust prediction model for screening of MDC.

Preparation and Scale Up

Once the prediction of MDC formation is completed, then the next step is preparation or synthesis of MDC. The conventional cocrystal preparation methods and methods used for MDC preparation are similar. As depicted in Table 1, conventional cocrystal preparation methods such as mechanical grinding (both neat and solvent-drop or liquid assisted), slow solvent evaporation and slurry mediated transformation can be used for MDC preparation. Apart from these conventional methods, other methods that are reported for formation of MDC include microfluidic approach, high-throughput screening, supercritical fluid technologies and ultrasound assisted solution cocrystallization. Figure 3 outlines the general preparation methods of

Figure 2. Different approaches for prediction of MDC formation

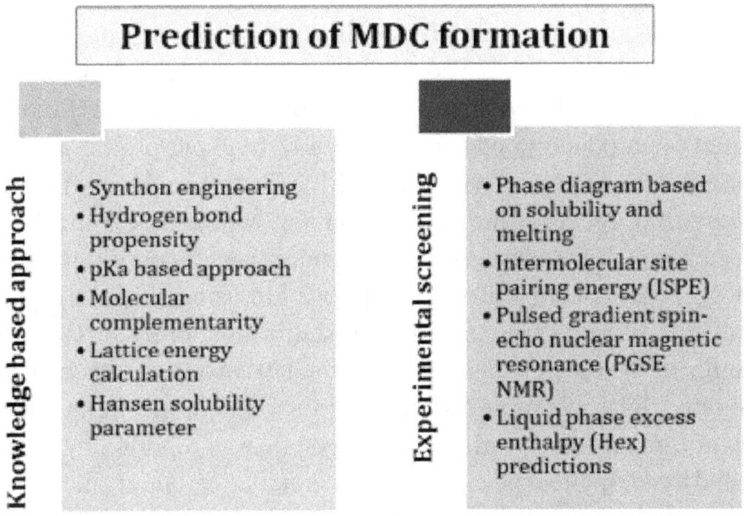

Figure 3. Preparation methods of cocrystals

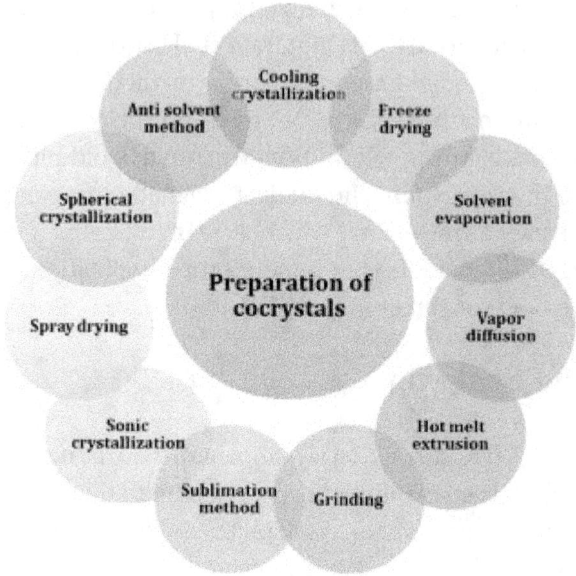

MDC. For more details on co-crystals preparation methods and their applications in the synthesis of MDC, interested readers may refer to previously published studies (Duggirala et al., 2016).

Scale up of MDC is a major challenge in pharmaceutical industry. Methods like solution crystallization, hot melt extrusion, spray drying, high shear granulation are scalable for cocrystals. Solution crystallization is preferred for scale up of cocrystals. However, a challenge of difference in solubility of drug and coformer in the selected solvent that may result in preferential crystallization of individual substances has to be addressed. Zhao et al., prepared cocrystal of α-lipoic acid with nicotinamide and scaled up it over 1 kg of solid co-crystals. Continuous oscillatory baffled crystallizer was employed for production of cocrystal at a throughput of 350 gm/hr yielding a purity of 99% of cocrystal (Zhao et al., 2014). In this scale up process, ternary phase diagram of drug, coformer and solvent was found to be critical as it give a cocrystal region to produce cocrystals. Leung et al., reported cocrystal of anti-diabetic molecule with benzoic acid and scaled up to 2 gm using solution crystallization (Leung et al., 2012). Apart from solution crystallization, other scalable techniques that are attempted by researchers include hot melt extrusion, spray drying, resonant acoustic mixing, high shear granulation etc. Utility of high shear granulation for the development of piracetam-tartaric acid co-crystals was reported by Rehder et al., Authors stated that impeller speed, amount of granulating liquid, and the excipients have significant impact on co-crystal formation (Allesø et al., 2009). Dhumal et al., in their research scaled up the cocrystal formation of ibuprofen and nicotinamide using hot melt extrusion up to 1 kg (Aher et al., 2010). Daurio et al., reported scale up of AMG 517–sorbic acid cocrystal by twin screw extrusion to 100 gm (Daurio et al., 2014). Nagaudi et al., reported scale up theophylline oxalic acid cocrystals up to 80 gm with 94% yield in resonant acoustic mixing by using design of experiment approach (Nagapudi et al., 2017).

Large scale production of MDC requires study of process parameters and their interactions. Additionally, researchers are exploring the continuous manufacturing techniques such as mixed-suspension mixed-product removal, continuous oscillatory baffled crystallizers, continuous anti-solvent crystallization, resonant acoustic mixing, hot melt extrusion and electrospray technique for cocrystal preparation. With a view to support the implementation of continuous manufacturing, USFDA recommends using a science and risk-based approach, while the regulatory requirement for the quality of the product remains the same as in batch processing. Interested readers can refer to a detailed review on continuous cocrystallization techniques by Chavan et al. (Chavan et al., 2018).

Characterization of Cocrystals

Prepared novel crystals are primarily characterized using techniques such as differential scanning calorimetry (DSC), powder x-ray diffraction (PXRD), single crystal X- ray diffraction, spectroscopic techniques (infrared spectroscopy, near infrared spectroscopy, Raman spectroscopy and tetra hertz spectroscopy), solid state nuclear magnetic resonance (ssMNR) and thermogravimetric analysis (TGA). As single crystals are not always available during initial stages of discovery, application of advanced spectroscopic techniques may help in determining the structure from the powder samples. Raman spectroscopy finds application in identifying cocrystal formation during high-throughput slurry screening (Kojima et al., 2010), discriminating a cocrystal and a physical mixture in formulated tablets (Burley et al., 2012) and also in quantifying the cocrystals from binary or ternary mixtures (Allesø et al., 2008). Near infrared spectroscopy has been reported for identification and quantification of cocrystals in binary or ternary mixtures and final finished dosage form (Mukherjee et al., 2013). Terahertz time-domain-spectroscopy has also been employed to differentiate among the chiral and racemic of cocrystals of theophylline with malic acid and tartaric acid. Use of ssNMR for characterization of cocrystals was explained by Vogt et al., who diagnosed hydrogen bonding and local conformational changes by ^{1}H–^{1}H, ^{1}H–^{13}C and ^{19}F–^{13}C coupling (Vogt et al., 2008). Brief overview of various characterization techniques has been provided in Figure 4.

Figure 4. Characterization tools used for MDC

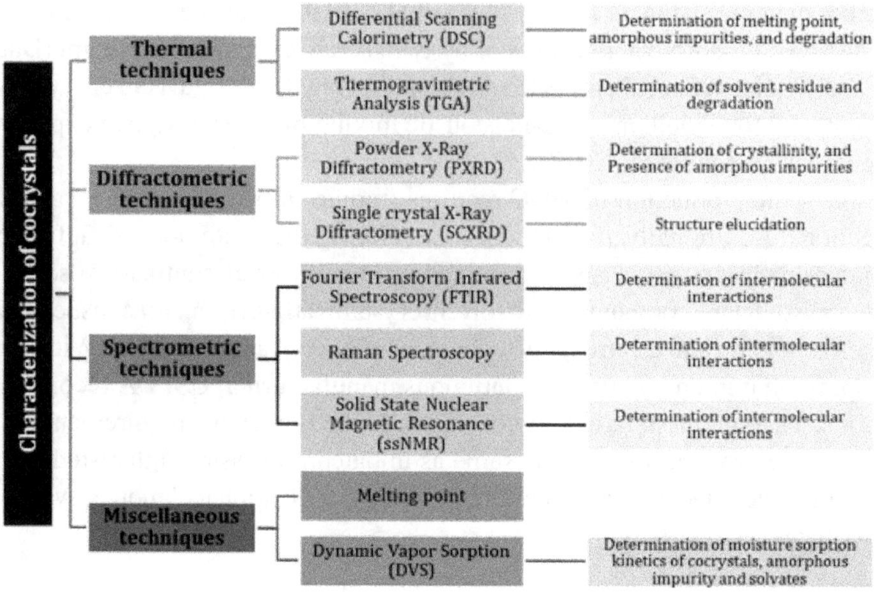

Evaluation of MDC

Major objective behind the development of MDC is to improve the therapeutic efficacy through synergistic or additive effect of second drug component of MDC, in addition to other pharmaceutical attributes (solubility, dissolution, stability and mechanical properties). Currently more than 30 articles on MDC have demonstrated improvement of solubility, stability and dissolution. As the MDC list is extensive, brief summary of articles published after 2015 have been provided in table 1. Wang et al., developed a cocrystal of vitamin D3 with vitamin D2 to address the chemical stability issue of vitamin D3. Vitamin D3 is widely used in the food and nutraceutical industries but is chemically unstable as it is susceptible to topochemical reaction. Due to unique packing arrangement in polymorphic form A of the developed cocrystal, extraordinary chemical and physical advantage was obtained over pure components (Wang et al., 2016). However, fewer reports are available on MDC that address the biopharmaceutical aspects of MDC (Table 1). Analysis of the reported pharmacokinetic data generated from the MDC suggests that an improvement in area under curve (AUC) can be mainly attributed to the solubility advantage of MDC. Impact of MDC on other pharmacokinetic parameters was also found to be significant by few authors. Cheney et al., developed meloxicam: aspirin MDC which showed significant improvement in bioavailability (4 fold) as compared to plain drug. Five and four fold enhancement in C_{max} and AUC was reported by the authors

Table 1. Reported drug-drug/drug-nutraceuticals cocrystal

Drug Combination	Preparation Method	Pharmaceutical Attributes	Therapeutic Category	Reference
Sildenafil–aspirin	Solvent evaporation	IDR	Antihypertensive and NSAID	(Žegarac et al., 2014)
Diclofenac and diflunisal with theophylline	Solvent drop grinding and solvent evaporation	Stability and dissolution	Anti-asthmatic and NSAID	(Surov et al., 2014)
Dapsone–sulfanilamide flavone, luteolin, caffeine and benzothiazolone	Solution crystallization	Stability and solubility	Anti-leprotic, antibacterial and antioxidants	(Jiang et al., 2014)
Sinapic acid-6-propyl-2-thiouracil	Solution crystallization	Stability	Anti-oxidant, anti-microbial, anti-inflammatory, anti-cancer, and anti-anxiety	(Sinha et al., 2015)
Gliclazide- metformin	Solvent evaporation	Solubility, dissolution and hygroscopicity	Antidiabetic	(Putra et al., 2016)
Vitamin D2 and D3	Solvent evaporation	Chemical stability	Hormonal therapy	(Wang et al., 2016)
Norfloxacin-sulfathiazole	Liquid assisted grinding	Solubility, diffusion and antimicrobial activity	Antibacterial and antimicrobial	(Gopi et al., 2016)
Telmisartan-atenolol	Liquid assisted grinding	Solubility, IDR, stability and in vivo pharmacodynamic activity	Antihypertensive	(Haneef et al., 2017b)
4-aminosalicylic acid-caffeine	Solvent evaporation	Solubility and thermo chemical stability	Anti-tuberculous and anti-asthmatic	(Drozd et al., 2017a)
Flufenamic acid-ethenzamide	Solvent evaporation	Solubility, stability	NSAID	(Nechipadappu et al., 2017)
Ethenzamide- gentisic acid	Solid state grinding	Compressibility, stability and solubility	NSAID, analgesic and antipyretic activity	(Sokal et al., 2017)
Caffeine- dapsone	Liquid-assisted grinding and spray drying	Solubility, in vitro cytotoxicity and in vitro permeability study	Pulmonary infection	(do Amaral et al., 2018)
Carbamazepine- para-amino salicylic acid	Solvent evaporation and grinding	Solubility and dissolution	Anti-tuberculosis	(Drozd et al., 2017b)
Tramadol HCl–celecoxib	Wet grinding	IDR and oversaturation study	Pain management	(Almansa et al., 2017)
Sulfathiazole with theophylline and sulfanilamide	Cooling cocrystallization	pH-dependent solubility, partition coefficient and moisture stability	Antibacterial	(Yeh et al., 2018)
Lamotrigine-phenobarbital	Solvent evaporation	pH-dependent solubility and IDR	Anticonvulsants	(Kaur et al., 2017)
Dapsone- caffeine	Liquid-assisted milling	Granulation on fluidized bed processor	Antibacterial	(Todaro et al., 2019)

continued on following page

Table 1. Continued

Drug Combination	Preparation Method	Pharmaceutical Attributes	Therapeutic Category	Reference
Olmesartan medoxomil-hydrochlorothiazide	Co-evaporation	Dissolution	Antihypertensive	(Abdelquader et al., 2019)
Theophylline- aspirin	Liquid assisted grinding and ball milling	Solubility	Pain management	(Darwish et al., 2018)
5-Fluorocytosine-5-Fluorouracil	Neat grinding and solvent drop grinding	Physical stability	Anti-cancer	(da Silva et al., 2018)
Apremilast with caffeine, and acetylsalicylic	Solvent evaporation	Solubility and IDR	Psoriasis	(Wang et al., 2018)
Ibuprofen-levetiracetam	Ball milling	Chiral purity	Pain management	(Harmsen et al., 2018)
Temozolomide-baicalein	Slurry crystallization	Dissolution, stability and oral bioavailability	Anti-cancer	(Li et al., 2018)
Emodin- berberine Chloride	Solvent evaporation	Solubility, dissolution and oral bioavailability	Anti-bacterial, anti-cancer, and anti-diabetic	(Deng et al., 2018)
Chrysin- berberine	Ball milling	Oral bioavailability	Antioxidant, anti-inflammatory, anti-tumor, anti-bacterial, and cardio protective effects.	(Sa et al., 2018)
Zonisamide- caffeine	Solvent evaporation	Solubility, dissolution and stability	Anti-epileptic	(ShanáChow, 2018)
Entacapone with isoniazid, pyrazinamide and theophylline	Liquid assisted grinding	Solubility, dissolution and permeability	Parkinson's disease	(Bommaka et al., 2018)
Mefenamic acid–paracetamol	Gas antisolvent process	Dissolution	Anti-inflammatory	(Wichianphong et al., 2018)
Resveratrol-isoniazid	CO2 antisolvent recrystallization	Dissolution	Antioxidant, anti-cancer, anti-microbial and cardio protective	(Pessoa et al., 2019)
Isoniazid-Protocatechuic acid	Solvent evaporation	Solubility and Stability	Anti-tuberculous, anti-oxidant and Anti-inflammatory	(Mashhadi et al., 2016)
5-Fluorocytosine-isoniazid	Mechanochemical synthesis and solvent evaporation	Solubility and stability	Anti-tuberculous	(Souza et al., 2018)
Quercetin-pyrazinamide	Solvent evaporation	IDR, oral bioavailability and in vivo hepatotoxicity study	Anti-tuberculous and Hepato-protective study	(Liu et al., 2018)
Riluzole-syringic acid and riluzole-ferulic acid	Solvent evaporation	Dissolution and in vivo hepatotoxicity study	Amyotrophic lateral sclerosis	(Yadav et al., 2018a)

(Cheney et al., 2011). Post 2017, a paradigm shift towards evaluation of MDC for oral bioavailability was observed, which is reflected through some interesting research papers on chrysin- berberine, quercetin- pyrazinamide, temozolomide- baicalein and Emodin- berberine Chloride MDC that have disclosed the improvement in oral bioavailability through formation of cocrystal.

However, an extensive literature search has revealed a near absence of reports on pharmacodynamic or efficacy studies of MDC, which is more crucial, as combination of two drugs in MDC can only prove beneficial once their pharmacological potential is evaluated and proven experimentally. Recently, Yadav et al., and Liu et al., have showcased the importance of nutraceutical coformers like syringic acid, ferulic acid and quercetin in reducing the hepatotoxicity side effects of pyrazinamide and riluzole through the formation of drug-nutraceutical cocrystals (Liu et al., 2018 and Yadav et al., 2018).

Regulatory Guidelines for Pharmaceutical Cocrystals

Recently, EMA published a reflection paper in May 2015, followed by Regulatory Classification of Pharmaceutical Co-Crystals guidance from US-FDA in February 2018 for co-crystal development which is expected to substantially promote their development. As per this recent guidance by FDA, co-crystals are distinguished from salts based on co-existence of drug and coformers in the co-crystal lattice with a defined stoichiometry that interact non-ionically. Instead, co-crystals are more similar to solvates, in that both contain more than one component in the lattice. From a physical chemistry and regulatory perspective, co-crystals can be viewed as a special case of solvates and hydrates, wherein the second component, the coformer, is not a solvent (including water), and is typically nonvolatile. A comparative overview of these two regulatory guidelines regarding co-crystal-based product development is provided in Table 2.

Market and Clinical Status of MDC

Currently, there are a few commercial pharmaceutical cocrystals approved by the FDA. The Entresto® cocrystal of valsartan with sacubitril was approved by FDA in July 2015 and by EMA in November 2015 to treat depression and generalized anxiety disorders. E-58425 a new MDC has also entered Phase III clinical trial. E-58425 is a novel ionic co-crystal composed of racemic tramadol hydrochloride and celecoxib in a 1:1 molecular ratio (Chavan et al., 2018). It was developed using innovative platforms and is based on complementary mechanisms of analgesic action

Table 2. Comparative analysis of US-FDA Guidance February 2018 and EMA Reflection Paper May, 2015 on cocrystal

Factor	US-FDA Guidance February 2018	EMA Reflection Paper May, 2015
Definitions	Co-crystals are crystalline materials composed of two or more different molecules, typically drug and co-crystal formers (coformers), in the same crystal lattice.	Homogenous (single phase) crystalline structures made up of two or more components in a definite stoichiometric ratio where the arrangement in the crystal lattice is not based on ionic bonds (as with salts).
Regulatory status	Considers co-crystals as polymorphs of active pharmaceutical ingredients	Considers co-crystals as active pharmaceutical ingredients
Regulatory considerations	Views co-crystals as a special case of solvates and hydrates, wherein the second component, the coformer, is non-volatile	Considers solvates including hydrates as subgroup of co-crystals and limits the definition of co-crystals by stating that the components of a co-crystal should exist as individual solids at ambient conditions
Sameness with the parent API	Same as API and is specifically not regarded as new active substance or new chemical entity	Same as API unless a different safety/ efficacy is demonstrated. If demonstrated, EMA allows new active substance or new chemical entity registration.

of both the drugs that are very relevant in pain. Nevertheless, current regulations for pharmaceutical cocrystals issued by the FDA and EMA need more international harmonization to boost the development of cocrystal drug products.

Nano-Cocrystal

In recent past, researcher coined new term “nano-cocrystal” by combining the nanocrystal and cocrystal approach to improve the pharmaceutical and biopharmaceutical attributes of poorly soluble drug. The nanoscaling of cocrystals may further enhance their performance because of the larger surface to volume ratio of nano-cocrystal. De Smet et al. developed itraconazole–adipic acid nano-cocrystal suspension with 549 nm particle size which improved the dissolution and oral bioavailability of itraconazole significantly compared to amorphous formulations (De Smet et al., 2014). Karashima et al. prepared a suspension of indomethacin–saccharin, carbamazepine–saccharin and furosemide–caffeine nano-cocrystal with less than 300 nm particle diameter to improve the dissolution (Karashima et al., 2016). Huang et al. reported the nano-cocrystal suspension of phenazopyridine drug with phthalimide for the treatment dysuria. Prepared nano-cocrystal with particle diameter of 21.4 ± 0.1 nm showed superior release rate and oral absorption as compared to the phenazopyridine hydrochloride salt and the original cocrystal (Huang et al., 2017). Pi et al., reported that development of baicalein-nicotinamide nano-cocrystal by high pressure homogenization method with mean particle size of 251.53 nm. Baicalein-nicotinamide nano-cocrystal showed 2.17-fold and 2.54-fold improvement in dissolution compared to plain drug in simulated gastric media FaSSIF-V2 and FaSSGF, respectively. During oral bioavailability study, nano-cocrystal of baicalein-nicotinamide demonstrated 6-fold enhancement in AUC_{0-t} compared to plain baicalein (Pi et al., 2018).

On preparation technique perspective, nano-cocrystal were developed using top down approaches like grinding (Liu et al., 2016), wet milling (Kojima et al., 2018) and high-pressure homogenization (Pi et al., 2018). Electro spraying, spray drying, sono-chemical synthesis (Liu et al., 2016), antisolvent precipitation (Mohammad et al., 2018) were reported for generation of nano-cocrystal.

CO-AMORPHOUS SYSTEM

Last few years has evidenced rapid growth of binary amorphous systems. This binary system referred as CAM are systems where drug is incorporated with small molecules instead polymers (Dengale et al., 2016). Co amorphous term was coined by Chieng et al. with an intention to differentiate amorphous mixture containing two small molecules from the term polymeric amorphous solid dispersion (PASD) (Chieng et al., 2009). CAM is defined as "a multi-component single phase amorphous solid system which lacks periodicity in lattice and is associated by weak and discrete intermolecular interactions between the components" (Suresh et al., 2014). They possess short-range interactions such as hydrogen bonding of carboxylic acids, phenols/alcohols and carboxamides similar to amorphous system of single component systems. However, this system differs from cocrystal, salt or eutectic primarily by its amorphous nature which is characterized by presence of broad hump ('amorphous halo') in the PXRD. Two types of co-amorphous systems have been proposed so far, namely drug–drug combinations and drug–excipient mixtures. Among these, drug-drug CAM have gained importance as two pharmacologically relevant drugs intended for multidrug therapies are combined to stabilize both the drugs in amorphous form. Both drugs thus act as an active component and a stabilizing excipient at the same time. As a result of the stable amorphous system, both drugs if poorly soluble achieve higher solubility and dissolution rate. Several drug-drug CAMs were reported after 2015 were listed out in Table 3. These systems are developed with an intention to improve solubility, dissolution rate and physical stability of amorphous form of drug. Apart from the advantage of stabilization, solubility and dissolution, CAM also offers a platform for the development of new combinational therapy. Combination of drugs from two different therapeutic categories helps in more efficient therapy. Generally CAM are produced in a molar ratio of 1:1, which may show improvement in stability as it is assumed that both components of CAM interact at molecular level through hydrogen bonds (Alleso et al., 2009; Lobmann et al., 2011; Suresh et al., 2014). In addition to the potential therapeutic advantage, co amorphous approach offers bioavailability enhancement as one of the drugs may act as dissolution-enhancing and amorphous stabilizing agent for the second drug (Dengale et al., 2014). To date, more than 30 drug-drug CAMs are reported, probably due to the limited availability of pharmacologically relevant drug pairs with glass forming ability that can be used in combination therapy.

Screening of Co-Former for Co-Amorphous System Preparation

Selection of right co-former is the biggest challenge in the development of CAM, since co-former decides the fate of the final product in terms of stability and pharmaceutical performance. Screening process involves systematic investigation of crystallization tendency of co-former. To make these processes easy and predictable, quantum mechanics can be used for assigning various molecular interactions in FTIR and Raman spectra to provide insights into the near range order of amorphous systems and help in identification of CAM formation via molecular interactions. Lobmann et al., investigated the formation of heterodimer in indomethacin and naproxen CAM through analysis of molecular interaction by quantum mechanics (Löbmann et al., 2013). Russo et al., further explored the applicability of quantum mechanics in evaluating intermolecular interactions between drug and co-former of CAM by studying the hydrogen bonding interactions between omeprazole and amoxicillin (Russo et al., 2016). The authors calculated the density functional theory (DFT) followed by quantum theory of atoms in molecules (QTAIM) and natural bond orbital (NBO) analysis to find out the formation of heterodimer at a molecular level between drug and coformer, these findings were further supported by spectroscopic experimental findings (Russo et al., 2016). Multivariate analysis (partial least squares discriminative analysis, PLS-DA) was also explored by Ueda et al., to study the contribution of physicochemical properties of co-former such as glass transition temperature (T_g), crystallization tendency, and molecular flexibility in the formation and stabilization of CAM. In conclusion of his study, the author stated that several physicochemical properties of coformer like glass forming ability, hydrogen bonding acceptor number, reduced glass transition temperature, area/volume and flexibility, topological polar surface area and polarizability play key role in its crystallization inhibitory potential (Ueda et al., 2016). Few studies also explored the applicability of other miscellaneous theoretical approaches such as miscibility, anti-plasticization effect etc., in screening of co-formers. Use of parameters like Flory-Huggins interaction parameter (Pajula et al., 2014) and solubility parameter to predict the miscibility of the components is well documented. However, mere understanding of stabilization potential of coformer is not sufficient to develop drug-drug CAM, because such combination might not provide any therapeutic benefits unless and until justifiable evidence about practical application of such combination in therapy or synergism or drug-drug interactions has not been provided. The prime objective of drug-drug CAMs which were reported to date was more focused towards the stabilization of amorphous form of drugs, improve the pharmaceutical attributes of the drugs and identification of mechanism for stabilization. As shown in Table 3, very few reports (atorvastatin- carvedilol and glibenclamide, curcumin- artemisinin, ritonavir- quercetin and talinolol- naringin) are available demonstrating therapeutic benefits of CAM. The scarcity of such reports can be attributed to the requirement of detailed clinical investigation.

Preparation and Characterization of Co-Amorphous System

Selection of viable preparation method is mainly governed by physicochemical properties of drug and co-former, among which melting point and thermal stability of these components play a key role in selection process of appropriate manufacturing method. Application of preparation techniques such as hot melt extrusion, spray drying, ball milling, rotary solvent evaporation techniques are well documented for generation of PASD. On the other hand, preparation techniques reported for CAM are still in infancy as most of the reported techniques are only applicable for lab scale production. These techniques are ideal for screening purpose but for large or industrial scale manufacturing, extensive research is required for checking their feasibility. Summary of the preparation techniques utilized for CAM are depicted in Figure 5. Scale up of CAM poses major challenge as existing preparation methods are suitable for making few milligrams to grams of CAM products.

Ball milling has already proven its scalability for single component amorphous systems. However, it faces few challenges such as high mechanical stress and difficulty in achieving a homogeneous mix of drug and coformer for large scale processes. Additionally, product obtained from milling possesses charge which cause aggregation and may aggravate the recrystallization tendency in the product. Such milled product due to charge development may stick to the wall of the milling chamber and create problem in product recovery from chamber. Milling temperature is one of the key operational parameter that has direct impact on the product. Heat generated during milling affects the stability of the product. If the temperature during operating process increased beyond T_g of the drug, then amorphous product may tend to crystallize. Similarly, this increased temperature enhances the molecular mobility of drug which may cause phase separation (Qi et al., 2014). Hence, application of this method should be restricted to thermally stable drugs and co-formers with higher T_g.

Scale up is not expected for melting methods which is widely used for screening or optimization of CAM. However, newer techniques such as hot melt extrusion (HME) which work on the same principle of melting of components has proved its efficacy in manufacturing of PASD products, with several PASDs available in market that are manufactured by HME process. HME may be extrapolated for CAM preparation due to the physical similarity of the end product desired. Advantages offered by HME includes continuous and solvent free processing with ease of scale-up due to availability of different equipment capacities to develop and optimize at bench and pilot plant level. This method also offers in-line monitoring advantage which help in achieving the maximum mixing efficiency, monitoring of in process degradation and to study the intermolecular interactions between drug and co-former. To reach a commercial viable scale, various process variables of HME and their impact on the performance of the final product need to be extensively studied (Qi et al., 2014; Vasconcelos et al., 2016).

Solvent evaporation is third most widely used technique for CAM preparation. Spray-drying is already an established technique for the production of stable amorphous glass solutions, as its robustness during scale up of solid dispersions is well documented (Qi et al., 2014). Recently, few reports have emerged where CAM products were produced by spray drying (Jensen et al., 2016) which were subsequently formulated into final dosage forms (Lenz et al., 2015). Jensen et al., have demonstrated the feasibility of spray drying for the preparation of drug-amino acid CAM formulations on a larger scale. Amorphous salt of indomethacin–arginine prepared by spray drying method exhibited comparable properties as that of the ball milled formulation (Jensen et al., 2016). As spray drying makes co amorphous indomethacin–arginine available in a larger amount, the further successful processing to a final drug product i.e. tablet form was reported by Lenz et al. (Lenz et al., 2015). Kasten et al., demonstrated the upscaling of spray drying process from lab to pilot scale for indomethacin-lysine co amorphous system using 2^2 full factorial design of experiments (DoE). The author optimized the critical process parameters (atomization gas flow rate and outlet temperature) against critical quality attributes of the co amorphous system i.e. amorphization, glass transition temperature, bulk density, yield, and particle size distribution (Kasten et al., 2019). Screening of solvent is the key factor as output of this method for large scale production may be hampered due to solvent loading capacity and solvent toxicity. Numerous issues which may arise during large scale production of CAM by spray drying includes yield, quality and morphology of the product, and various safety issues such as boiling point of the solvent and solubilization capacity. Factors which are important for large scale production by using this technique involve thermal stability of drugs/ excipients, molecular mixing, phase separation, temperature, solvent induced recrystallization, solvent toxicity, and amorphous to crystalline ratio in final product, need careful deliberation and study. Solvent evaporation technique in addition may pose environmental challenges (Paudel et al., 2013).

Characterization of Co-Amorphous System

To understand the stability and performance of CAM, different advanced characterization tools are utilized. These analytical tools help in determination of molecular interactions, crystallinity, miscibility, molecular mobility, phase separation, moisture or solvent residue, surface chemistry and morphology of CAM at qualitative or quantitative level. However, use of simultaneous estimation tools or hyphenated techniques has increased for collecting the integrated information with a spatiotemporal resolution. Analytical tools utilized for CAM characterization are categorized based on the application in CAM and depicted in Figure 6.

Biopharmaceutical Aspects

As discussed earlier, CAM is a newer approach to solve the stability and dissolution related issues of amorphous system. However, limited studies have been published on *in vivo* performance of these systems. Results of reported pharmacokinetic studies

Figure 5. Techniques available for preparation of co-amorphous system

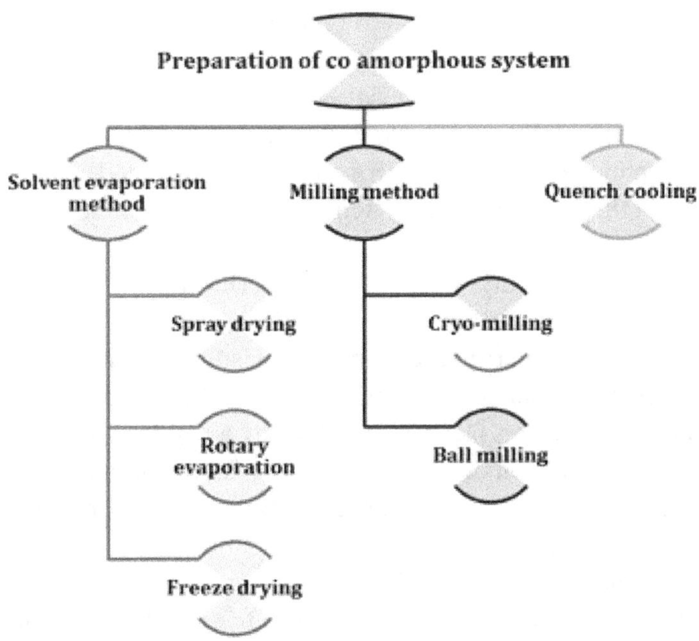

Figure 6. Analytical tools used for characterization of co-amorphous system

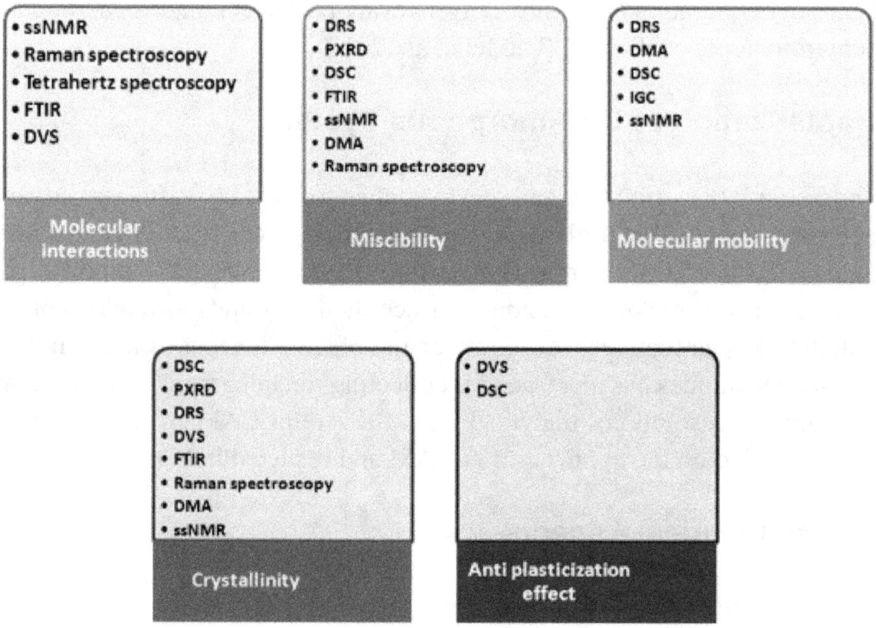

of co amorphous system provide a general conclusion that enhanced AUC is likely due to improved solubility. Most of the CAM showed significant improvement in C_{max} and AUC. Improvement in C_{max} ranged from around 1.3 to 30-fold increase (Suresh et al., 2014) while AUC showed enhancements of nearly 1 to 5 folds. In addition, significant reduction in T_{max} of CAM was documented in literature which was mainly attributed to the solubility advantage of these systems (Dengale et al., 2015). Haneef et al., performed in vivo pharmacodynamic study of irbesartan-atenolol co amorphous system and confirmed that systolic blood pressure decreased significantly with the co amorphous system in comparison to the physical mixture (Haneef et al., 2017a).

Apart from poor solubility, poor intestinal permeability is also a significant contributor to poor bioavailability of drugs. Physicochemical properties of the drug molecule (size and polarity) are found to be responsible for poor permeability of drug. Similarly, intestinal efflux pumps also contribute to poor permeability of drug across the intestine. This factor is found to be crucial for drugs which are P-gp substrate because permeation of such drugs across GI membrane might have been compromised due to poor solubility of drug, which limits the concentration of drug penetrating into the enterocyte by preventing the saturation of efflux transporters. It is well known that these P-gp efflux transporters are amenable to saturation; hence solubility advantage of CAM might solve the problem by maintaining the

Table 3. Reported drug-drug/drug-nutraceutical CAM, PK- Pharmacokinetic

CAM	Preparation Method	Solubility	Dissolution	Stability	PK	Ref.
Curcumin- artemisinin	Solvent evaporation method	✓	-	-	✓	(Suresh et al., 2014)
Ritonavir- indomethacin	Solvent evaporation method	✓	✓	-	-	(Dengale et al., 2014)
Ritonavir- quercetin	Solvent evaporation method	✓	-	-	✓	(Dengale et al., 2015)
Ezetimibe- indapamide	Quench cooling	-	-	✓	-	(Knapik et al., 2015)
Nateglinide- metformin HCl	Ball milling	✓	✓	-	-	(Wairkar et al., 2015)
Talinolol- naringin	Quench cooling	✓	-	-	✓	(Teja et al., 2015)
Glipizide- atorvastatin	Cryo milling	-	✓	✓	-	(Renuka et al., 2015)
Indomethacin–cimetidine and naproxen–cimetidine	quench cooling, co-evaporation and ball milling	-	-	✓	-	(Lim et al., 2016)
Tranilast-diphenhydramine HCl	Quench cooling	-	-	✓	-	(Ueda et al., 2017)
Glipizide- atorvastatin	Cryomilling	-	✓	✓	-	(Renuka et al., 2017)
Naproxen–indomethacin		-	-	-	-	(Radi, et al., 2016)
Naproxen-indomethacin	melt-quenching	-	-	-	-	(Beyer, Grohganz, et al., 2016)
Naproxen-indomethacin		-	-	-		(Beyer et al., 2017)
Irbesartan-atenolol	Grinding	✓	✓	✓	✓	(Haneef et al., 2017a)
Docetaxel-bicalutamide	Ball milling	-	✓	✓	✓	(Bohr et al., 2019)
Valsartan- cilnidipine	Quench cooling	-	✓	✓	-	(Lodagekar et al., 2018)
Nifedipine-cimetidine and nimesulide-Carvedilol	Quench cooling	-	-	-	-	(Martínez et al., 2016)
Simvastatin-Nifedipine	Melt-quenching	✓	✓	✓	-	(Martínez et al., 2018)
Nifedipine-nimodipine	Quench cooling	-	-	-	-	(Knapik et al., 2018)
Ritonavir- lopinavir	Quench cooling	✓	✓	✓	✓	(Anand et al., 2018)

higher luminal concentration of drug which will result into saturation of transporters thus leading to enhanced absorption of drug across GIT. Additionally, use of P-gp inhibitors in combination with the P-gp substrate drug may help in overcoming such permeability issues due to efflux transporters and multiply the effect of CAM for improving the bioavailability of such poorly soluble and permeable drugs. Teja et al.

applied a similar hypothesis for improving the bioavailability issue of P-gp substrate drug talinolol by combining it with P-gp inhibitor drug naringin for development of co amorphous formulation. Using this approach, they were able to improve the dissolution rate with simultaneous enhancement in absorption of talinolol through efflux pump inhibition by the co-administered naringin. The bioavailability study of talinolol in Wister rat showed nearly 5.4-fold enhancement in AUC of talinolol. In order to evaluate the role of naringin on improvement of permeability of talinolol, permeability study was conducted using *in situ* intestinal closed loop method. Outcome of this permeability studies confirmed the effect of naringin on P-gp inhibition wherein the permeability of talinolol was increased to 3.16×10^{-5} cm/s in contrast to 2.48×10^{-5} cm/s in absence of naringin (Teja et al., 2015). Similar observation were reported by Bohr et al., wherein a 15 fold enhancement in the oral bioavailability of efflux substrate anti-cancer drug, docetaxel was attributed to its the drug-drug co amorphous system with efflux inhibitor bicalutamide drug (Bohr et al., 2019). Conversely, Dengale et al., reported that increased permeation of ritonavir through enterocyte after oral administration of ritonavir- quercetin co amorphous system to rats might be due to solubility advantage of co amorphous system and not because of P-gp inhibition (Dengale et al., 2015).

Recently, Anand et al., performed the *in vitro* and *ex vivo* study using a semipermeable membrane and intestinal everted sac method to evaluate diffusion behavior of the drugs from ritonavir- lopinavir co amorphous system. The author studied the supersaturation generation and precipitation inhibitory potential of co amorphous system and concluded that co amorphous system has the potential to generate a supersaturated state. However, the reduction in the amorphous solubility was observed for both the drug(s) and the degree of reduction was found proportionate with the mole fraction of the compound in the co amorphous system (Anand et al., 2018).

Regulatory Issues

Few patents have been granted to CAM in last few decades. These patents satisfy all three preliminary requisite (novelty, non-obviousness and utility) for issuing of patents. Such intellectual property protection helps in life cycle management of drug products. CAM is comprised of amorphous form of drug, hence face similar regulatory challenges as that of PASD wherein the key risk factor is to prove the stability of amorphous form during manufacturing and shelf life, in order to fulfill quality requirement (Rahman et al., 2014). Hence, during the final product development, monitoring and controlling the stability of amorphous based system is a crucial regulatory challenge. This is due to the fact that such products normally meet the quality specifications at the time of release but fails in quality control testing such as dissolution on aging of the product during storage. Recrystallization of amorphous drug during storage may lead to similar type of discrepancy in quality control testing. However, market existence of numerous PASD based products may help in clearing a path for commercialization of CAM as both CAM and PASD are conceptual similar. This will also assist a formulator in applying the same principles for regulatory documentation. However, multifold concern has been raised for drug-drug CAM since pharmacological relevancy creates big challenge for patient safety. This highlights major regulatory constraint of administering more than one drug in a fixed ratio between the two drugs which need to be addressed.

MULTI-DRUG EUTECTICS

The Greek term eutectics means easy melting (eu=easy and teksis= melting). Well known definition of eutectic state that these are the solid materials which possess low melting point in comparison to their individual counterparts. Eutectics are differed from co crystal, based on their unit cell integrity (cocrystal shows the different x ray diffraction pattern whereas eutectics shows similar diffraction pattern of their parent molecules). As per IUPAC Gold Book, eutectic formation is defined as "an isothermal, reversible reaction between two (or more) solid phases during the heating of a system, as a result of which a single liquid phase is produced" (Cherukuvada et al., 2014). However, Cherukuvada and Nangia recently redefined the eutectics as conglomerates of solid solution (Cherukuvada et al., 2014). As per the solid dispersion classification, eutectic can be defined as 1st generation crystalline solid dispersion system which consist of two crystalline phases (biphasic system) and differ from solid solution which is a single phase system (Dengale et al., 2016; Vo et al., 2013). Comparison of eutectics, solid solution and cocrystals has been provided in Table 4.

Table 4. Difference between eutectics, solid solution and cocrystal (Cherukuvada et al., 2014)

Solid Form	Phases Involved	Nature of Component	Lattice Structure	Nature of Interaction	Example
Eutectic	2	Can be similar or dissimilar	Similar to components	Predominantly cohesive	Curcumin–hydroquinone
Solid solution	1	Isomorphous	Similar to components ensemble of solid solutions (Cherukuvada et al., 2014)	Cohesive	Benzoic acid–4-fluorobenzoic acid
Cocrystal	1	Can be similar or dissimilar	Different from components	Predominantly adhesive	Curcumin–resorcinol

Literature suggest that eutectics are the undesired/desired fruits during the screening of cocrystals which can be ascribed to a straight tussle between the molecules to reach the stable supramolecular assembly through various non-covalent interaction (Thipparaboina et al., 2017). Eutectic systems are classified into three classes based upon volume fraction of each phase involved, viz. rounded rod (the interphase surface energy for phases of eutectic isotropic and volume fraction of second phase less than 0.28), lamellar rod (surface energy for phases of eutectic anisotropic, volume of second phase more than 0.28) and faceted rod (conjugation of the several planes of eutectic phase with low energy). Recently Jain et al., further classified the eutectic system based on entropy of fusion of component into three classes mainly lamellar or rod shape with coupled growth, irregular or regular complex structure and irregular structure without coupled growth (Table 5) (Jain et al., 2014).

Apart from drug excipient eutectics system, researchers have explored drug-drug eutectic systems for improving pharmaceutical attributes to achieve the therapeutic benefits. First report on drug-drug eutectics emerged in 1985, where eutectic systems of local anesthetics were prepared for improving the permeation of drug. Recently, our group has reported eutectics of etodolac with paracetamol and propranolol hydrochloride for improving the pharmaceutical attributes such as dissolution, compressibility and biopharmaceutical properties (Thipparaboina et al., 2017). Repurposed activity of etodolac was improved due to synergistic action of paracetamol. To date less than 12 drug-drug eutectic systems are reported, among them only few were focused towards improving the therapeutic efficacy of the drugs (Table 6).

Methods for preparation of eutectics are similar to cocrystal preparation, ranging from solution crystallization to co grinding and slow solvent evaporation. However, major challenge in development of eutectic is its characterization, as they share some of the properties with solid solution (similar lattice structure) and cocrystal (similar or dissimilar nature of component). Various conventional characterization tools such as thermal (DSC, hot stage microscopy), microscopic (confocal laser scanning microscopy, optical and polarized microscopy and scanning electron

Table 5. Classification of eutectics proposed by Jain et al, (Jain et al., 2014)

Entropy of Fusion	Eutectic Mixture
Both components have low entropies of fusion (< 2 J/gK)	Lamellar or rod shape, couple growth
One component has low entropy of fusion (< 2 J/gK)	Irregular or regular complex structure
Both components have high entropies of fusion (> 2 J/gK)	Irregular structure no couple growth, grow near each other

microscopy) and spectroscopic techniques (IR, FT-Raman and ssNMR) along with PXRD are used for identification of eutectic systems, but have limited capacity to distinguish between the eutectics and cocrystal. Novel characterization techniques such as atomic pair distribution function (atomic arrangement measurement and local structural ordering determination), structure determination from powder diffraction (determine the microstructure based on solid-solid solubility) and total scattering PDF (differentiation of internal structural of eutectics) are promising approach for thorough characterization of the eutectic system in addition to conventional characterization tools.

As discussed under MDC, motivation behind drug-drug or drug- nutraceutical MDC or eutectics is to improve the pharmaceutical or biopharmaceuticals attributes. Apart from solubility and dissolution improvement, drug-drug eutectics have shown significant enhancement in pharmacokinetic and pharmacodynamic parameters. Among the reported eutectics (Table 5), simvastatin- aspirin and etodolac-paracetamol/ propranolol hydrochloride demonstrated synergistic/ additive effect when evaluated for their respective pharmacological action. In addition to improved fast dissolving capability, etodolac paracetamol eutectics showed improvement in hardness values thus making them suitable for tableting. This system has shown significant reduction of inflammatory markers such as TNF-α, IL-6 and COX-2 in cell culture analysis

Although reported drug eutectics fulfill the desired goal such as enhanced physicochemical properties, the design of these systems are still semi-empirical or by trial-and-error instead of chemical and deliberate. Eutectics are not popular as that of cocrystals or solid dispersions in spite their proven efficiency for improving various pharmaceutical and biopharmaceutical attributes. There will be always a few down-side issues with any technology, and eutectics are no exception. The concern with eutectics in the pharmaceutical industry might be due to the lack of proper understanding of their microstructures and difficulties in their complete characterization.

CLINICAL PERSPECTIVE TO MULTI-DRUG SOLID FORMS

In development of multi drug solid forms the most important consideration should be to demonstrate the pharmacology of drug-drug combinations. The best example when due importance is not provided to this consideration is the one faced by the Indian pharmaceutical market. The Indian scenario is currently facing a massive regulatory problem due to the approval of several multi drug formulations that lack evidence or are un-safe or irrational. Hence, it is the duty of the researchers to ensure that the drugs do not interact through antagonism or potentially dangerous

Table 6. Reported drug-drug eutectics

Drug Components	Ratio	Pharmaceutical Attributes Addresses	Preparation Methods	Therapeutic Indication	Ref.
Aspirin-paracetamol	53:47	Improvement in compressibility, tabletability and compaction behavior	Solvent evaporation	NSAIDs	(Jain et al., 2014)
Pyridoxine-isoniazid	3:1 and 4:1	-	Co grinding	Vitamin and anti-tubercular activity	(Ganduri et al., 2015)
Hydrochlorothiazide-atenolol	0.3:0.7	Solubility, dissolution and stability	Co grinding	Anti-hypertensive	(Haneef et al., 2017b)
Posaconazole-benznidazole	80:20 wt%	Solubility and dissolution	Evaporative crystallization, hot melt and cooling	In Chagas disease treatment and anti-fungal activity	(Figueirêdo et al., 2017)
Etodolac-paracetamol and etodolac-propranolol HCl	-	Solubility, dissolution, mechanical properties and *in vitro* cytotoxicity study	Co grinding	Prostate cancer and inflammatory conditions osteoarthritis	(Thipparaboina et al., 2017)
Paracetamol–caffeine, and paracetamol–aspirin	-	-	-	Migraine headache pain	(Dichi et al., 2018)
Hydrochloride salts of lidocaine and prilocaine	4: 1	Stability	-	anesthetic agent	(Wojnarowska et al., 2018)
Irbesartan with syringic acid, ascorbic acid and nicotinic acid	1:1	Solubility, dissolution, oral bioavailability and anti-hypertensive activity	Liquid assisted grinding	Anti-hypertensive	(Haneef et al., 2018)
Febuxostat-aspirin and Febuxostat-paracetamol	1:2.5 and 1:3	Compressibility and compactibility	Solvent drop grinding	Gout	(Yadav et al., 2018b)

synergy, by appropriate clinical studies of the proposed drug combinations. There is need to apply powerful computational techniques and vital research in computer sciences such as in silico drug screening tool for identifying drug candidates, and providing their in vitro and in vivo fate. Along with this, application of high-throughput screening for drug target identification should be directed to identify new drug synergies for incorporation into multi drug solid forms. Additionally, through multi drug therapy or multidrug solid forms, success can be achieved for new and existing small molecule and biopharmaceuticals previously shelved due to delivery problems, by enhancing their bioavailability and therefore clinical impact. The ideal drug-drug combination should be comprised of complementary drugs which can treat different aspects of the disease state. For achieving such success there is a need to collaborate the knowledge of multidisciplinary scientific teams (solid state chemist, clinician, formulation scientist and pharmacologist).

FUTURE PERSPECTIVES AND CONCLUDING REMARK

Novel solid forms such as cocrystals, CAM and eutectics can modulate various pharmaceutical attributes (solubility, permeability, dissolution and pharmacokinetic parameters such as T_{max}, C_{max} and AUC for drugs with poor solubility) and tackle many challenges involved in delivery of therapeutic agents. Progress in the field of multi component solid forms is growing by leaps and bounds and is found promising, as numerous reports on drug-drug/ drug-nutraceutical cocrystals, CAM and eutectics have emerged in recent past with demonstrated potential to provide alternative to existing FDC or multi drug therapy. These multi component solid forms by enhancing the therapeutic activity may prove to be singularly advantageous over existing therapy by improving various pharmaceutical attributes. For successful development of multi component solid forms, selection of appropriate drug combination is a challenging task which requires careful consideration of key factors such as therapeutic applications, differential solubility, and drug–drug interactions. Drug-nutraceutical based combinations may tackle the bioavailability and stability issues of the nutraceutical with an added advantage of providing new therapeutic hybrids with a unique combination of pharmaceuticals and therapeutically effective nutraceutical for synergistic benefits and reduced adverse effects. From regulatory point of view, these solid forms are considered novel, non-obvious with potential utility and hence can be protected by composition of matter patents. To date, the existing work in this field is more focused towards coformer screening, preparation and characterization of multi component solid form, formation mechanism, stability and evaluation of pharmaceutical attributes. However, pharmacokinetics and pharmacodynamic of multi component solid forms are largely unexplored and represent a potential avenue for further studies. Similarly, the scale up related challenges needs to be addressed to ensure successful commercialization. Meanwhile, with marketing approval granted for Entresto and Ertugliflozin cocrystal in clinical development stage, one might be justified in expecting a bright future for multi component solid forms.

ACKNOWLEDGMENT

The authors acknowledge the financial support from the Department of Pharmaceuticals (DoP), Ministry of Chemicals and Fertilizers, Govt. of India.

REFERENCES

Abdelquader, M. M., Essa, E. A., & El Maghraby, G. M. (2019). Inhibition of Co-Crystallization of Olmesartan Medoxomil and Hydrochlorothiazide for Enhanced Dissolution Rate in Their Fixed Dose Combination. *AAPS PharmSciTech*, *20*(1), 3. doi:10.120812249-018-1207-9 PMID:30560314

Aher, S., Dhumal, R., Mahadik, K., Paradkar, A., & York, P. (2010). Ultrasound assisted cocrystallization from solution (USSC) containing a non-congruently soluble cocrystal component pair: Caffeine/maleic acid. *European Journal of Pharmaceutical Sciences*, *41*(5), 597–602. doi:10.1016/j.ejps.2010.08.012 PMID:20801215

Aitipamula, S., Banerjee, R., Bansal, A. K., Biradha, K., Cheney, M. L., Choudhury, A. R., ... Duggirala, N. (2012). Polymorphs, salts, and cocrystals: What's in a name? *Crystal Growth & Design*, *12*(5), 2147–2152. doi:10.1021/cg3002948

Aitipamula, S., Cadden, J., & Chow, P. S. (2018). Cocrystals of zonisamide: Physicochemical characterization and sustained release solid forms. *CrystEngComm*, *20*(21), 2923–2931. doi:10.1039/C8CE00084K

Alleso, M., Chieng, N., Rehder, S., Rantanen, J., Rades, T., & Aaltonen, J. (2009). Enhanced dissolution rate and synchronized release of drugs in binary systems through formulation: Amorphous naproxen–cimetidine mixtures prepared by mechanical activation. *Journal of Controlled Release*, *136*(1), 45–53. doi:10.1016/j.jconrel.2009.01.027 PMID:19331842

Allesø, M., Chieng, N., Rehder, S., Rantanen, J., Rades, T., & Aaltonen, J. (2009). Enhanced dissolution rate and synchronized release of drugs in binary systems through formulation: Amorphous naproxen–cimetidine mixtures prepared by mechanical activation. *Journal of Controlled Release*, *136*(1), 45–53. doi:10.1016/j.jconrel.2009.01.027 PMID:19331842

Allesø, M., Velaga, S., Alhalaweh, A., Cornett, C., Rasmussen, M. A., Berg, F., ... Rantanen, J. (2008). Near-infrared spectroscopy for cocrystal screening. A comparative study with Raman spectroscopy. *Analytical Chemistry*, *80*(20), 7755–7764. doi:10.1021/ac8011329 PMID:18798651

Almansa, C., Mercè, R., Tesson, N., Farran, J., Tomàs, J., & Plata-Salamán, C. R. (2017). Co-crystal of tramadol hydrochloride–celecoxib (ctc): A novel API–API co-crystal for the treatment of pain. *Crystal Growth & Design*, *17*(4), 1884–1892. doi:10.1021/acs.cgd.6b01848

Anand, V. S. K., Sakhare, S. D., Sree, K. N., Nair, A. R., Varma, K. R., Gourishetti, K., & Dengale, S. J. (2018). The relevance of co-amorphous formulations to develop supersaturated dosage forms: In-vitro, and ex-vivo investigation of Ritonavir-Lopinavir co-amorphous materials. *European Journal of Pharmaceutical Sciences*, *123*, 124–134. doi:10.1016/j.ejps.2018.07.046 PMID:30048798

Beyer, A., Grohganz, H., Löbmann, K., Rades, T., & Leopold, C. S. (2016). Influence of the cooling rate and the blend ratio on the physical stability of co-amorphous naproxen/indomethacin. *European Journal of Pharmaceutics and Biopharmaceutics*, *109*, 140–148. doi:10.1016/j.ejpb.2016.10.002 PMID:27746228

Beyer, A., Grohganz, H., Löbmann, K., Rades, T., & Leopold, C. S. (2017). Improvement Of The Physicochemical Properties Of Co-amorphous Naproxen-indomethacin By Naproxen-sodium. *International Journal of Pharmaceutics*, *526*(1-2), 88–94. doi:10.1016/j.ijpharm.2017.04.011 PMID:28392278

Beyer, A., Radi, L., Grohganz, H., Löbmann, K., Rades, T., & Leopold, C. S. (2016). Preparation and recrystallization behavior of spray-dried co-amorphous naproxen–indomethacin. *European Journal of Pharmaceutics and Biopharmaceutics*, *104*, 72–81. doi:10.1016/j.ejpb.2016.04.019 PMID:27130786

Bhatt, P. M., Azim, Y., Thakur, T. S., & Desiraju, G. R. (2008). Co-crystals of the anti-HIV drugs lamivudine and zidovudine. *Crystal Growth & Design*, *9*(2), 951–957. doi:10.1021/cg8007359

Bohr, A., Nascimento, T. L., Harmankaya, N., Weisser, J. J., Wang, Y., Grohganz, H., ... Löbmann, K. (2019). Efflux Inhibitor Bicalutamide Increases Oral Bioavailability of the Poorly Soluble Efflux Substrate Docetaxel in Co-Amorphous Anti-Cancer Combination Therapy. *Molecules (Basel, Switzerland)*, *24*(2), 266. doi:10.3390/molecules24020266 PMID:30642009

Bommaka, M. K., Mannava, M. C., Suresh, K., Gunnam, A., & Nangia, A. (2018). Entacapone: Improving Aqueous Solubility, Diffusion Permeability, and Cocrystal Stability with Theophylline. *Crystal Growth & Design*, *18*(10), 6061–6069. doi:10.1021/acs.cgd.8b00921

Burley, J. C., Alkhalil, A., Bloomfield, M., & Matousek, P. (2012). Transmission Raman spectroscopy for quality control in model cocrystal tablets. *Analyst (London)*, *137*(13), 3052–3057. doi:10.1039/c2an35216h PMID:22617192

Chavan, R. B., Thipparaboina, R., Yadav, B., & Shastri, N. R. (2018). Continuous manufacturing of co-crystals: Challenges and prospects. *Drug Delivery and Translational Research*, *8*(6), 1726–1739. doi:10.100713346-018-0479-7 PMID:29352367

Cheney, M. L., Weyna, D. R., Shan, N., Hanna, M., Wojtas, L., & Zaworotko, M. J. (2011). Coformer selection in pharmaceutical cocrystal development: A case study of a meloxicam aspirin cocrystal that exhibits enhanced solubility and pharmacokinetics. *Journal of Pharmaceutical Sciences*, *100*(6), 2172–2181. doi:10.1002/jps.22434 PMID:21491441

Cherukuvada, S., & Nangia, A. (2014). Eutectics as improved pharmaceutical materials: Design, properties and characterization. *Chemical Communications (Cambridge)*, *50*(8), 906–923. doi:10.1039/C3CC47521B PMID:24322207

Chieng, N., Aaltonen, J., Saville, D., & Rades, T. (2009). Physical characterization and stability of amorphous indomethacin and ranitidine hydrochloride binary systems prepared by mechanical activation. *European Journal of Pharmaceutics and Biopharmaceutics*, *71*(1), 47–54. doi:10.1016/j.ejpb.2008.06.022 PMID:18644443

Childs, S. L., Stahly, G. P., & Park, A. (2007). The salt– cocrystal continuum: The influence of crystal structure on ionization state. *Molecular Pharmaceutics*, *4*(3), 323–338. doi:10.1021/mp0601345 PMID:17461597

Conway, D., & Cohen, J. A. (2010). Combination therapy in multiple sclerosis. *Lancet Neurology*, *9*(3), 299–308. doi:10.1016/S1474-4422(10)70007-7 PMID:20170843

Cruz-Cabeza, A. J. (2012). Acid–base crystalline complexes and the p K a rule. *CrystEngComm*, *14*(20), 6362–6365. doi:10.1039/c2ce26055g

da Silva, C. C., de Melo, C. C., Souza, M. S., Diniz, L. F., Carneiro, R. L., & Ellena, J. (2018). 5-Fluorocytosine/5-Fluorouracil Drug-Drug Cocrystal: A New Development Route Based on Mechanochemical Synthesis. *Journal of Pharmaceutical Innovation*, *14*(1), 50–56.

Darwish, S., Zeglinski, J., Krishna, G. R., Shaikh, R., Khraisheh, M., Walker, G. M., & Croker, D. M. (2018). A New 1: 1 Drug-Drug Cocrystal of Theophylline and Aspirin: Discovery, Characterization, and Construction of Ternary Phase Diagrams. *Crystal Growth & Design*, *18*(12), 7526–7532. doi:10.1021/acs.cgd.8b01330

Daurio, D., Nagapudi, K., Li, L., Quan, P., & Nunez, F.-A. (2014). Application of twin screw extrusion to the manufacture of cocrystals: Scale-up of AMG 517–sorbic acid cocrystal production. *Faraday Discussions*, *170*, 235–249. doi:10.1039/C3FD00153A PMID:25406487

De Smet, L., Saerens, L., De Beer, T., Carleer, R., Adriaensens, P., Van Bocxlaer, J., ... Remon, J. P. (2014). Formulation of itraconazole nanococrystals and evaluation of their bioavailability in dogs. *European Journal of Pharmaceutics and Biopharmaceutics*, *87*(1), 107–113. doi:10.1016/j.ejpb.2013.12.016 PMID:24388913

Delori, A., Galek, P. T., Pidcock, E., Patni, M., & Jones, W. (2013). Knowledge-based hydrogen bond prediction and the synthesis of salts and cocrystals of the anti-malarial drug pyrimethamine with various drug and GRAS molecules. *CrystEngComm*, *15*(15), 2916–2928. doi:10.1039/c3ce26765b

Deng, Y., Zhang, Y., Huang, Y., Zhang, M., & Lou, B. (2018). Preparation, Crystal Structures, and Oral Bioavailability of Two Cocrystals of Emodin with Berberine Chloride. *Crystal Growth & Design*, *18*(12), 7481–7488. doi:10.1021/acs.cgd.8b01257

Dengale, S. J., Grohganz, H., Rades, T., & Löbmann, K. (2016). Recent advances in co-amorphous drug formulations. *Advanced Drug Delivery Reviews*, *100*, 116–125. doi:10.1016/j.addr.2015.12.009 PMID:26805787

Dengale, S. J., Hussen, S. S., Krishna, B., Musmade, P. B., Shenoy, G. G., & Bhat, K. (2015). Fabrication, solid state characterization and bioavailability assessment of stable binary amorphous phases of Ritonavir with Quercetin. *European Journal of Pharmaceutics and Biopharmaceutics*, *89*, 329–338. doi:10.1016/j.ejpb.2014.12.025 PMID:25542681

Dengale, S. J., Ranjan, O. P., Hussen, S. S., Krishna, B., Musmade, P. B., Shenoy, G. G., & Bhat, K. (2014). Preparation and characterization of co-amorphous Ritonavir–Indomethacin systems by solvent evaporation technique: Improved dissolution behavior and physical stability without evidence of intermolecular interactions. *European Journal of Pharmaceutical Sciences*, *62*, 57–64. doi:10.1016/j.ejps.2014.05.015 PMID:24878386

Dichi, E., Sghaier, M., & Guiblin, N. (2018). Reinvestigation of the paracetamol–caffeine, aspirin–caffeine, and paracetamol–aspirin phase equilibria diagrams. *Journal of Thermal Analysis and Calorimetry*, *131*(3), 2141–2155. doi:10.100710973-017-6855-6

do Amaral, L. H., do Carmo, F. A., Amaro, M. I., de Sousa, V. P., da Silva, L. C. R. P., de Almeida, G. S., ... Cabral, L. M. (2018). Development and characterization of dapsone cocrystal prepared by scalable production methods. *AAPS PharmSciTech*, *19*(6), 2687–2699. doi:10.120812249-018-1101-5 PMID:29968042

Drozd, K. V., Manin, A. N., Churakov, A. V., & Perlovich, G. L. (2017a). Drug-drug cocrystals of antituberculous 4-aminosalicylic acid: Screening, crystal structures, thermochemical and solubility studies. *European Journal of Pharmaceutical Sciences*, *99*, 228–239. doi:10.1016/j.ejps.2016.12.016 PMID:28011126

Drozd, K. V., Manin, A. N., Churakov, A. V., & Perlovich, G. L. (2017b). Novel drug–drug cocrystals of carbamazepine with para-aminosalicylic acid: Screening, crystal structures and comparative study of carbamazepine cocrystal formation thermodynamics. *CrystEngComm*, *19*(30), 4273–4286. doi:10.1039/C7CE00831G

Duggirala, N. K., Perry, M. L., Almarsson, Ö., & Zaworotko, M. J. (2016). Pharmaceutical cocrystals: Along the path to improved medicines. *Chemical Communications (Cambridge)*, *52*(4), 640–655. doi:10.1039/C5CC08216A PMID:26565650

Etter, M. C., MacDonald, J. C., & Bernstein, J. (1990). Graph-set analysis of hydrogen-bond patterns in organic crystals. *Acta Crystallographica. Section B, Structural Science*, *46*(2), 256–262. doi:10.1107/S0108768189012929 PMID:2344397

Figueirêdo, C. B. M., Nadvorny, D., de Medeiros Vieira, A. C. Q., Sobrinho, J. L. S., Neto, P. J. R., Lee, P. I., & Soares, M. F. L. R. (2017). Enhancement of dissolution rate through eutectic mixture and solid solution of posaconazole and benznidazole. *International Journal of Pharmaceutics*, *525*(1), 32–42. doi:10.1016/j.ijpharm.2017.04.021 PMID:28412452

Ganduri, R., Cherukuvada, S., & Guru Row, T. N. (2015). Multicomponent Adducts of Pyridoxine: An Evaluation of the Formation of Eutectics and Molecular Salts. *Crystal Growth & Design*, *15*(7), 3474–3480. doi:10.1021/acs.cgd.5b00546

Gopi, S. P., Ganguly, S., & Desiraju, G. R. (2016). A Drug–Drug Salt Hydrate of Norfloxacin and Sulfathiazole: Enhancement of in Vitro Biological Properties via Improved Physicochemical Properties. *Molecular Pharmaceutics*, *13*(10), 3590–3594. doi:10.1021/acs.molpharmaceut.6b00320 PMID:27580175

Haneef, J., & Chadha, R. (2017a). Drug-drug multicomponent solid forms: Cocrystal, coamorphous and eutectic of three poorly soluble antihypertensive drugs using mechanochemical approach. *AAPS PharmSciTech*, *18*(6), 2279–2290. doi:10.120812249-016-0701-1 PMID:28101724

Haneef, J., & Chadha, R. (2017b). Drug-Drug Multicomponent Solid Forms: Cocrystal, Coamorphous and Eutectic of Three Poorly Soluble Antihypertensive Drugs Using Mechanochemical Approach. *AAPS PharmSciTech*, 18(6), 2279-2290. PMID:28101724

Haneef, J., & Chadha, R. (2018). Antioxidant-Based Eutectics of Irbesartan: Viable Multicomponent Forms for the Management of Hypertension. *AAPS PharmSciTech*, 19(3), 1191-1204. PMID:29247285

Harmsen, B., & Leyssens, T. (2018). Enabling Enantiopurity: Combining Racemization and Dual-Drug Co-crystal Resolution. *Crystal Growth & Design*, *18*(6), 3654–3660. doi:10.1021/acs.cgd.8b00438

Huang, Y., Li, J., Lai, Z. H., Wu, J., Lu, T. B., & Chen, J. M. (2017). Phenazopyridine-phthalimide nano-cocrystal: Release rate and oral bioavailability enhancement. *European Journal of Pharmaceutical Sciences*, *109*, 581–586. doi:10.1016/j.ejps.2017.09.020 PMID:28917964

Issa, N., Karamertzanis, P. G., Welch, G. W., & Price, S. L. (2008). Can the formation of pharmaceutical cocrystals be computationally predicted? I. Comparison of lattice energies. *Crystal Growth & Design*, *9*(1), 442–453. doi:10.1021/cg800685z

Jain, H., Khomane, K. S., & Bansal, A. K. (2014). Implication of microstructure on the mechanical behaviour of an aspirin–paracetamol eutectic mixture. *CrystEngComm*, *16*(36), 8471–8478. doi:10.1039/C4CE00878B

Jensen, K. T., Blaabjerg, L. I., Lenz, E., Bohr, A., Grohganz, H., Kleinebudde, P., ... Lobmann, K. (2016). Preparation and characterization of spray-dried co-amorphous drug–amino acid salts. *The Journal of Pharmacy and Pharmacology*, *68*(5), 615–624. doi:10.1111/jphp.12458 PMID:26245703

Jiang, L., Huang, Y., Zhang, Q., He, H., Xu, Y., & Mei, X. (2014). Preparation and solid-state characterization of dapsone drug–drug co-crystals. *Crystal Growth & Design*, *14*(9), 4562–4573. doi:10.1021/cg500668a

Karashima, M., Kimoto, K., Yamamoto, K., Kojima, T., & Ikeda, Y. (2016). A novel solubilization technique for poorly soluble drugs through the integration of nanocrystal and cocrystal technologies. *European Journal of Pharmaceutics and Biopharmaceutics*, *107*, 142–150. doi:10.1016/j.ejpb.2016.07.006 PMID:27393561

Kasten, G., Duarte, Í., Paisana, M., Löbmann, K., Rades, T., & Grohganz, H. (2019). Process Optimization and Upscaling of Spray-Dried Drug-Amino acid Co-Amorphous Formulations. *Pharmaceutics*, *11*(1), 24. doi:10.3390/pharmaceutics11010024 PMID:30634423

Kaur, R., Cavanagh, K. L., Rodríguez-Hornedo, N., & Matzger, A. J. (2017). Multidrug cocrystal of anticonvulsants: Influence of strong intermolecular interactions on physiochemical properties. *Crystal Growth & Design*, *17*(10), 5012–5016. doi:10.1021/acs.cgd.7b00741

Knapik, J., Wojnarowska, Z., Grzybowska, K., Jurkiewicz, K., Tajber, L., & Paluch, M. (2015). Molecular dynamics and physical stability of co-amorphous ezetimib and indapamide mixtures. *Molecular Pharmaceutics*, *12*(10), 3610–3619. doi:10.1021/acs.molpharmaceut.5b00334 PMID:26301858

Knapik-Kowalczuk, J., Tu, W., Chmiel, K., Rams-Baron, M., & Paluch, M. (2018). Co-stabilization of amorphous pharmaceuticals-the case of nifedipine and nimodipine. *Molecular Pharmaceutics*, *15*(6), 2455–2465. doi:10.1021/acs.molpharmaceut.8b00308 PMID:29738666

Kojima, T., Karashima, M., Yamamoto, K., & Ikeda, Y. (2018). Combination of NMR Methods To Reveal the Interfacial Structure of a Pharmaceutical Nanocrystal and Nanococrystal in the Suspended State. *Molecular Pharmaceutics*, *15*(9), 3901–3908. doi:10.1021/acs.molpharmaceut.8b00360 PMID:30059624

Kojima, T., Tsutsumi, S., Yamamoto, K., Ikeda, Y., & Moriwaki, T. (2010). High-throughput cocrystal slurry screening by use of in situ Raman microscopy and multi-well plate. *International Journal of Pharmaceutics*, *399*(1), 52–59. doi:10.1016/j.ijpharm.2010.07.055 PMID:20696223

Lenz, E., Jensen, K. T., Blaabjerg, L. I., Knop, K., Grohganz, H., Lobmann, K., ... Kleinebudde, P. (2015). Solid-state properties and dissolution behaviour of tablets containing co-amorphous indomethacin–arginine. *European Journal of Pharmaceutics and Biopharmaceutics*, *96*, 44–52. doi:10.1016/j.ejpb.2015.07.011 PMID:26197392

Leung, D. H., Lohani, S., Ball, R. G., Canfield, N., Wang, Y., Rhodes, T., & Bak, A. (2012). Two novel pharmaceutical cocrystals of a development compound–screening, scale-up, and characterization. *Crystal Growth & Design*, *12*(3), 1254–1262. doi:10.1021/cg201270s

Li, J.-M., Dai, X.-L., Li, G.-J., Lu, T.-B., & Chen, J.-M. (2018). Constructing Anti-Glioma Drug Combination with Optimized Properties through Cocrystallization. *Crystal Growth & Design*, *18*(8), 4270–4274. doi:10.1021/acs.cgd.8b00807

Lim, A. W., Löbmann, K., Grohganz, H., Rades, T., & Chieng, N. (2016). Investigation of physical properties and stability of indomethacin–cimetidine and naproxen–cimetidine co-amorphous systems prepared by quench cooling, coprecipitation and ball milling. *The Journal of Pharmacy and Pharmacology*, *68*(1), 36–45. doi:10.1111/jphp.12494 PMID:26663364

Liu, F., Wang, L.-Y., Li, Y.-T., Wu, Z.-Y., & Yan, C.-W. (2018). Protective Effects of Quercetin against Pyrazinamide Induced Hepatotoxicity via a Cocrystallization Strategy of Complementary Advantages. *Crystal Growth & Design*, *18*(7), 3729–3733. doi:10.1021/acs.cgd.8b00576

Liu, M. Y., Hong, C., Li, G. W., Ma, P., & Xie, Y. (2016). The generation of myricetin–nicotinamide nanococrystals by top down and bottom up technologies. *Nanotechnology*, *27*(39), 395601. doi:10.1088/0957-4484/27/39/395601 PMID:27535365

Lobmann, K., Laitinen, R., Grohganz, H., Gordon, K. C., Strachan, C., & Rades, T. (2011). Coamorphous drug systems: Enhanced physical stability and dissolution rate of indomethacin and naproxen. *Molecular Pharmaceutics*, *8*(5), 1919–1928. doi:10.1021/mp2002973 PMID:21815614

Löbmann, K., Laitinen, R., Grohganz, H., Strachan, C., Rades, T., & Gordon, K. C. (2013). A theoretical and spectroscopic study of co-amorphous naproxen and indomethacin. *International Journal of Pharmaceutics*, *453*(1), 80–87. doi:10.1016/j.ijpharm.2012.05.016 PMID:22613066

Lodagekar, A., Chavan, R. B., Chella, N., & Shastri, N. R. (2018). Role of Valsartan as an Antiplasticizer in Development of Therapeutically Viable Drug–Drug Coamorphous System. *Crystal Growth & Design*, *18*(4), 1944–1950. doi:10.1021/acs.cgd.8b00081

Martínez, L. M., Videa, M., Sosa, N. G., Ramírez, J. H., & Castro, S. (2016). Long-Term Stability of New Co-Amorphous Drug Binary Systems: Study of Glass Transitions as a Function of Composition and Shelf Time. *Molecules (Basel, Switzerland)*, *21*(12), 1712. doi:10.3390/molecules21121712 PMID:27983640

Martínez-Jiménez, C., Cruz-Angeles, J., Videa, M., & Martínez, L. (2018). Co-Amorphous Simvastatin-Nifedipine with Enhanced Solubility for Possible Use in Combination Therapy of Hypertension and Hypercholesterolemia. *Molecules (Basel, Switzerland)*, *23*(9), 2161. doi:10.3390/molecules23092161 PMID:30154310

Mashhadi, S. M. A., Yunus, U., Bhatti, M. H., Ahmed, I., & Tahir, M. N. (2016). Synthesis, characterization, solubility and stability studies of hydrate cocrystal of antitubercular Isoniazid with antioxidant and anti-bacterial Protocatechuic acid. *Journal of Molecular Structure*, *1117*, 17–21. doi:10.1016/j.molstruc.2016.03.057

Mohammad, I. S., He, W., & Yin, L. (2018). A Smart Paclitaxel-Disulfiram Nanococrystals for Efficient MDR Reversal and Enhanced Apoptosis. *Pharmaceutical Research*, *35*(4), 77–95. doi:10.100711095-018-2370-0 PMID:29488114

Mohammad, M. A., Alhalaweh, A., & Velaga, S. P. (2011). Hansen solubility parameter as a tool to predict cocrystal formation. *International Journal of Pharmaceutics, 407*(1), 63–71. doi:10.1016/j.ijpharm.2011.01.030 PMID:21256944

Mukherjee, A., Tothadi, S., Chakraborty, S., Ganguly, S., & Desiraju, G. R. (2013). Synthon identification in co-crystals and polymorphs with IR spectroscopy. Primary amides as a case study. *CrystEngComm, 15*(23), 4640–4654. doi:10.1039/c3ce40286j

Nagapudi, K., Umanzor, E. Y., & Masui, C. (2017). High-throughput screening and scale-up of cocrystals using resonant acoustic mixing. *International Journal of Pharmaceutics, 521*(1), 337–345. doi:10.1016/j.ijpharm.2017.02.027 PMID:28229947

Nakao, S., Fujii, S., Sakaki, T., & Tomita, K. I. (1977). The crystal and molecular structure of the 2: 1 molecular complex of theophylline with phenobarbital. *Acta Crystallographica. Section B, Structural Science, 33*(5), 1373–1378. doi:10.1107/S0567740877006116

Nechipadappu, S. K., Tekuri, V., & Trivedi, D. R. (2017). Pharmaceutical Co-Crystal of Flufenamic Acid: Synthesis and Characterization of Two Novel Drug-Drug Co-Crystal. *Journal of Pharmaceutical Sciences, 106*(5), 1384–1390. doi:10.1016/j.xphs.2017.01.033 PMID:28185907

Pajula, K., Wittoek, L., Lehto, V.-P., Ketolainen, J., & Korhonen, O. (2014). Phase Separation in Coamorphous Systems: In Silico Prediction and the Experimental Challenge of Detection. *Molecular Pharmaceutics, 11*(7), 2271–2279. doi:10.1021/mp400712m PMID:24824610

Paudel, A., Worku, Z. A., Meeus, J., Guns, S., & Van den Mooter, G. (2013). Manufacturing of solid dispersions of poorly water soluble drugs by spray drying: Formulation and process considerations. *International Journal of Pharmaceutics, 453*(1), 253–284. doi:10.1016/j.ijpharm.2012.07.015 PMID:22820134

Pessoa, A. S., Aguiar, G. P. S., Oliveira, J. V., Bortoluzzi, A. J., Paulino, A., & Lanza, M. (2019). Precipitation of resveratrol-isoniazid and resveratrol-nicotinamide cocrystals by gas antisolvent. *The Journal of Supercritical Fluids, 145*, 93–102. doi:10.1016/j.supflu.2018.11.014

Pi, J., Wang, S., Li, W., Kebebe, D., Zhang, Y., Zhang, B., ... Liu, Z. (2018). *A nano-cocrystal strategy to improve the dissolution rate and oral bioavailability of baicalein*. Asian J Pharm Sci; doi:10.1016/j.ajps.2018.04.009

Putra, O. D., Furuishi, T., Yonemochi, E., Terada, K., & Uekusa, H. (2016). Drug–Drug Multicomponent Crystals as an Effective Technique to Overcome Weaknesses in Parent Drugs. *Crystal Growth & Design, 16*(7), 3577–3581. doi:10.1021/acs.cgd.6b00639

Qi, S., McAuley, W. J., Yang, Z., & Tipduangta, P. (2014). Physical stabilization of low-molecular-weight amorphous drugs in the solid state: A material science approach. *Therapeutic Delivery, 5*(7), 817–841. doi:10.4155/tde.14.39 PMID:25287388

Rahman, Z., Siddiqui, A., Gupta, A., & Khan, M. (2014). *Regulatory considerations in development of amorphous solid dispersions. In Amorphous Solid Dispersions* (pp. 545–563). Springer.

Renuka, S., Singh, S. K., Gulati, M., & Narang, R. (2017). Stable amorphous binary systems of glipizide and atorvastatin powders with enhanced dissolution profiles: Formulation and characterization. *Pharmaceutical Development and Technology, 22*(1), 13–25. doi:10.3109/10837450.2015.1125921 PMID:26708555

Russo, M. G., Sancho, M. I., Silva, L. M., Baldoni, H. A., Venancio, T., Ellena, J., & Narda, G. E. (2016). Looking for the interactions between omeprazole and amoxicillin in a disordered phase. An experimental and theoretical study. *Spectrochimica Acta. Part A: Molecular and Biomolecular Spectroscopy, 156*, 70–77. doi:10.1016/j.saa.2015.11.021 PMID:26654963

Sa, R., Zhang, Y., Deng, Y., Huang, Y., Zhang, M., & Lou, B. (2018). Novel salt cocrystal of chrysin with berberine: Preparation, characterization, and oral bioavailability. *Crystal Growth & Design, 18*(8), 4724–4730. doi:10.1021/acs.cgd.8b00696

Shin, H.-C., Alani, A. W., Rao, D. A., Rockich, N. C., & Kwon, G. S. (2009). Multi-drug loaded polymeric micelles for simultaneous delivery of poorly soluble anticancer drugs. *Journal of Controlled Release, 140*(3), 294–300. doi:10.1016/j.jconrel.2009.04.024 PMID:19409432

Sinha, A. S., Khandavilli, U. R., O'Connor, E. L., Deadman, B. J., Maguire, A. R., & Lawrence, S. E. (2015). Novel co-crystals of the nutraceutical sinapic acid. *CrystEngComm, 17*(26), 4832–4841. doi:10.1039/C5CE00777A

Sokal, A., Pindelska, E., Szeleszczuk, L., & Kolodziejski, W. (2017). Pharmaceutical properties of two ethenzamide-gentisic acid cocrystal polymorphs: Drug release profiles, spectroscopic studies and theoretical calculations. *International Journal of Pharmaceutics, 522*(1), 80–89. doi:10.1016/j.ijpharm.2017.03.004 PMID:28274662

Souza, M. S., Diniz, L. F., Vogt, L., Carvalho, P. S. Jr, D'vries, R. F., & Ellena, J. (2018). Mechanochemical Synthesis of a Multicomponent Solid Form: The Case of 5-Fluorocytosine Isoniazid Codrug. *Crystal Growth & Design*, *18*(9), 5202–5209. doi:10.1021/acs.cgd.8b00647

Suresh, K., Mannava, M. C., & Nangia, A. (2014). A novel curcumin–artemisinin coamorphous solid: Physical properties and pharmacokinetic profile. *RSC Advances*, *4*(102), 58357–58361. doi:10.1039/C4RA11935E

Surov, A. O., Voronin, A. P., Manin, A. N., Manin, N. G., Kuzmina, L. G., Churakov, A. V., & Perlovich, G. L. (2014). Pharmaceutical cocrystals of diflunisal and diclofenac with theophylline. *Molecular Pharmaceutics*, *11*(10), 3707–3715. doi:10.1021/mp5004652 PMID:25184906

Teja, A., Musmade, P. B., Khade, A. B., & Dengale, S. J. (2015). Simultaneous improvement of solubility and permeability by fabricating binary glassy materials of Talinolol with Naringin: Solid state characterization, in-vivo in-situ evaluation. *European Journal of Pharmaceutical Sciences*, *78*, 234–244. doi:10.1016/j.ejps.2015.08.002 PMID:26253355

Thipparaboina, R., Chavan, R. B., Kumar, D., Modugula, S., & Shastri, N. R. (2015). Micellar carriers for the delivery of multiple therapeutic agents. *Colloids and Surfaces. B, Biointerfaces*, *135*, 291–308. doi:10.1016/j.colsurfb.2015.07.046 PMID:26263217

Thipparaboina, R., Kumar, D., Chavan, R. B., & Shastri, N. R. (2016). Multidrug co-crystals: Towards the development of effective therapeutic hybrids. *Drug Discovery Today*, *21*(3), 481–490. doi:10.1016/j.drudis.2016.02.001 PMID:26869329

Thipparaboina, R., Thumuri, D., Chavan, R., Naidu, V., & Shastri, N. R. (2017). Fast dissolving drug-drug eutectics with improved compressibility and synergistic effects. *European Journal of Pharmaceutical Sciences*, *104*, 82–89. doi:10.1016/j.ejps.2017.03.042 PMID:28366649

Todaro, V., Worku, Z. A., Cabral, L. M., & Healy, A. M. (2019). In Situ Cocrystallization of Dapsone and Caffeine during Fluidized Bed Granulation Processing. *AAPS PharmSciTech*, *20*(1), 28. doi:10.120812249-018-1228-4 PMID:30603811

Ueda, H., Kadota, K., Imono, M., Ito, T., Kunita, A., & Tozuka, Y. (2017). Co-amorphous formation induced by combination of tranilast and diphenhydramine hydrochloride. *Journal of Pharmaceutical Sciences*, *106*(1), 123–128. doi:10.1016/j.xphs.2016.07.009 PMID:27539557

Ueda, H., Muranushi, N., Sakuma, S., Ida, Y., Endoh, T., Kadota, K., & Tozuka, Y. (2016). A strategy for co-former selection to design stable co-amorphous formations based on physicochemical properties of non-steroidal inflammatory drugs. *Pharmaceutical Research, 33*(4), 1018–1029. doi:10.100711095-015-1848-2 PMID:26700604

Vasconcelos, T., Marques, S., das Neves, J., & Sarmento, B. (2016). Amorphous solid dispersions: Rational selection of a manufacturing process. *Advanced Drug Delivery Reviews, 100*, 85–101. doi:10.1016/j.addr.2016.01.012 PMID:26826438

Vo, C. L.-N., Park, C., & Lee, B.-J. (2013). Current trends and future perspectives of solid dispersions containing poorly water-soluble drugs. *European Journal of Pharmaceutics and Biopharmaceutics, 85*(3), 799–813. doi:10.1016/j.ejpb.2013.09.007 PMID:24056053

Vogt, F. G., Clawson, J. S., Strohmeier, M., Edwards, A. J., Pham, T. N., & Watson, S. A. (2008). Solid-state NMR analysis of organic cocrystals and complexes. *Crystal Growth & Design, 9*(2), 921–937. doi:10.1021/cg8007014

Wairkar, S., & Gaud, R. (2015). Co-Amorphous Combination of Nateglinide-Metformin Hydrochloride for Dissolution Enhancement. *AAPS PharmSciTech*, 17(3), 673-681. PMID:26314243

Wang, F.-Y., Zhang, Q., Zhang, Z., Gong, X., Wang, J.-R., & Mei, X. (2018). Solid-state characterization and solubility enhancement of apremilast drug–drug cocrystals. *CrystEngComm, 20*(39), 5945–5948. doi:10.1039/C8CE00689J

Wang, J.-R., Yu, Q., Dai, W., & Mei, X. (2016). Drug–drug co-crystallization presents a new opportunity for the development of stable vitamins. *Chemical Communications (Cambridge), 52*(17), 3572–3575. doi:10.1039/C5CC10297A PMID:26845759

Wichianphong, N., & Charoenchaitrakool, M. (2018). Application of Box–Behnken design for processing of mefenamic acid–paracetamol cocrystals using gas anti-solvent (GAS) process. *J. CO2 Utilization, 26*, 212-220.

Wojnarowska, Z., Smolka, W., Zotova, J., Knapik-Kowalczuk, J., Sherif, A., Tajber, L., & Paluch, M. (2018). The effect of electrostatic interactions on the formation of pharmaceutical eutectics. *Physical Chemistry Chemical Physics, 20*(43), 27361–27367. doi:10.1039/C8CP05905E PMID:30357184

Yadav, B., Balasubramanian, S., Chavan, R. B., Thipparaboina, R., Naidu, V., & Shastri, N. R. (2018a). Hepatoprotective Cocrystals and Salts of Riluzole: Prediction, Synthesis, Solid State Characterization, and Evaluation. *Crystal Growth & Design, 18*(2), 1047–1061. doi:10.1021/acs.cgd.7b01514

Yadav, J. P. A., Bansal, A. K., & Jain, S. (2018b). Molecular Understanding and Implication of Structural Integrity in the Deformation Behavior of Binary Drug–Drug Eutectic Systems. *Molecular Pharmaceutics*, *15*(5), 1917–1927. doi:10.1021/acs.molpharmaceut.8b00077 PMID:29620908

Yeh, K. L., & Lee, T. (2018). Intensified Crystallization Processes for 1: 1 Drug–Drug Cocrystals of Sulfathiazole–Theophylline, and Sulfathiazole–Sulfanilamide. *Crystal Growth & Design*, *18*(3), 1339–1349. doi:10.1021/acs.cgd.7b01197

Žegarac, M., Lekšić, E., Šket, P., Plavec, J., Bogdanović, M. D., Bučar, D.-K., ... Meštrović, E. (2014). A sildenafil cocrystal based on acetylsalicylic acid exhibits an enhanced intrinsic dissolution rate. *CrystEngComm*, *16*(1), 32–35. doi:10.1039/C3CE42013B

Zhao, L., Raval, V., Briggs, N. E., Bhardwaj, R. M., McGlone, T., Oswald, I. D., & Florence, A. J. (2014). From discovery to scale-up: α-lipoic acid: nicotinamide co-crystals in a continuous oscillatory baffled crystalliser. *CrystEngComm*, *16*(26), 5769–5780. doi:10.1039/C4CE00154K

This research was previously published in the Journal of Nanotoxicology and Nanomedicine (JNN), 3(1); edited by Bakhtiyor Rasulev, pages 23-48, copyright year 2018 by IGI Publishing (an imprint of IGI Global).

Chapter 5 OpTrak: Tracking Opioid Prescriptions via Distributed Ledger Technology

Peng Zhang
Vanderbilt University, USA

Douglas C Schmidt
Vanderbilt University, USA

Breck Stodghill
Vanderbilt University, USA

Jules White
Vanderbilt University, USA

Cory Pitt
Vanderbilt University, USA

Alan Pitt
Barrow Neurological Institute, USA

Cavin Briody
Vanderbilt University, USA

Kelly Aldrich
Center for Medical Interoperability, USA

ABSTRACT

This article describes the structure and functionality of OpTrak, a decentralized app implemented using the Ethereum blockchain that targets the opioid epidemic currently plaguing the United States. Over-prescription and distribution of opioids cost the national healthcare system over $78 billion every year. Problems persist in every stage of the process, from doctors prescribing the medication to the pharmacists fulfilling prescriptions. These problems arise from a combination of factors, including lack of accountability, transparency, and reliability in the current prescription drug monitoring programs. This work provides three key contributions to research on a technical approach to mitigate the opioid epidemic. First, the authors pinpoint key problems in the current opioid prescription system. Second, they propose an integrated approach for addressing the problems by leveraging distributed ledgers, focusing on blockchain technology. Third, the authors describe the structure and functionality of OpTrak that allows a consortium of care providers to exchange patient prescription data securely.

DOI: 10.4018/978-1-7998-1680-5.ch005

INTRODUCTION

Emerging Trends and Challenges

It is widely known that the United States (US) is in the midst of an opioid epidemic. Opioids are a class of drugs that consists of heroin, as well as legal pain relievers like oxycodone, hydrocodone, codeine, and morphine. Pain relieving opioids can be safe when prescribed for the right reasons and duration. These opioids can easily be misused, however, due to the production of euphoria and the relief of pain. Due to these effects, regular use (even through valid prescriptions) can yield dependence and addiction. In turn, the abuse of pain relievers often leads to overdose and death (National, 2018).

Every day in the United States, over 115 Americans die after overdosing on opioids (CDC/NCHS, 2017). Moreover, the DEA states that up to 80% of heroin addictions begin with the misuse of prescription opioids (Bresnick, 2017). By calculating the costs of healthcare, addiction treatment, lost productivity, and criminal justice involvement, The US Centers for Disease Control and Prevention estimates that prescription opioid misuse has a total economic burden of $78.5 billion per year on the United States (CDC/NCHS, 2017).

Many efforts are attempting to address this crisis, as shown by The Drug Supply Chain Safety Act (DSCSA) (Center, 2013), the establishment of the President's Commission on Combating Drug Addiction and the Opioid Crisis (Madras, 2018), and numerous prescription awareness campaigns (CDC, 2017). Unfortunately, the current prescription tracking system in the US lacks the technical infrastructure to address this crisis effectively. In particular, the prescription opioid marketplace is rife with data hoarding, doctor shopping, provider ignorance, vulnerable and centralized data, and over-prescription (Laxmaiah, 2012).

Attacking the opioid crisis in the US requires an approach to prescription monitoring that not only makes prescriptions safer, but also incentivizes providers to write fewer prescriptions. Providers today are economically incentivized to prescribe opioids to patients. As a result, providers often spend less face-time with patients, thereby lowering costs associated with patient treatment, while increasing their financial returns. Similarly, pharmacies today are incentivized to produce and distribute opioids because the more opioids sold, the greater their revenue, which also increases shareholder value.

Patients themselves are also incentivized to consume opioids. For example, physical therapy in the treatment of pain can be extremely frustrating and filled with disappointment. Opioids provide short-term relief, though they often lead to patient addiction (Van, 1999). This self-reinforcing cycle can be ameliorated by a technical approach that realigns incentives for providers, pharmacies, and patients.

Our Contribution

The OpTrak decentralized app (DApp) that tracks opioid prescription using distributed ledger technology. To provide a technical platform for more effective sharing of opioid-related activities, we have developed OpTrak, which is a distributed ledger technology (DLT)-based DApp designed to operate within a networked consortium of healthcare professionals. OpTrak allows a trusted network of stakeholders (e.g., hospitals and pharmacies) to store opioid transaction records in a secure and accountable manner. By securely disseminating knowledge that a prescription has been filled by a patient, OpTrak helps remedy various problems in the current US opioid system, such as lack of communications between providers causing duplicated opioid orders of the same patient (Goldman, 2017).

Opioid data in OpTrak is shared with the networked consortium in a secure fashion with no single point of failure that could corrupt the entire system. Healthcare professionals, such as providers and pharmacists, are incentivized to participate in the consortium through access to data that will increase the quality and transparency of care. In turn, proper analysis of this data enables patients to receive care that is more appropriate to their condition(s).

OpTrak can also create personalized logs for each individual patient to help them identify past prescription activities. These logs can help steer patients away from the dangers of opioid addiction by encouraging them to adopt more effective long-term treatment actions. For patients who have genuine needs for opioid prescriptions, OpTrak helps make a safer marketplace.

Paper Organization

The remaining of this article is organized as follows: the Background and Challenges section describes the context of our work on opioid tracking via blockchain. The Structure and Functionality of OpTrak section describes the design and implementation of a prototype OpTrak DApp we developed using the Ethereum blockchain platform. The Addressing Key Opioid Misuse Challenges via OpTrak section presents key considerations we applied when developing our OpTrak DApp to address each of the challenges facing current opioid prescription tracking systems. The Related Work section compares our research on OpTrak with other work related to understanding drug prescriptions, as well as applications of distributed ledger technology in healthcare. Finally, the Concluding Remarks section summarizes key lessons learned from our work on OpTrak.

BACKGROUND AND CHALLENGES

This section presents an overview of blockchain technologies used by OpTrak and describes key challenges faced by current approaches to addressing opioid misuse.

Summary of Blockchain Concepts and Capabilities Used by OpTrak

A blockchain is an append-only ledger of a digital asset, such as digital currency or a piece of data. Transactions tracking the ownership of the assets are maintained by a number of nodes in a decentralized network. The ledger is not stored in a single location, but instead is replicated across the entire network and continually reconciled to present consistent and verifiable information. This distributed ledger achieves consensus through a process called mining, which has different implementations for different blockchains. The Ethereum blockchain, which underlies our OpTrak DApp, uses Proof of Work in its public incarnation, where network nodes compete to solving a difficult cryptographic puzzle, with the "winner" having their block be the first appended to the blockchain. Mining nodes are incentivized to complete the puzzle with some cryptocurrency award.

The Ethereum blockchain also provides a more generalized blockchain framework with its programmable "smart contracts" (Buterin, 2014). A smart contract is a piece of software that enables autonomous code execution when certain predefined conditions are met. It also supports data storage as state variables that can be updated based on access and conditions defined in the smart contract.

Interactions with an Ethereum smart contract are always deterministic and are recorded on the distributed ledger as transactions in a network-wide sequential order. All transactions are verifiable and are very hard to modify due to the decentralization nature of blockchain. These mechanisms render data and data operations on the blockchain immutable and non-reputable, thereby attracting significant interest from healthcare IT researchers as a framework to enable more interoperable clinical exchanges without a third-party intermediary (Blockchain 2018). Below we describe how OpTrak leverages this decentralized blockchain technology to mitigate the challenges related to opioid misuse.

Key Challenges Faced by Current Approaches to Addressing Opioid Misuse

OpTrak is designed to address key challenges in healthcare related to accurately tracking prescription opioid medication. As described in the Introduction section, the United States currently faces a national epidemic involving the abuse and misuse of opioids.

With the widespread problem of opioid misuse in the United States, federal, state, and local governments have begun efforts to implement prescription drug monitoring programs (PDMPs) (Finklea, 2013). For example, according to the National Alliance for Model State Drug Laws (NAMSDL) (National, n.d.), states are implementing PDMP electronic databases that collect designated data on substances dispensed in the state. The agency responsible for administration of the PDMP varies by state and includes state's regulatory, administrative, and law enforcement agencies. These agencies then distribute data to entities authorized by state law who use the information for their profession, such as physicians and pharmacies (Diversion, 2016).

Despite the implementation of these programs in recent years, current evidence does not indicate that PDMPs are highly effective in combating drug abuse (Office, 2013; US, 2016), due to a variety of factors, such as the fact that they still do not fix the fundamental problems with how doctors and others are incentivized regarding opioids (Reuben, 2015). Some studies have shown improvement, such as the CDC's statement that the "Evaluations of PDMPs have illustrated changes in prescribing behaviors, use of multiple providers by patients, and decreased substance abuse treatment admissions" (Center, 2017), but there has not been clear and concrete highly successful outcomes. Despite these signs of progress, however, there is also substantial room for improvement in more timely responses of opioid prescription reporting, interoperability across states, and more accurate approaches to identify patients. Figure 1 shows the current status of prescription tracking, where providers within the same state may be able to exchange prescription history of a patient via statewide PDMPs.

Figure 1. Traditional prescription tracking system with little interoperability across different states

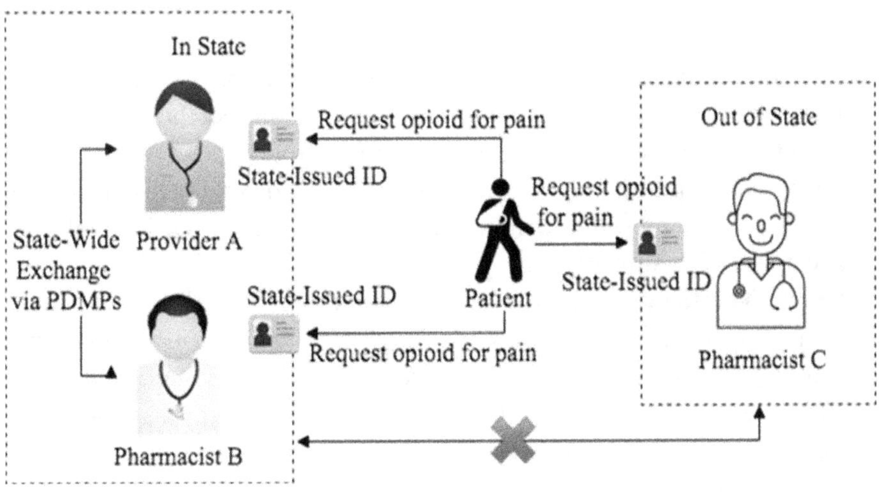

Figure 1 depicts a scenario where a patient attempts to request opioid prescription (e.g., for pain management). In this conventional approach, the patient is required to present a state-issued ID as proof of their identity. Providers (Provider A and Pharmacist B) within the same state are able to exchange prescription data of the same patient using their provided ID through case reporting enabled by state-wide PDMPs. The state-by-state siloed implementation of PDMPs, however, limits interoperability across state lines. As a result, when the same patient visits another provider (Pharmacist C), Pharmacist C is unaware of the patient's previous prescription activities, which creates a loophole in the system that patients with opioid addiction can exploit to doctor shop across states and obtain more than the required opioid dosage.

Although PDMPs provide an important contribution in the fight against opioid abuse, the following challenges remain largely unresolved:

1. **Lack of Interoperability Between States:** PDMPs create one statewide electronic database to contain data related to the dispensing of particular substances (Diversion, 2016). While these databases are a necessary first step, their state-by-state implementation restricts the interoperability of states. In particular, with states siloing their own data, there is a significant loss in potential sharing of prescription data across state lines. Physicians, pharmacies, states, and the federal government are therefore limited in the scope of data they can analyze to identify trends and draw valid conclusions.
2. **Vulnerability of Centralized Databases:** Maintaining one central database introduces the risk of losing all data in one incident or cyber-attack. Moreover, if any malicious actor succeeds in manipulating the database—e.g., by supplying false information, changing information, or erasing information (Theoharidou, 2005)—the centralized database will be unable to remedy the information without cross referencing individual databases that have previously contributed to its information (if such sub-databases even exist). In conventional prescription monitoring approaches, states have the option to contract the responsibility of transaction recording to private organizations (Appriss, n.d.) who are utilized in many states and store information in a centralized system. If that centralized database was compromised in some way, it would be hard to validate the correctness of its information.
3. **Identity Verification:** Conventional methods of prescribing and fulfilling prescriptions only require an individual to provide valid identification, typically through a state driver license (National, 2013). These material licenses can be falsified, thus rendering the identity verification process inadequate. In cases where genuine identifications are provided by patients, errors (such as

mismatching patients using aliases or failing to link prescriptions to the correct patients (McDonald, 2013)) may still surface due to the lack of interoperable medical identity management system.

4. **Reliability and Consistency of Information:** Physicians using current PDMP databases are often dissatisfied with data reliability and consistency (Grossman, 2011) due to several issues, including frequency and timeliness of data entry and the limited scope of the data. Different entities input their data at different intervals, e.g., some states require monthly data entry while only one state provides real-time data reporting (Prescription, 2012). Without a system that provides immediate entry of data related to dispensing medication, physicians will not have the proper real-time information to draw valid conclusions. Moreover, current databases typically only contain prescription data of patients within their state. It would thus be helpful to disseminate knowledge and increase physician awareness for authorized entities to access data from neighboring states (Lopez, 2017).

Section Addressing Key Opioid Misuse Challenges via OpTrak describes how the OpTrak DApp applied blockchain technologies to address each of the challenges described above.

THE STRUCTURE AND FUNCTIONALITY OF OPTRAK

This section first provides an overview of our OpTrak prototype, which is a blockchain-based web app we developed to provide an opioid prescription tracking system. We then describe the functionality and technical components of OpTrak.

OpTrak Architecture Overview

OpTrak is designed as a web app built atop an Ethereum blockchain alongside existing provider databases (simulated for the prototype), as shown in Figure 2. OpTrak's smart contracts accept messages (e.g., a prescription transaction or a request to view a patient's prescription history) from OpTrak web app. OpTrak then persists and/or delivers data (e.g., data related to shared access or a specific data access request) used for prescription tracking.

The Optrak web app provides a portal for care provider users, with its server component handling and encapsulating all blockchain communications. Each provider database is registered into the blockchain consortium if it sets up or connects to an OpTrak server. OpTrak's design enables the connection of traditionally siloed provider databases with each other in a decentralized manner, regardless of the

Figure 2. Components in the OpTrak architecture

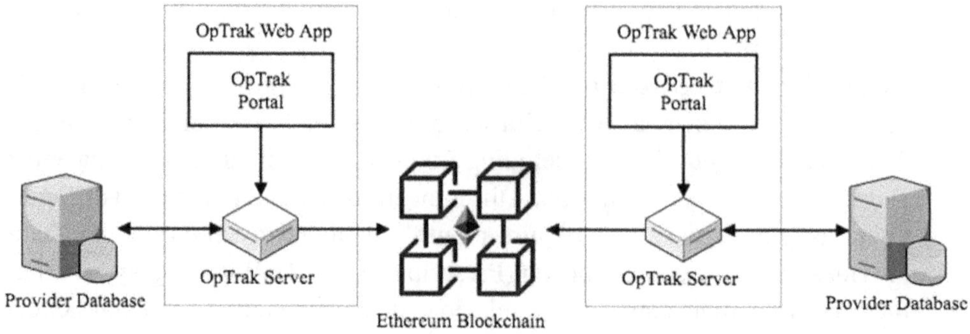

physical location of the database owner entity. The OpTrak web app was written largely in Python and HTML and the smart contract was implemented with Solidity, which is the programming model Ethereum provides to write smart contracts. Two Postgres databases are used to simulate two provider databases.

Technical Components of OpTrak

OpTrak is comprised of three key components: (1) a standardized Postgres database simulator with API keys to permission access, (2) an Ethereum smart contract to log access requests and responses on the blockchain, and (3) a Python-based web app to provide users with familiar experience. As shown in Figure 3, each block contains a bundle of requests and responses and is chained in a network-wide sequential order. When a provider needs to access a patient's prescription information, a data request is sent to each provider in the registry with that patient's biometric-based identifier. Each provider responds with a binary (i.e., "yes" or "no") message indicating whether they possess data for the corresponding patient. Each "yes" response will also contain an API access key that grants the requesting provider temporary access to that patient's data in the responder's database.

Standardized Database

To facilitate the frictionless exchange of data between providers, OpTrak standardizes how prescription data is recorded. It can be costly to exchange data that is not uniformly recorded in a standardized manner. Fortunately, 43 of the 50 states in the US use the centralized Appriss database to centrally storeopioid prescription data. Rather than rely on Appriss to provide central storage of prescription data, however, OpTrak works alongside each provider's local data server. When a provider in the system requests access to another external provider's database, a new API access keycan be generated

Figure 3. Detailed OpTrak workflow diagram and technical components

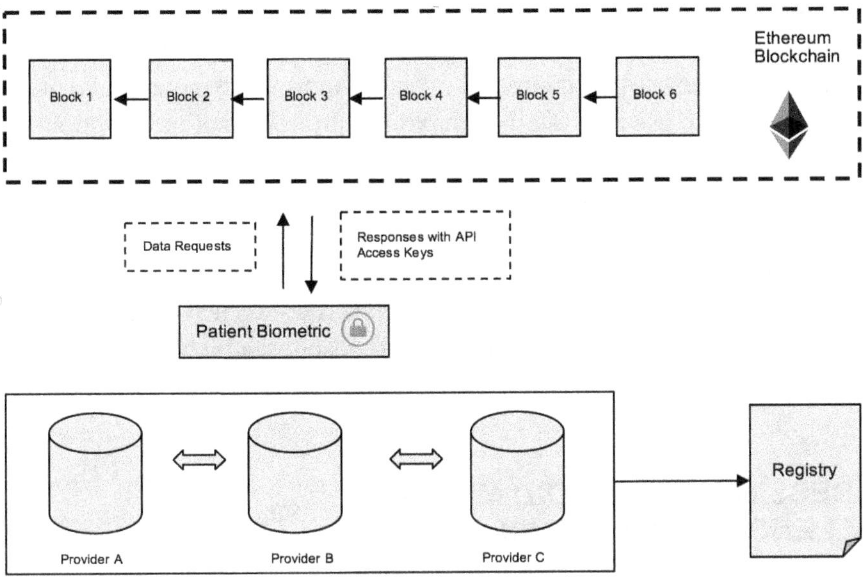

granting them temporary access (Appriss, 2016; Controlled, 2018). Since data is standardized, this information can be easily understood by the receiving provider and thus leveraged to recognize a genuine patient request for opioid prescriptions.

Ethereum Smart Contract

We designed an Ethereum smart contract to log all data requests and responses on the Ethereum blockchain. When a provider requests data on a patient, it sends a data request to each provider in the registry, which is also simultaneously recorded on the Ethereum blockchain with a timestamp. Each provider then sends a response that is also logged on the blockchain. If the provider holds data related to the requested patient an encrypted API access key is attached to the response. Only the requesting provider can decrypt this key to retrieve the data. Maintaining the history of each data request and response on the blockchain allows OpTrak to track which provider has accessed another provider's database at any given time (Buterin, 2014).

Python Web App

All services offered by OpTrak are wrapped in a Python web app implemented via the Django web framework to provide users with familiar web experience (Django, n.d.). We allow users to register or sign in to the system via a user-friendly portal according to their role (i.e., patient or provider). This web service is responsible for all communications with the blockchain, thereby avoiding any additional technical burden to users. OpTrak's Python web app interacts with the Ethereum smart contract via the JavaScript remote procedure call (web3.js, n.d.). Both patients and providers can be on-boarded to use the system to maximize awareness of prescription-related activities. The web app also allows providers to request data on a patient once the correct biometric-based identifier of that patient has been provided. When a data request has been transmitted through the web app portal, the web server instantiates a new request object in the smart contract component, which is in turn saved on the Ethereum blockchain. The request is then broadcasted to each provider registered in the system and their responses are logged into response objects saved in the same smart contract.

ADDRESSING KEY OPIOID MISUSE CHALLENGES VIA OPTRAK

OpTrak is designed to address the key challenges described in the Background and Challenges section above. In particular, it creates a system for stakeholders to securely monitor and track patient opioid prescription data across state lines. It therefore increases provider access to prescription-related data and ensures the integrity of all parties involved in each prescription transaction and legitimacy of opioid prescriptions to prevent opioid misuse. Figure 3 presents the functionality of OpTrak that addresses the limitations of traditional system shown in Figure 1 using the same scenario, i.e., a patient attempts to request opioid from different providers within and across state line.

Figure 4 shows how OpTrak enables providers to verify patient identity via a biometric-based authentication mechanism that maps to a network-wide unique patient identifier. Upon authenticating the patient, all providers in this scenario can then securely share prescription activities of that patient (given proper authorization) through the smart contact log of OpTrak's decentralized design. This approach better equips providers with knowledge about the patient's prescription request and fulfillment history in (near) real-time, thereby helping determine whether it is safe to prescribe opioids to the patient.

The remainder of this section discusses how OpTrak addresses each of the four challenges facing current opioid tracking systems.

Figure 4. OpTrak prescription tracking system creating interoperability across state lines

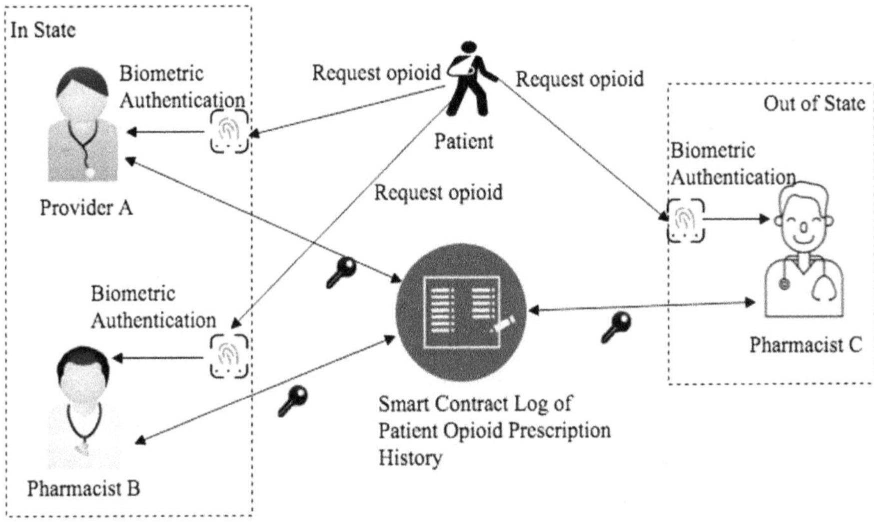

Addressing Problem 1: Lack of Interoperability Between States

OpTrak addresses the lack of interoperability between states, which is a key problem prevalent in current medical practice that partially fosters the opioid epidemic. The Drug Supply Chain Safety Act (DSCSA) was put into effect to improve drug security, and by 2023 the law requires that all prescription drugs are trackable across the supply chain via an interoperable system (Center, 2013). The DSCSA, however, does not account for the need of an interoperable system regarding actual drug prescriptions.

Through lack of interoperability, patients can manipulate the medical system by doctor shopping across state borders, playing ignorant in writing scripts, etc., thereby creating less collaborative and less effective medical practices. OpTrak improve interoperability through enabling providers residing in different states with a new way to share prescription information. In particular, rather than permanently sharing all data, OpTrak enables the distribution of temporary API access tokens. Data can then be supplied from the local provider via OpTrak's secure APIs, thereby enabling more interoperable data sharing.

To achieve these goals, OpTrak acts as a pipeline for the transmission of prescription data to appropriate and relevant parties within a consortium of providers, such as hospitals, insurance agencies, pharmaceutical distributors, etc. The membership of each additional provider (or their organization representative) must be approved by the existing consortium to ensure that they are a known and accountable entity, thereby ensuring that each network node is responsible for any action they perform.

Addressing Problem 2: Vulnerability of Centralized Databases

Rather than storing records of prescription transactions in a centralized global database, OpTrak allows providers to maintain control of the data they generate. Even if corrupted data enters a single local database, the collection of databases as a whole will remain untainted. This design minimizes the scope of any issue that jeopardizes the consistency of the overall database.

An alternative approach is to simply distribute each provider's database to the entire network, which would allow immediate remediation of any data corruption of data. We rejected this approach in OpTrak, however, for the following reasons:

- **Decentralization Prevents Mistakes in Data Records:** People quite often make mistakes. By distributing the entire database using blockchain, any modification of past recorded data will be impossible or hard due to blockchain's decentralized architecture and tamper-aware properties. While one could update data, each update event is permanently and immutably recorded.
- **Authorization to Access Data may be Bypassed that Violates Regulation:** To comply with healthcare information privacy and security regulations (i.e., HIPAA, Health Insurance Portability and Accountability Act) (US, 2003), data should only be viewable by relevant and authorized parties. Just because a patient has visited Hospital A, that transaction may not be permitted viewable by Hospital B unless authorization to view that specific information is granted or needed by the patient.
- **Market Competition Becomes Disincentives to Participation:** Medical data is a form of leverage. Providers within the consortium will likely not be incentivized to share their full datasets with each other or their competitors, which leads to OpTrak's permissioned viewing.

Instead of storing patient data in OpTrak's blockchain component, it only stores timestamped records of transactions. The fact that a transaction took place will be immutable and permanent, rather than storing actual information about what the transaction was (i.e., some event occurred that was relevant to Patient X and Provider Y). This design enables OpTrak to grant providers permissioned viewing.

By distributing a record of transactions involving certain parties have taken place, OpTrak can alert any provider that pertinent patient information may exist and where it would be to retrieve the actual, detailed prescription information. Given that provider data is still locally stored, external providers in the consortium will not have access to that data unless it is granted by the provider that stores it locally. Through the use of temporary authentication tokens, each local provider can then grant temporary access to a patient's information if it is deemed appropriate via disintermediation with OpTrak's blockchain component. OpTrak ensures that request for patient data access is only deemed appropriate if that patient is indeed under the care of the external provider by an immutable log that can be verified by the patient and provider at any point in time.

Addressing Problem 3: Identity Verification

The decentralization property of blockchain technology can facilitate the identity verification process by standardizing identity representations. Smart contract-based public key infrastructure (PKI) has been proposed as a useful mechanism to create and manage identities (Al-Bassam, 2017) and has been preliminarily prototyped as a global registry (Zhang, White, 2017). PKI (Housley, 1998) is widely used by Internet services and applications to secure communications, including authentication of client requests via Secure Socket Layer (SSL) (Bhiogade, 2002) and encryption of email messages using Secure/Multipurpose Internet Mail Extensions (S/MIME) (Ramsdell, 2010). PKI uses a pair of mathematically linked public and private keys to encrypt data and verify digital signatures. The mechanism generating the key pair ensures it is computationally infeasible to derive the private key (which owners keep private and secure) from the public key (which owners are free to share with others to encrypt data and verify digital signature).

For provider users, OpTrak employs PKI-based identifiers in conjunction with a registry model created via a smart contract component to enable authenticated and encrypted communications between providers (Zhang, White, 2017). The public and private keys can be managed by each provider's parent organization and encapsulated to the providers by using a traditional username/password authentication scheme on top of a key management software, such as a software wallet or key vault. To identify patient users, however, our design incorporates a biometric-based identity (Pitt, 2012) verification process because PKI-based key management would incur significant technical challenges (such as technical knowledge, management limitations, etc.) in this much larger population, thereby impeding wide-range adoption. OpTrak therefore uses patient biometric data that are securely encrypted and stored with their provider(s), along with a hashed value of the data used to identify the patient.

Addressing Problem 4: Reliability and Consistency of Information

Many current Prescription Drug Monitoring Programs (PDMPs) suffer from the issue of providers submitting their data in a timely fashion (Rutkow, 2015). By allowing local providers to store their generated data, OpTrak enables data updates as soon as it is recorded in the local system. thereby eliminating a step in submitting prescription records. In addition to streamlining the process by logging transactions, providers will now be more accountable for transactions that do occur., which will have the following two-part effect:

- Prescribing doctors (or their surrogate) will feel more responsible for the transactions they sign off on. Providers will likewise be more precautious in writing a prescription for opioids if they believe each transaction can be observed and audited in a tamper-proof manner. The number and frequency of prescriptions can also be utilized to alert when doctors abuse their licenses.
- If doctors are more precautious in writing opioid prescriptions they may be less inclined to write as many opioid scripts. In turn, this reduction in scripts will lower the number of opioids in legal circulation and hopefully incentivize safer medical practices.

RELATED WORK

There are few discussions in the academic literature on systems for opioid prescription monitoring using a distributed and shared ledger, such as blockchain technologies. Given the opportunities that these technologies present, however, there are many projects underway aimed at revolutionizing the healthcare industry. Many of these projects are focused on solving problems including data fragmentation, interoperability, and audit tracking. This section describes the most relevant of these projects to characterize the current digital health landscape and understand how blockchain technologies can improve it.

MediLedger (MediLedger, n.d.) intends to utilize the blockchain to solve interoperability issues between drug manufacturers, distributors, and dispensers. Their platform aims to improve compliance of track and trace regulations, reduce the cost and effort involved in regulatory adherence, improve drug quality and security, and improve overall business operations of the pharmaceutical supply chain. Appriss Health (Appriss, n.d.) aims to help providers, pharmacies, and state governments identify, prevent, and manage substance use disorders. They provide a suite of data analytics platforms that integrate with EHR workflows to identify at-risk patients and the resources necessary to support them. MedRec (Azaria, 2016) applies smart contracts on the Ethereum blockchain to create a decentralized content-management system for patient's healthcare data. The authentication log, similar to OpTrak's permission management schema, governs medical record access, while providing means for auditability and data sharing. MedRec aims to integrate with providers' local EHR database solutions to give patients a "one-stop-shop" platform with access to all of their medical records. MedRec is being developed by researchers at the MIT Media Lab.

ScriptDrop (ScriptDrop, 2017) integrates a delivery service, a pharmacy focused EHR, and a blockchain backend to provide better prescription drug access to patients. ScriptDrop also aims to utilize daily medication reminders to provide a two-way communication with the patient, and identify which patients are not in compliance with adherence programs. Recent research by Zhang et al. focused on recommending design practice (Zhang, White, 2017) and evaluation metrics (Zhang, Walker, 2017) for creating and assessing blockchain-based healthcare apps. Moreover, we identified a number of plausible applications for using distributed ledger technology in healthcare, one of which discussed its potential for monitoring opioid prescription (Zhang, Schmidt, 2018). They also proposed FHIRChain (Zhang, White, 2018) as a more generic health IT system for securely exchanging clinical data by analyzing a subset of technical requirements that would comply with security and privacy regulations.

CONCLUSION

This paper motivated the need to address the problem of opioid misuse and abuse in the US and described how the blockchain technology used in the OpTrak DApp can serve as a promising solution. OpTrak is well-suited for a Prescription Drug Monitoring Program (PDMP) that tracks prescriptions at the national level. The blockchain technology underlying OpTrak enables any provider across the United States to exchange and access their patients' prescription records regardless of when or where they were prescribed, thereby helping to reduce prescription fraud. The following are key lessons we learned from developing and evaluating the OpTrak DApp thus far:

- **A decentralized and shared permissioned blockchain allows loosely coupled providers to access data silos without the need of centralized trust**. A consortium of providers that use the OpTrak technology act as an oracle, i.e., external verifiable data feed to the smart contract for providing secure data retrieval service. The consortium must agree to add new providers to the OpTrak system. Stakeholders within the system (hospitals, government agencies, etc.) are incentivized to add new members to the consortium because with each additional member, they can form a more complete picture with a broader distributed dataset. Each patient's prescription record grows longitudinally as more time points are referenced by temporary access API queries. Likewise, the data becomes more layered as more information about the prescriptions are logged in a shared ledger.

- **OpTrak has no centralized data store, which provides some benefits compared with centralized architectures.** A key benefit is that providers using OpTrak do not actually have to give up rights to their coveted data sets. This benefit overcomes a common challenge in the healthcare industry: how does an organization facilitate beneficent data sharing between providers that do not trust each other (Galli, 2018)? The answer comes in the form of a peer-to-peer API protocol that references a permissioned blockchain backend. With conventional prescription tracking technology, it is not feasible and too hard to expand past a local setting. In contrast, however, tracking and accessing prescriptions nationally with OpTrak would akin to tracking them on a local level and could be done with ease and speed. Moreover, a simple biometric-based identity approach is useful to look up a patient's information from any location that is part of the consortium. OpTrak provides a less expensive, more efficient, and more secure approach to facilitate prescription drug distribution.
- **The speed of blockchain technology provides a significantly more efficient method for tracking opioid prescriptions.** Today, the existence of any centralized form of tracking prescriptions necessitates the need for manual methods of input and updating. With these methods, the main source of tracking prescriptions is not updated as prescriptions are filled and are never really up-to-date. OpTrak would enforce and update tracking in (near) real-time across the entire chain, meaning that as soon as a prescription is entered into the system it is also entered into the chain and hence updated on every entity's system. This approach provides a more efficient, feasible solution to prescription tracking and the prevention of opioid abuse. Without real-time updates, it is easy to over-prescribe opioids to a patient with little opportunity for recourse.
- **OpTrak minimizes adoption overhead by working alongside existing systems.** The introduction of any new platform may cause changes in medical practice, thereby impeding adoption. The DEA, however, already requires the medical field to track and record every opioid that they prescribe. Allowing OpTrak to work side-by-side with existing systems in hospitals or doctor offices incurs minimal adoption overhead since opioid prescriptions can be entered onto the blockchain and provider databases simultaneously. Incorporating OpTrak into existing systems would therefore incur little additional time and would be easy to use since doctors would observe little/ no differences from their existing systems. Opioid prescriptions would be

entered onto the shared blockchain simply behind the scenes and would be unnoticeable to every participant. The provider themselves would never need to (1) see a private or public key, (2) understand how to run a node, and/or (3) learn an entirely new platform. OpTrak is thus an efficient solution to opioid prescription tracking that adds little/no overhead for entities adopting it.

In future work, we are exploring the practicality of OpTrak via a case study to evaluate various metrics in terms of real-time performance in addition to analyze the implementation effort required. These metrics include transaction throughput and turnaround time of a prescription transaction being available across the network. Moreover, we are extending the work presented in this paper to provide more patient-centric permissions that allow patient family members to access their prescriptions on demand and also consider monitoring adjustments for users with varying degrees of opioid dependencies, e.g., new opioid patients versus patients with higher risks of addiction.

ACKNOWLEDGMENT

This work was funded in part by Varian Medical Systems and by the Vanderbilt University School of Engineering's Summer Undergraduate Research Program. The authors would like to thank Mason Hall, Jared Rothstein, and Colleen Gruendel for their participation and contribution to this research.

REFERENCES

Al-Bassam, M. (2017, April). SCPKI: A smart contract-based PKI and identity system. In *Proceedings of the ACM Workshop on Blockchain, Cryptocurrencies and Contracts* (pp. 35-40). ACM. 10.1145/3055518.3055530

Appriss, Inc. (2016, January). *Tennessee Controlled Substance Collection Database Data Collection Manual*. Retrieved from https://www.tnrxreport.com/docs/DataReportingManualforTN.pdf

Appriss, Inc. (n.d.). *PMP Aware*. Retrieved from https://apprisshealth.com/solutions/pmp-awarxe/

Azaria, A., Ekblaw, A., Vieira, T., & Lippman, A. (2016, August). Medrec: Using blockchain for medical data access and permission management. In *International Conference on Open and Big Data (OBD)* (pp. 25-30). IEEE.

Bhiogade, M. S. (2002, June). Secure socket layer. In *Computer Science and Information Technology Education Conference* (pp. 85-90).

Blockchain in Healthcare: The Case for Pragmatic Innovation. (2018, April 23). Retrieved from https://www.himss.org/news/blockchain-healthcare-case-pragmatic-innovation

Bresnick, J. (2017, August 07). DOJ Leverages Big Data Analytics to Combat Opioid Fraud, Abuse. *HealthITAnalytics*. Retrieved from https://healthitanalytics.com/news/doj-leverages-big-data-analytics-to-combat-opioid-fraud-abuse

Buterin, V. (2014). A next-generation smart contract and decentralized application platform (white paper).

CDC. (2013, June). *Menu of State Prescription Drug Identification Laws*. Retrieved from https://www.cdc.gov/phlp/docs/menu-pdil.pdf

CDC/NCHS, National Vital Statistics System, Mortality. (2017). *CDC Wonder*. Retrieved from https://wonder.cdc.gov

Center for Drug Evaluation and Research. (2013). *Drug Supply Chain Security Act (DSCSA)*. Retrieved from https://www.fda.gov/Drugs/DrugSafety/DrugIntegrityandSupplyChainSecurity/DrugSupplyChainSecurityAct/

Centers for Disease Control and Prevention. (2017, October 03). *Opioid Overdose*. Retrieved from https://www.cdc.gov/drugoverdose/pdmp/states.html

Controlled Substance Monitoring Database Committee. (2018, March). *Controlled Substance Monitoring Database: 2018 Report to the 110th Tennessee General Assembly*. Retrieved from https://www.tn.gov/content/dam/tn/health/healthprofboards/csmd/2018ComprehensiveCSMDAnnual Report.pdf

Diversion Control Division. (2016, June). *State Prescription Drug Monitoring Programs*. Retrieved from https://www.deadiversion.usdoj.gov/faq/rx_monitor.htm

Django. (n.d.). Retrieved from https://www.djangoproject.com/

Finklea, K. M., Bagalman, E., & Sacco, L. N. (2013, January). *Prescription drug monitoring programs*. Washington, DC: Library of Congress, Congressional Research Service.

Galli, B. (2018). Ethics of Electronic Health Record (EHR) Systems. *International Journal of Information Systems and Social Change*, *9*(3), 53–69. doi:10.4018/IJISSC.2018070104

Goldman, A. B. (2017, October 24). *How Health Care Providers Can Help End the Overprescription of Opioids*. Retrieved from https://hbr.org/2017/10/how-health-care-providers-can-help-end-the-overprescription-of-opioids

Grossman, J. M., Boukus, E. R., Gross, D. A., & Cohen, G. R. (2011). *Physician practices, e-prescribing and accessing information to improve prescribing decisions*. Washington, DC: Center for Studying Health System Change.

Housley, R., Ford, W., Polk, W., & Solo, D. (1998). *Internet X. 509 public key infrastructure certificate and CRL profile* (No. RFC 2459).

López, V., Urgelés, D., Sánchez, Ó., & Valverde, G. (2017). Big Data in Healthcare and Social Sciences: Bip4Cast as a CAD system. *International Journal of Information Systems and Social Change*, *8*(3), 1–16. doi:10.4018/IJISSC.2017070101

Madras, B. K. (2018). The President's Commission on Combating Drug Addiction and the Opioid Crisis: Origins and Recommendations. *Clinical Pharmacology and Therapeutics*, *103*(6), 943–945. doi:10.1002/cpt.1050 PMID:29570781

Manchikanti, L., Helm, S., Fellows, B., Janata, J.W., Pampati, V., Grider, J.S. & Boswell, M.V. (2012). Opioid epidemic in the United States. *Pain Physician*, *15*, 2150–1149. PMID:22786464

McDonald, D. C., & Carlson, K. E. (2013). Estimating the prevalence of opioid diversion by "doctor shoppers" in the United States. *PLoS One*, *8*(7), e69241. doi:10.1371/journal.pone.0069241 PMID:23874923

MediLedger. (n.d.). MediLedger - Blockchain solutions for Pharma companies. Retrieved from https://www.mediledger.com/

National Alliance for Model State Drug Laws. (2013). *States That Require an ID from a Recipient Prior to Dispensing Prescriptions*. Santa Fe, NM: The National Alliance for Model State Drug Laws.

National Alliance for Model State Drug Laws. (n.d.). Retrieved from http://www.namsdl.org/

National Institute on Drug Abuse. (2018, June 07). *Prescription Opioids*. Retrieved from https://www.drugabuse.gov/publications/drugfacts/prescription-opioids

Newsroom, C. D. C. (2017, September 25). *CDC launches campaign to help states fight prescription opioid epidemic*. Retrieved from https://www.cdc.gov/media/releases/2017/p0925-rx-awareness-campaigns.html

Pitt, A. M., Partovi, S., & Rosati, K. (2012). *U.S. Patent No. 8,320,638*. Washington, DC: U.S. Patent and Trademark Office.

Prescription Monitoring Program Center of Excellence at Brandeis. (2012, January). *Real Time Reporting: Oklahoma's Pioneering PMP*. Notes from the Field. Retrieved from http://www.pdmpassist.org/pdf/Resources/ok_real_time_data_nff_11912.pdf

Ramsdell, B., & Turner, S. (2010). Secure/multipurpose internet mail extensions (S/MIME) version 3.2 message specification (No. RFC 5751).

Reuben, D. B., Alvanzo, A. A., Ashikaga, T., Bogat, G. A., Callahan, C. M., Ruffing, V., & Steffens, D. C. (2015). National Institutes of Health Pathways to Prevention Workshop: The role of opioids in the treatment of chronic pain. *Annals of Internal Medicine*, *162*(4), 295–300. doi:10.7326/M14-2775 PMID:25581341

Rutkow, L., Turner, L., Lucas, E., Hwang, C., & Alexander, G. C. (2015). Most primary care physicians are aware of prescription drug monitoring programs, but many find the data difficult to access. *Health Affairs*, *34*(3), 484–492. doi:10.1377/hlthaff.2014.1085 PMID:25732500

ScriptDrop. (2017). *ScriptDrop - At the Intersection of Healthcare & Blockchain*. Retrieved from https://github.com/masonicGIT/ico-whitepapers/blob/master/scriptdrop-white-paper.pdf

Theoharidou, M., Kokolakis, S., Karyda, M., & Kiountouzis, E. (2005). The insider threat to information systems and the effectiveness of ISO17799. *Computers & Security*, *24*(6), 472–484. doi:10.1016/j.cose.2005.05.002

US Department of Health and Human Services. (2003). *Summary of the HIPAA privacy rule*. Washington, DC.

US Department of Health and Human Services. (2016). Facing addiction in America: The Surgeon General's report on alcohol, drugs, and health.

Van Ree, J. M., Gerrits, M. A., & Vanderschuren, L. J. (1999). Opioids, reward and addiction: An encounter of biology, psychology, and medicine. *Pharmacological Reviews*, *51*(2), 341–396. PMID:10353987

Web3.js - Ethereum JavaScript API. (n.d.). Retrieved from https://web3js.readthedocs.io/en/1.0/

Zhang, P., Schmidt, D. C., White, J., & Lenz, G. (2018). Blockchain Technology Use Cases in Healthcare. In G. Deka (Ed.), *Blockchain Technology: Platforms, Tools, and Use Cases*. Elsevier. doi:10.1016/bs.adcom.2018.03.006

Zhang, P., Walker, M. A., Schmidt, D. C., White, J., & Lenz, G. (2017, October). Metrics for assessing blockchain-based healthcare decentralized apps. In *2017 IEEE 19th International Conference on e-Health Networking, Applications and Services (Healthcom)* (pp. 1-4). IEEE.

Zhang, P., White, J., Schmidt, D. C., & Lenz, G. (2017, October). Design of Blockchain-Based Apps Using Familiar Software Patterns with a Healthcare Focus. *Paper accepted by and presented at the 24th Pattern Languages of Programming conference*, Vancouver, Canada, October 22-25, 2017.

Zhang, P., White, J., Schmidt, D. C., Lenz, G., & Rosenbloom, S. T. (2018). FHIRChain: Applying blockchain to securely and scalably share clinical data. *Computational and Structural Biotechnology Journal*, *16*, 267–278. doi:10.1016/j.csbj.2018.07.004 PMID:30108685

This research was previously published in the International Journal of Information Systems and Social Change (IJISSC), 10(2); edited by John Wang and Jungwoo Lee, pages 45-61, copyright year 2019 by IGI Publishing (an imprint of IGI Global).

Section 3
ICTs, Mobile Applications, and Online Programs

Chapter 6
An Innovative, Information and Communication Technology Supported Approach, Towards Effective Chronic Pain Management

Haridimos Kondylakis
Institute of Computer Science (ICS), Greece

Santiago Hors-Fraile
Salumedia Tecnologías, Spain

Lefteris Koumakis
Institute of Computer Science (ICS), Greece

Angelina Kouroubali
Institute of Computer Science (ICS), Greece

George Notas
University of Crete, Greece

Alejandro Rivero-Rodriguez
Salumedia Tecnologías, Spain

Prodromos Sidiropoulos
University of Crete, Greece

Panagiotis Simos
University of Crete, Greece

Dimitrios G. Katehakis
Institute of Computer Science (ICS), Greece

ABSTRACT

Chronic pain is one of the most common health problems affecting daily activity, employment, relationships and emotional functioning. Unfortunately, the lack of specialized health care personnel, and the high heterogeneity in terms of clinical manifestation and treatment results contribute in failure to manage efficiently and effectively pain. Information and communication technology (ICT) can be a valuable

DOI: 10.4018/978-1-7998-1680-5.ch006

tool, enabling patients and healthcare professional empowerment and better self-management of pain. To this direction, this article reports on the design of a novel technical infrastructure to support effectively and efficiently chronic pain management, based on an Intelligent Personal Health Record platform on top of already available ICT tools. The designed platform targets, among others, at improving the knowledge on the patient data, effectiveness and adherence to treatment and providing effective communication channels between patients and healthcare professionals.

INTRODUCTION

Chronic pain is one of the most common health problems worldwide (Elliott et al., 1999) and a common cause for patients consulting a doctor (Breivik et al., 2005; Eriksen et al., 2003). Pain is defined as being chronic or long-term when it lasts for longer than 3 to 6 months, or beyond the normal healing time of an injury. Classifying pain is helpful to guide assessment and treatment whereas, there are many ways to classify pain and classifications may overlap (International Association for the Study of Pain, 2011). People with chronic pain often experience high levels of disability (Blyth et al., 2003) and are adversely affected on areas including daily activity, employment, relationships, and emotional functioning (Breivik et al., 2005). Impairment due to chronic pain leads to high levels of work absence and dramatically increases health care needs. In addition, pain imposes a huge financial and psychosocial burden on patients, their families and society (Andersson, 2009; Gore et al. 2012; Gustavsson at al. 2012; Nitter, 2013; Waddell & Nordlund 2000). According to (Elliott et al., 1999) patients suffering from chronic nonmalignant pain constitute a heterogeneous population in terms of clinical presentation and treatment results.

Chronic pain is associated with many different diagnostic entities ranging from diseases like, e.g. osteoarthritis, low-back pain and other musculoskeletal conditions to neuropathic pain conditions like painful diabetic polyneuropathy and pain following a stroke or multiple sclerosis. Due to this, treatment also varies from patient to patient and may include pharmacological treatments, neuromodulation, physiotherapy, multimodal rehabilitation. According to (Kroenke et al. 2009) pain and depression are the most common physical and psychological symptoms in primary care. Parallel assessment and treatment of psychiatric comorbidities and sleep disorders combined with traditional rehabilitation, i.e. physical activation and cognitive reorganization are imperative for improved outcomes.

Pain management is one of the most neglected aspects of health care. Chronic pain management is often limited. Pain specialists are able to manage very few patients, while almost half of the patients with chronic pain receive inadequate pain management. Failure to adequately address chronic pain is a major driver of its economic and social burden. Inappropriate and ineffective management and treatment generate repetitive visits to primary care physicians and referrals to specialists. The International Association for the Study of Pain (https://www.iasp-pain.org/) has identified significant problems with waiting times and access to pain services, issues that often result in significant deterioration of patient's health. Evidence suggests that patients should receive treatment as soon as possible, to avoid deterioration in the quality of life, psychological well-being and depression. Clinicians need to work with patients to establish the best course of treatment. Enhancement of communication between clinicians and patients is one of the most important elements to establish an optimal pain treatment and quality pain self-management support. Improvement of chronic pain management in a large patient population, with limited resources, requires the development of tools for self-management, therapeutic control, and documentation of effects (Phillips, 2000). Such tools can encourage patients in taking an active involvement in their treatment while facilitating care providers to assist patients in a cost-effective manner.

Most chronic pain patients are actually managed by primary care physicians but, in several severe cases, optimal care can only be designed and implemented by special pain units. These units usually do not have the capacity to absorb all (or even most) of the severe chronic pain cases. Tools that can assist in the improvement of their capacity are urgently needed. Such tools should focus on reducing the effort needed for the evaluation of patients, the design and the implementation of their therapeutic plan and their follow-up. The scientific community has widely accepted Information and Communication technologies as useful tools for chronic pain self-management (Buhman, 2016). Chronic pain rehabilitation is very costly (Dagenais et al. 2008), and internet-based treatments could be used as a cost-effective complement or even a first-hand primary intervention, as highlighted in the case of the management of anxiety disorders (Hedman et al. 2011). According to (Buhrman et al. 2015) an individualized guided internet-delivered treatment based on cognitive-behaviour therapy can be effective for persons with chronic pain comorbid emotional distress. ICT for chronic pain has to address several challenges including the provision of tools to support the efficient organization and availability of existing information before the visit to a pain specialist, the consistent follow-up monitoring in between visits, and the support for adherence to treatment. Key features for patient-empowerment include a) personalized support such as personalized information material about non-pharmacological approaches (Hysing et al. 2017) and personalized education with quality content, b) effective communication between patients and clinicians, c) access to social networks with chronic patients having the same conditions, and d) secure data transfer for research purposes.

As already described in (Katehakis et al. 2017), technical challenges have mostly to do with issues relevant to interoperability, device connectivity, security, compliance with national and international legislation regulation, as well as with local policies, usability and accessibility from different devices by users with different profiles.

The aim of this work is to describe a platform for chronic pain management to support patient-centered care, self-management and effective use of health care resources. The platform will be dynamically adapted according to patient preferences and medical history, and incorporates intelligent alerts, recommendations, motivation and other personalized features, aiming towards promoting efficient patient-physician communication.

More specifically the contributions of this paper are twofold:

- We present the requirements' elicitation methodology and results collected out of a variety of sources including related research projects, three pain clinics and a local medical advisory group. To this direction we provide an end-to-end scenario, capturing the full journey of the patient before his first visit to a pain clinic ending with the release of the patient from the clinic. We proceed further to identify 14 use-cases out of this scenario, which is transformed then to a technical infrastructure proposal.
- We subsequently present the technical architecture of this platform that is able to support disease self-management. The platform includes an intelligent personal health record, apps specifically for monitoring and managing pain, high-quality recommendations, smart, analytical data services, a central decision support and guidance system, means of synchronous and asynchronous communication, tools for lifestyle monitoring and digital behavioral change support and a ticketing system for the helpdesk.

To the best of our knowledge, the designed platform is the only one offering all these functionalities required for the efficient and effective management of pain. The specific pain types and medical contents and details for each pain type will be incorporated in a later stage of the development process and are not described at this time.

The rest of the paper is structured as follows: Section 2 presents related ICT tools for pain management. Then, Section 3 describes requirements elicitation, following input from three different sites in Europe, and a high-level description of a real world, end-to-end scenario. Section 4 presents a description of the proposed architecture and its core components. Finally, Section 5 discusses open issues and outlines the roadmap towards implementation.

BACKGROUND

Applications for chronic pain, according to a recent review (Portelli & Eldred, 2016), are divided into those that address pain in general, and those that focus on specific conditions, such as arthritis, back pain, migraine, and others. Self-management interventions are mostly absent from these applications that focus more on monitoring and data collection (de la Vega et al., 2014). Although an increase in the availability of applications for pain management, evaluation of their effectiveness and efficiency is uncommon (Dario et al., 2017; Portelli & Eldred, 2016). For specific conditions, such as low back pain, application use in combination with other interventions has been shown to be superior to minimal interventions improving functionality and quality of life for people with chronic pain (del Pozo-Cruz, Borja, et al., 2013; Irvine et al., 2015). However, poor patient engagement and adherence to advice may compromise the potential benefits of technology engagement. (Eysenbach, 2005; Singh et al., 2016).

Pain applications have been divided into three categories (Rosser and Eccleston, 2011): 1) pain information, symptom identification, and treatment planning (approximately 55% of available apps); 2) assessment of pain, and medication and appointment reminders (about 25%); 3) self-management interventions for the management of pain (less than 20% of available apps). Applications reviewed combine some of these functionalities, but no application combines all of them. More specifically, pain apps have a variety of purposes/goals and include several elements/techniques, although only a few try to incorporate multiple goals and strategies (Dario et al., 2017; Portelli & Eldred, 2016, Singh et al., 2016; Sundararaman, Edwards, Ross, & Jamison, 2017). The main features that have been identified are combined in the following list:

1. Information about pain in various formats including documents, videos, or avatars.
2. Self-monitoring tools for assessment and evaluation of pain, frequency, severity and identification of consequences. The self- reported monitoring takes place in the format of a diary, single questions or formal questionnaires. In some cases, pain-related factors, such as psychological distress, treatment adherence, drug use, and others are also assessed.
3. Physical activity monitoring through activity trackers.
4. Text messaging for reminders (e.g. appointments) and/or motivation.
5. Self-management and stress-management strategies including features for goal setting, reinforcement, cognitive appraisal and restructuring, problem-solving, positive activity scheduling, healthy lifestyle tips and relaxation techniques.

6. Medication modules for keeping track of drug intake/dosage, and information about interactions, contraindications, side-effects, and others.
7. Connection with peers through online chat.
8. Communication between healthcare providers and patients.

It is interesting to note that less than 2% of these applications have modules that enable communication with healthcare providers and connection with peers through patient groups. Also, the majority of these apps are not designed by health care providers with only 25-30% confirmed the participation of a health care provider (Lallo et al., 2015; Wallace & Dhingra, 2014). In addition, self-management features and education about psychological implications of chronic pain can be found in only 15% of the available applications (Lallo et al., 2015). Finally, Sundararaman et al. (2017) have pointed out that no application combines all five main functionalities of self-monitoring, goal setting, skills acquisition, education, and provision of social support.

Other important aspects that need to be taken into consideration include the potential benefits of remote digital diagnostics and corresponding devices/wearables, the need to increase users' engagement and motivation, the need to increase person-centered and individual tailored care, and the need to assess mHealth literacy and promote ease of use (Sundararaman et al., 2017; Lin & Bautista, 2017). A validated theoretical context for self-management in chronic illness is also important for establishing a solid background for application features.

Based on these suggestions and the relevant literature, applications that provide a holistic approach to chronic pain management will have the following features:

- Short presentation of application features and functionalities using multimedia to facilitate user familiarization with the application.
- A self-management assessment to identify patient's beliefs and knowledge about their condition, goals and action plans for physical and emotional outcomes (e.g., the Common Sense Model (Leventhal, Halm, Horowitz, Leventhal, & Ozakinci, 2005)).
- Information about chronic pain, including psycho-emotional aspects, in multimedia format, tailored to user conditions and needs.
- Self-monitoring and assessment of pain characteristics including severity, frequency, impact, and pain-related variables including physical functioning.
- Tailored suggestions and motivational messages for improving chronic pain and adhering to therapies (e.g., text messaging of corresponding self-management techniques).
- Individualized goal setting and action planning.

- Self-management strategies to achieve goals (e.g., the pacing of activity, reinforcement, problem-solving, positive activity scheduling, healthy life-style tips).
- Stress management strategies (e.g., breathing and other easy to implement relaxation techniques).
- Tailored reminders (e.g., through text messaging and/or emails) of drug dosing and relevant information.
- Interaction and online chat with other members of support groups, such as chronic pain or specific illness patient associations (if possible).
- Interaction with healthcare providers based on predefined criteria for frequency and type of interaction.

In addition to taking into consideration, the inclusion of all key characteristics for a holistic pain management application, the design and development phases of such applications should also include clinicians and patients. The inclusion of key stakeholders will support the identification of the relevant functional characteristics that will benefit patient care in real life conditions. Pain management applications may offer an opportunity to establish mutually beneficial conditions for patients and physicians targeting specific needs at the point of care. The pain management application that is presented in this paper addresses this issue. Pain experts have coupled with technology experts to deliver the necessary modules and tools that will provide the most support to patients as well as physicians involved in chronic pain.

Review of related work has provided the key characteristics of applications for a holistic approach to pain management. In addition, an exploration of real-life scenarios was undertaken to identify the actual needs of physicians and patients. It has been determined that a self-management application for chronic pain need to include both patients and physicians and to have the capacity for integration with existing systems such as electronic health records. The specific requirement elicitation is further described below.

REQUIREMENT ELICITATION

To analyze the future environment and perform a deep requirement elicitation necessary for building such an environment we relied on the following:

- input received by three pain clinics (at Cordoba, Uppsala and Paris)
- input received by a local medical advisory group from the University Hospital of Heraklion in Crete

- Relevant Personal Health Tools available already, implemented in the context of several, related EU research project. Some are indicative of the following:
    - iManageCancer (H2020) for the self-management of cancer patients
    - MyHealthAvatar (FP7) for a complete virtual representation of citizens/ patients
    - EURECA (FP7) linking research and hospital information systems
    - P-Medicine (FP7) personalized management for a cancer patient
    - SmokeFreeBrain (H2020) for assessing the effectiveness of a multi-level variety of interventions aiming at smoking cessation.
    - CATCH (H2020) to activate technology in bridging the gap between cancer survivors' reduced physical activity and emotional state, and their ultimate ability to return to a fully functional societal role through technology-supported physical exercise.

To this direction, we created initially, an end-to-end scenario, starting before the visit of the patient to the pain clinic and finishing when the patient is released from the clinic – and his/her data are available to be used for research purposes. Since the first contact point of a chronic pain patient with the healthcare system is his primary care physician we have created a primary chronic pain screening tool that can be used to increase awareness of primary care physicians regarding chronic pain and to help them choose patients eligible for treatment in specialized chronic pain units. Therefore, once the patient has been found eligible for referral to a chronic pain management unit, the scenario supported by the designed tool includes all the information that will need to be collected throughout the different stages that the patient engages with the pain clinic. The scenario starts once the patient has been referred to the pain clinic and has booked an appointment for a specified date and time. The patient is provided with access to the platform to input all his/ her relevant information. The scenario describes information gathering from the time before the first visit to the pain clinic until the release of the patient from the clinic.

The patient is able to report a complete patient history in a structured, guided way and to provide their personal story about their pain before their first visit. Valuable information relevant to chronic pain includes Characteristics of the pain – location, intensity, and duration, how the pain feels like and what comforts or aggravates the pain. Relevant pain specific questionnaires can be completed before the patient's first visit. An intelligent algorithm adapted to the clinic's policies and based on patient input presents to the patient the relevant questions to be answered. Personal goals and objectives for successful treatment are decided such as reduced anxiety, increased mobility, days at work, daily activities and others. Success indicators are not so much focused on relieving pain completely but improving the quality of life.

During the first visit, the physician will review and validate the patient input, and include all new input based on the physical examination and the proposed treatments. For all treatments, there will be an information component describing what the treatment is about, side effects, success rates and other relevant details. The system will support the pain clinic in appointment management as well as providing an asynchronous communication channel with the pain clinic. Based on the treatment plan, the system will be able to support a smart decision aid that will help the patient implement the treatment plan. The physician will specify some rules that will appear to the patient as alerts or reminders.

In between visits, patients will be able to input in a structured way the characteristics of their pain, the efficacy of treatment, side effects, and impact on quality of life. The patients will be able to monitor and report their outcomes. Patients will be provided with the tools for self-management and will be prompted to monitor their progress. Self-management activities include physical exercise, diet, relaxation & mindfulness techniques and medication dosage adaptation based on a specified set of rules as provided by the clinic. The application will be able to track physical activity and sleep. Self-management will be enhanced with motivational messages and advice that will prompt the patient to follow up with activities, assigned tasks, and encourage change. The physician and the patient will decide the frequency of collecting relevant information based on the type of treatment the patient has had and the selected questionnaires between visits.

Based on the aforementioned scenario 14 use-cases were identified and developed, creating the corresponding use-case diagrams, identifying the actors, the trigger, the pre-conditions, the post-conditions and capturing the high-level basic flow. They are listed in Table 1.

Out of this analysis, some system requirements were identified requesting several modules to be implemented.

PROPOSED ARCHITECTURE

Based on the aforementioned analysis and requirements, a high-level architecture of the proposed solution was specified, as depicted in Figure 1.

As we can see at the top of Figure 1, the core models of the Personal Health Record (PHR) (blue boxes) are complemented with pain specific modules (orange boxes). The modular architecture of the PHR makes the platform easily expandable to other diseases/ phenotypes.

The proposed solution will provide a multilingual disease self-management platform designed accordingly to the specific needs of patient groups and focusing on the pain management of the patient with special emphasis on adherence, healthy

Table 1. Identified use cases

Use Case	Title	Purpose
1	Data collection of patient demographics and medical history	To record patient's demographics and medical history, as well as information related to expectations & goal settings, pain characteristics and history. Members of the care team may share captured data.
2	Self-reported questionnaires	To be filled by the patient regularly, based on questionnaires selected by the healthcare professionals from existing templates
3	Review of the patient's available information	The physician is able to review all information available for the patient.
4	Medication plan & treatment monitoring	Members of the care team (including patients) are able to insert medication plan to the medication application, as well as update medication intakes. The patient can set up reminders for the medication intakes, and the application will inform the patient with detected irregularities and report adverse events.
5	Non-pharmacological treatments	Healthcare professionals may upload videos suggesting specific non-pharmacological treatment, while the patient may watch them and rate the experience. Patients may record information regarding physical activity and nutrition and check their progress.
6	Patient education	Registering high-quality content created by subject matter experts. Patients should be able to find information relevant to their condition.
7	Personalized recommendations	Automatic identification of content relevant to one's profile.
8	Forum & Social Network	Patients are able to communicate with social networks and peers and share information with healthcare professionals.
9	Motivational messages	To keep the patient engaged in an endurable behavioral change.
10	Recommendations for medication update	A decision aid based on rules set by the clinic and the doctors guides patients into changing the dosage of medication or switching to alternative medication in case of side effects.
11	Scheduling visits	For online scheduling of visits. Support provided for rescheduling visits in case of emergency or good course of treatment.
12	Communication with the pain clinic (emergency & triaging)	Asynchronous communication of the patient with the clinic, in cases of emergency.
13	Sharing data for research	Patients may give their consent for the use of their data for research purposes.
14	Data analysis and data mining	An overview of the available data for the whole set of patients sharing information with the healthcare professional using various visualization techniques, such as charts, plots, bubble charts, parallel coordinates. The end user can select specific features and set inclusion/exclusion criteria in order to create a new cohort. The system applies data analysis for the new cohort(s). The end user can select one or more patients and plot patient's data in conjunction with average values of the specific cohort(s). If significant differences appear, the researcher is informed.

Figure 1. High-level architecture

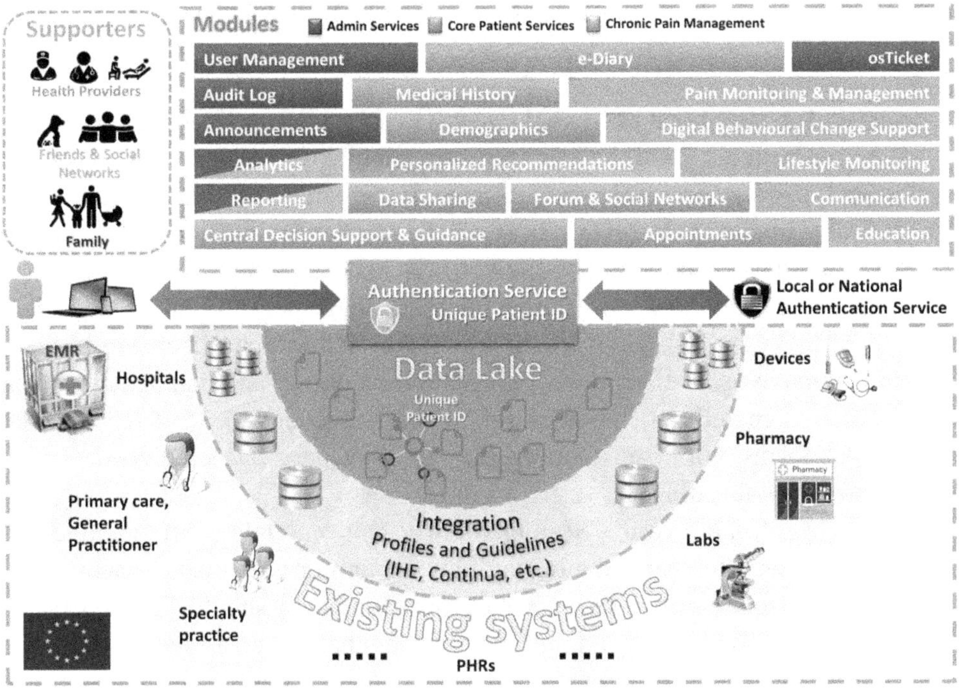

lifestyle, patient education and treatment. The platform is centered on a Personal Health Record for the individual patient surrounded by m-health applications. It is designed to encourage the patient to become more involved in his/her treatment, enhance clinician-patient communication, maximize compliance to therapy, predict, detect and manage side effects and contribute to pain management through minimization of patient anxiety and provision of motivational support for achieving specific goals and durable change. The project builds upon open architecture components to maximize the benefits of combining technologies from the partners and organizations in the regions of interest. Short iterations during implementation will help to keep quality under control by driving to a releasable state frequently, which will prevent the consortium from collecting a large backlog of defect correction work. The proposed solution focuses on the combination of a group of services into one technology while the core models of the platform are complemented with disease-specific (pain management) modules making the platform easily expandable to other diseases/ conditions. Apart from the modular architecture and the integration solution, a privacy and security layer wraps the whole architecture, data flow and interactions. The proposed solution enables privacy and security technologies and ensures that the data sharing constraints of each data source are respected at all times.

Based on the site visits, the proposed modules have been modified to map what has been requested by the end users. As such, the main components of the platform are the following:

- **iPHR**: The intelligent Personal Health Record (iPHR) is the central point for a citizen/patient. It will be optimized for mobile devices and will allow the patient registration and the management of the patient profile through a user-friendly Graphical User Interface (GUI). Using the Application Programming Interfaces (APIs) provided by the PHR database and the activity database it will enable individual profile creation and management. All apps, individual functionality etc. will be served through this system which will ensure efficient and effective user registration, information recording and management. The iPHR will include all modules for recording patient medical record. The various forms will be customized for pain management including treatment plans and goal setting.
- **Pain Monitoring and Management**: This module will include all questionnaires for pain monitoring and the appropriate management tools. The end users can decide on which questionnaires should be used based on specific conditions and individual patients. An Artificial Intelligence (AI) mechanism will automatically fill-in specific questions based on past experience. The patients will be able to record their own experience regarding their pain. In addition, this tool will enable monitoring the psycho-emotional status of the patient.
- **High-Quality Intelligent Recommendations to Patients (PHIR)**: This module targets on the education of the patients based only on verified high-quality documents and internet sources selected by experts (Iatraki et al. 2018; Kondylakis et al., 2015; Stratigi et al. 2017). Furthermore, it takes advantage of the personal information stored in the iPHR and provides personalized results (Potamias et al., 2005). A health care provider can upload text and multimedia (educational and/or practical) content relevant to pharmacological, pain or non-pharmacological treatments such as exercise and relaxation content. A search engine allows patients to look for personalized information based on their pain condition. A Frequently Asked Question (FAQ) section will also be available with information about pain conditions, treatments and other relevant information.
- **Smart Analytical Data Services**: The analytical services will be used to identify patterns and reveal trends in data in order to gain knowledge from the available health data sources (Koumakis et al. 2017) The smart analytical data services module will also support a mechanism to export anonymized data and provide basic statistical functionalities and machine learning approaches (Potamias et al.

2005) for secondary use. It will also offer readily available cohort analysis based on specific rules such as a cohort of patients with similar treatments, a cohort of patients of particular age groups, employment status and others. The system will offer the possibility to design own rules for data analysis.

- **Central Decision Support and Guidance System**: This module will act mainly as an intelligent calendar for the patient where rules for alerting will be available triggering various messages through the communication system, able to reschedule visits and inform the patient about actions, appointment and tasks. The module will also support a set of interrelated tools that focus on specific aspects of patient's decision process.
- **Patient Communication**: This module will provide the option to the user to publish information in the internal forum of the iPHR, connect him/her to legitimate social networks available through the platform and peer with patients experiencing similar conditions. In addition, the patient will be able to share information with other users such as family members and health providers. Finally, this module will include asynchronous communication methods with the clinic.
- **Digital Behavioral Change Support**: This tool will be a digital behavioral change support service aimed at improving adherence to pharmacological and non-pharmacological treatment, and promote lifestyle changes. Although simple reminders via SMS and phone calls have been proven to be effective in previous studies for medication adherence (Franklin et al., 2003), our approach will consist on using messages to foster a behavior change as other studies have already done (Cole-Lewis & Kershaw, 2010). Specifically, we will opt for a more tailored approach grounded in behavioral change models. Evidence shows that these techniques may produce better results (Noar et al. 2007). In our case, we will use the I-Change behavioral change model (De Vriea, 2017). This behavioral change model proposes that their several determinants influence people to transition towards an effective behavior change. By knowing the user profile, and with a health recommender system, we will be able to recommend users with tailored pieces of advice tackling those determinants. These recommendations will provide personalized coaching, motivation and support for adherence to treatment, including physical activities and rehabilitation exercises.
- **Lifestyle Monitoring**: Physical activity levels and sleep quality are two key elements for assessing a patient quality of life. Our solution will offer a monitoring module to capture that information. The filling frequency pattern will be limited so that it does not become a tedious and repetitive activity. All this gathered data will be summarized and accessible to healthcare professionals in web dashboards to support their decision making.

- **osTicket – Customer support ticket system**: Using this module user will be able to create tickets via the helpdesk website. In addition, it will support the management, organization and archive of all the support requests.

The infrastructure will be supported by a data management layer ensuring the effective and efficient management of the various types of data collected and their subsequent processing.

In the proposed solution, we intend to exploit several interlinking ontologies as a global schema to integrate all internal and external data – a task that has been successfully already implemented in relevant European projects. Personal health information will be stored in a central repository, which will then be combined with a semantic integration solution on top to integrate both internal and external data. Established models and terminologies (SNOMED CT, ICD, MeSH, LOINC etc.) will be also used as much as possible in order to ensure future linking to existing systems, whereas the integration with existing systems will be based on standardized middleware components (IHE profiles) as well as de-facto industrial standards such as Health Level-7 (HL7), while at the same time it allows exporting some of the output data to the Electronic Medical Records (EMRs) and/ or other available ICT tools.

Developing an innovative ICT platform for the management of pain includes acquisition and use of health-related personal data. Therefore, the proposed solution will comply not only with legal, but also with ethical requirements, and will take all necessary measures to protect the rights of the data subjects involved. As such, all subjects storing their data in the platform should have provided a valid consent and processing of personal data will be forbidden, except the subject has given valid consent as well. In addition to all necessary aspects for the effectiveness of the informed consent by the data subjects (such as the necessary moment of giving consent, voluntariness, renewal, and possibility of revoking consent at any time), other important aspects that will be considered include the lawful use of sensitive health-related data as well as appropriate anonymization techniques. The whole platform will be in accordance to all security and privacy regulations and guidelines including the General Data Protection Regulation (GDPR), whereas all access to information will be regulated providing efficient and effective state of the art mechanisms for authentication and authorization. The real owner of the data is the person (participant) themselves in compliance with the European legislation, and therefore she/he has immediate access to the personal data, and notification of any processing, or even the right to object any further preservation, sharing, and processing of them.

Finally, the proposed solution will accomplish all usability standards. It has already been developed with a user-centered design approach involving local clinical experts and end users. In the next phase user involvement will be escalated to include local patients as well more in-depth discussions with and users at the clinical sites.

CONCLUSION

The paper presented a novel, technical infrastructure for chronic pain self-management. The introduced platform provides innovative functionalities through open source tools, facilitates effective interactions between patients and health professionals, and provides an integration framework for accessing third party electronic medical record systems, facilitating the collection of clinical data for research purposes. It offers psychological and emotional assessment and encouragement tools and promotes health-related behaviors through personalized recommendations. Finally, it has the potential to improve health literacy and digital competence and increase the participation of the patient in the decision-making process. Additional communication features facilitate the interaction with peers and carers to support patient empowerment.

The proposed holistic patient centered platform for pain management does not replace medical practice but rather enhances and facilitates patient management. As a facilitator, the platform supports more effective management of chronic conditions and their psycho-emotional aspects. Further work needs to be conducted, in order for the proposed architecture to be in a position to better fit available methodologies and treatments, as well as local configuration needs. Other challenges to be further addressed include the complexity related to interoperability and security issues, and patient motivation to introduce valuable data. Further specifications on key characteristics are being investigated including the provision of timely feedback, tailored educational material to patient needs and comprehension capabilities, patient guidance to relevant connections, effective communication support between patients and clinicians, filtering of relevant information, and usage of data for research purposes.

Adaptive management of chronic pain depends to a large degree on how patients choose to cope with pain and its impact. Still, there is a need to determine whether (and which) motivation enhancement interventions increase active participation in self-management treatment programs for chronic pain (Jensen et al., 2003). User satisfaction with the information technology solution remains a key challenge, to be addressed at a later stage.

The ability to facilitate seamless integration with existing systems, as depicted at the bottom of Figure 1, is very important. Work relevant to interoperable Electronic Health Record (EHR) exchange is still ongoing. Standardization organizations such as HL7 already work towards the development of functional models to improve providers' workflows to support the timely transition of relevant clinical information at each point of care (HL7 Service Functional Model, 2017). This requires a systems engineering perspective which considers all parts of the ecosystem and collaborative activity between care team members, where the patient and designated family caregivers are considered as members of the care team. Protocols such as Fast Healthcare Interoperability Resources (FHIR), profiles such as the ones developed by IHE, and design guidelines such as those from PCHAlliance Continua help towards the delivery of standards-based, open specifications that can support the flow of data from the point they are captured into EHRs in the same format and coded content. Key issues include not matching semantic standards, quality needs and safe data exchange techniques. These limit the opportunities to reuse these data for research and better healthcare since they are usually kept in data silos.

The introduction of apps and tools, as public services to support chronic pain self-management, is expected to have a significant impact on the quality of life and overall cost to individuals and the society. Besides better management of the condition and more direct interaction towards more efficient treatment, public authorities and healthcare providers should also consider a sustainable business model for the systematic introduction of innovative services, such as the ones we described for chronic pain management, in an efficient and trustworthy manner.

ACKNOWLEDGMENT

Work presented in the paper is part of the RELIEF project that has received funding from the European Union's Horizon 2020 Research and Innovation Programme. Any opinions, results, conclusions, and recommendations expressed in this material are those of the authors and do not necessarily reflect the views of RELIEF or the European Commission.

REFERENCES

Andersson, H. I. (2009). Increased mortality among individuals with chronic widespread pain relates to lifestyle factors: A prospective population-based study. *Disability and Rehabilitation*, *31*(24), 1980–1987. doi:10.3109/09638280902874154

Blyth, F. M., March, L. M., Nicholas, M. K., & Cousins, M. J. (2003). Chronic pain, work performance and litigation. *Pain*, *103*(1-2), 41–47. doi:10.1016/S0304-3959(02)00380-9

Breivik, H., Collett, B., Ventafridda, V., Cohen, R., & Gallacher, D. (2006). Survey of chronic pain in Europe: Prevalence, impact on daily life, and treatment. *European Journal of Pain (London, England)*, *10*(4), 287–287. doi:10.1016/j.ejpain.2005.06.009

Buhrman, M., Gordh, T., & Andersson, G. (2016). Internet interventions for chronic pain including headache: A systematic review. Internet Interventions, 4, 17–34. doi:10.1016/j.invent.2015.12.001

Buhrman, M., Syk, M., Burvall, O., Hartig, T., Gordh, T., & Andersson, G. (2015). Individualized guided Internet-delivered cognitive-behavior therapy for chronic pain patients with comorbid depression and anxiety: A randomized controlled trial. *The Clinical Journal of Pain*, *31*(6), 504–516. doi:10.1097/AJP.0000000000000176

Cole-Lewis, H., & Kershaw, T. (2010). Text messaging as a tool for behavior change in disease prevention and management. *Epidemiologic Reviews*, *32*(1), 56–69. doi:10.1093/epirev/mxq004

Dagenais, S., Caro, J., & Halderman, S. (2008). A systematic review of low back pain cost of illness studies in the United States and internationally. *Spine*, *8*(1), 8–20. doi:10.1016/j.spinee.2007.10.005

Dario, A. B., Cabral, A. M., Almeida, L., Ferreira, M. L., Refshauge, K., Simic, M., ... Ferreira, P. H. (2017). Effectiveness of telehealth-based interventions in the management of non-specific low back pain: A systematic review with meta-analysis. *The Spine Journal*, *17*(9), 1342–1351. doi:10.1016/j.spinee.2017.04.008

de la Vega, R., Roset, R., Castarlenas, E., Sánchez-Rodríguez, E., Solé, E., & Miró, J. (2014). Development and testing of painometer: A smartphone app to assess pain intensity. *The Journal of Pain*, *15*(10), 1001–1007. doi:10.1016/j.jpain.2014.04.009

De Vries, H. (2017). An integrated approach for understanding health behavior; The i-change model as an example. Psychology and Behavioral Science International Journal, 2(2), 1–4. doi:10.19080/PBSIJ.2017.02.555585

del Pozo-Cruz, B., Gusi, N., del Pozo-Cruz, J., Adsuar, J. C., Hernandez-Mocholí, M., & Parraca, J. A. (2013). Clinical effects of a nine-month web-based intervention in subacute non-specific low back pain patients: A randomized controlled trial. *Clinical Rehabilitation*, *27*(1), 28–39. doi:10.1177/0269215512444632

eCancer Medical Science. (2018). International Association for the Study of Pain (IASP), Classification of Chronic Pain, Descriptions of Chronic Pain Syndromes and Definitions of Pain Terms (2nd rev. ed.). Retrieved May 08, 2018, from https://www.iasp-pain.org/PublicationsNews/Content.aspx?ItemNumber=1673

Elliott, A. M., Smith, B. H., Penny, K. I., Smith, W. C., & Chambers, W. A. (1999). The epidemiology of chronic pain in the community. *Lancet*, *354*(9186), 1248–1252. doi:10.1016/S0140-6736(99)03057-3

Eriksen, J., Jensen, M. K., Sjøgren, P., Ekholm, O., & Rasmussen, N. K. (2003). Epidemiology of chronic non-malignant pain in Denmark. *Pain*, *106*(3), 221–228. doi:10.1016/S0304-3959(03)00225-2

Eysenbach, G. (2005). The law of attrition. *Journal of Medical Internet Research*, *7*(1), e11. doi:10.2196/jmir.7.1.e11

Franklin, V., Waller, A., Pagliari, C., & Greene, S. (2003). "Sweet Talk": Text messaging support for intensive insulin therapy for young people with diabetes. *Diabetes Technology & Therapeutics*, *5*(6), 991–996. doi:10.1089/152091503322641042

Gore, M., Sadosky, A., Stacey, B. R., Tai, K. S., & Leslie, D. (2012). The burden of chronic low back pain: Clinical comorbidities, treatment patterns, and health care costs in usual care settings. *Spine*, *37*(11), E668–E677. doi:10.1097/BRS.0b013e318241e5de

Gustavsson, A., Bjorkman, J., Ljungcrantz, C., Rhodin, A., Rivano-Fischer, M., Sjolund, K. F., & Mannheimer, C. (2012). Socio-economic burden of patients with a diagnosis related to chronic pain–Register data of 840,000 Swedish patients. *European Journal of Pain (London, England)*, *16*(2), 289–299. doi:10.1016/j.ejpain.2011.07.006

HL7 Service Functional Model. (2017). Coordination of Care (CCS), Standard for Trial Use (STU) Release 1, Retrieved May 08, 2018, from http://www.hl7.org/implement/standards/product_brief.cfm?product_id=452

Hedman, E., Andersson, E., Ljótsson, B., Andersson, G., Rück, C., & Lindefors, N. (2011). Cost-effectiveness of Internet-based cognitive behavior therapy vs. cognitive behavioral group therapy for social anxiety disorder: Results from a randomized controlled trial. *Behaviour Research and Therapy*, *49*(11), 729–736. doi:10.1016/j.brat.2011.07.009

Hysing, E. B., Smith, L., Thulin, M., Karlsten, R., Butler, S., & Gordh, T. (2017). Identifying characteristics of the most severely impaired chronic pain patients treated at a specialized inpatient pain clinic. *Scandinavian Journal of Pain*, *17*(1), 178–185. doi:10.1016/j.sjpain.2017.09.008

Iatraki, G., Kondylakis, H., Koumakis, L., Chatzimina, M., Marias, K., & Tsiknakis, M. (n.d.). Personal Health Information Recommender: A Tool for the Empowerment of Cancer Patients,

Irvine, A. B., Russell, H., Manocchia, M., Mino, D. E., Glassen, T. C., & Morgan, R. … Ary, D. V. (2015). Mobile-Web app to self-manage low back pain: Randomized controlled trial. Journal of Medical Internet Research, 17(1), e1. doi:10.2196/jmir.3130

Jensen, M. P., Nielson, W. R., & Kerns, R. D. (2003). Toward the development of a motivational model of pain self-management. *The Journal of Pain*, *4*(9), 477–492. doi:10.1016/S1526-5900(03)00779-X

Katehakis, D. G., Kondylakis, H., Koumakis, L., Kouroubali, A., & Marias, K. (2017). Integrated Care Solutions for the Citizen: Personal Health Record Functional Models to support Interoperability. [EJBI]. *European Journal for Biomedical Informatics*, *13*(1), 51–58.

Kondylakis, H., Bucur, A., Dong, F., Renzi, C., Manfrinati, A., & Graf, N. … Kiefer, S. (2017, June). iManagecancer: developing a platform for empowering patients and strengthening self-management in cancer diseases. In *2017 IEEE 30th International Symposium on Computer-Based Medical Systems (CBMS)* (pp. 755-760). IEEE.

Kondylakis, H., Koumakis, L., Kazantzaki, E., Chatzimina, M., Psaraki, M., Marias, K., & Tsiknakis, M. (2015). *Patient Empowerment through Personal Medical Recommendations* (p. 1117). MedInfo.

Koumakis, L., Kondylakis, H., Katehakis, D. G., Iatraki, G., Argyropaidas, P., Hatzimina, M., & Marias, K. (2018). A Content-Aware Analytics Framework for Open Health Data. In *Precision Medicine Powered by pHealth and Connected Health* (pp. 59–64). Singapore: Springer; . doi:10.1007/978-981-10-7419-6_10

Kroenke, K., Bair, M. J., Damush, T. M., Wu, J., Hoke, S., Sutherland, J., & Tu, W. (2009). Optimized antidepressant therapy and pain self-management in primary care patients with depression and musculoskeletal pain: A randomized controlled trial. *Journal of the American Medical Association*, *301*(20), 2099–2110. doi:10.1001/jama.2009.723

Lalloo, C., Jibb, L. A., Rivera, J., Agarwal, A., & Stinson, J. N. (2015). "There's a pain app for that": Review of patient-targeted smartphone applications for pain management. *The Clinical Journal of Pain*, *31*(6), 557–563. doi:10.1097/AJP.0000000000000171

Leventhal, H., Halm, E., Horowitz, C., Leventhal, E. A., & Ozakinci, G. (2004). Living with chronic illness: A contextualized, self-regulation approach. In *The Sage Handbook of Health Psychology* (pp. 197–240). Sage.

Lin, T. T., & Bautista, J. R. (2017). Understanding the Relationships between mHealth Apps' Characteristics, Trialability, and mHealth Literacy. *Journal of Health Communication*, *22*(4), 346–354. doi:10.1080/10810730.2017.1296508

Nitter, A. K., & Forseth, K. Ø. (2013). Mortality rate and causes of death in women with self-reported musculoskeletal pain: Results from a 17-year follow-up study. *Scandinavian Journal of Pain*, *4*(2), 86–92. doi:10.1016/j.sjpain.2012.12.002

Noar, S. M., Benac, C. N., & Harris, M. S. (2007). Does tailoring matter? Meta-analytic review of tailored print health behavior change interventions. *Psychological Bulletin*, *133*(4), 673–693. doi:10.1037/0033-2909.133.4.673

Phillips, D. M. (2000). JCAHO pain management standards are unveiled. *Journal of the American Medical Association*, *284*(4), 428–429. doi:10.1001/jama.284.4.423b

Portelli, P., & Eldred, C. (2016). A quality review of smartphone applications for the management of pain. *British Journal of Pain*, *10*(3), 135–140. doi:10.1177/2049463716638700

Potamias, G., Koumakis, L., & Moustakis, V. (2005). Mining XML Clinical Data: The HealthObs System. Ingénierie des Systèmes d'Information, 10(1), 59–79. doi:10.3166/isi.10.1.59-79

Potamias, G., Koumakis, L., & Moustakis, V. S. (2005). Enhancing web based services by coupling document classification with user profile. In *The International Conference on Computer as a Tool EUROCON 2005* (Vol. 1, pp. 205–208). IEEE; . doi:10.1109/EURCON.2005.1629896

Rosser, B. A., & Eccleston, C. (2011). Smartphone applications for pain management. *Journal of Telemedicine and Telecare*, *17*(6), 308–312. doi:10.1258/jtt.2011.101102

Singh, K., Drouin, K., Newmark, L. P., Rozenblum, R., Lee, J., & Landman, A. … Bates, D. W. (2016). Developing a framework for evaluating the patient engagement, quality, and safety of mobile health applications. Issue Brief (Commonwealth Fund), 5(1), 11.

Stratigi, M., Kondylakis, H., & Stefanidis, K. (2017). Fairness in Group Recommendations in the Health Domain. In *2017 IEEE 33rd International Conference on Data Engineering (ICDE)* (pp. 1481-1488). IEEE.

Sundararaman, L. V., Edwards, R. R., Ross, E. L., & Jamison, R. N. (2017). Integration of Mobile Health Technology in the Treatment of Chronic Pain: A Critical Review. *Regional Anesthesia and Pain Medicine*, *42*(4), 488–498. doi:10.1097/AAP.0000000000000621

Waddell, G., & Norlund, A. I. (2000). Review of social security systems. *Neck and Back Pain: The Scientific Evidence of Causes. Diagnosis and Treatment*, *1*, 427–471.

Wallace, L. S., & Dhingra, L. K. (2014). A systematic review of smartphone applications for chronic pain available for download in the United States. *Journal of Opioid Management*, *10*(1), 63–68. doi:10.5055/jom.2014.0193

This research was previously published in the International Journal of Reliable and Quality E-Healthcare (IJRQEH), 8(1); edited by Anastasius Moumtzoglou, pages 23-39, copyright year 2019 by IGI Publishing (an imprint of IGI Global).

Chapter 7
Participant Perspectives on Benefits and Challenges of Engaging in an Online Pain Self-Management Program

Marian Wilson
Washington State University, USA

Michele R. Shaw
Washington State University, USA

ABSTRACT

The purpose of this study was to evaluate participants' perspectives after engaging in an 8-week online pain self-management program. Unexplored qualitative data for this analysis were collected via secure online surveys distributed during a previously published randomized controlled trial. Participants for the present study were 47 adults prescribed opioid medicines for chronic pain. A qualitative descriptive approach using content analysis methods was used to identify common themes regarding online participation. Three themes described the benefits of the program and included: positive reframing, improved accountability, and feeling supported. Two themes described how participants would like to improve the program experience and included: ease of use and desire for personalizing. Participants' insights can assist health care providers and program developers in understanding how online programs may improve chronic disease self-management for a multitude of health problems.

DOI: 10.4018/978-1-7998-1680-5.ch007

INTRODUCTION

Innovations are needed to provide people with chronic pain access to evidence-based options for managing symptoms. Cognitive and behavioral therapies that are known to assist pain control are not always accessible due to costs, insurance reimbursement structures, and stigma and receptivity related to psychological care (National Academies Press, 2011). Online programs show promise in delivering cognitive behavioral therapy (CBT) approaches that teach people to recognize relationships between thoughts, feelings and behaviors. Unfortunately, CBT has been underutilized and participants with pain do not always engage to the fullest extent, thereby lessening the effectiveness (Knoerl et al., 2016; Wilson et al., 2015). Treatment-seeking adults with chronic pain in the United States are most likely to receive pharmacological interventions and less likely to access psychologically-based treatments (National Academies Press, 2011). Such practices increase risks related to opioid medicine use and reduce opportunities to improve symptom management.

Limited qualitative research has been conducted to fully understand participants' experiences and improve online pain self-management program delivery. Therefore, this qualitative study was nested within a randomized controlled trial (RCT) that was previously published. The prior study reported on the quantitative effects for participants engaged in the online "Chronic Pain Management Program" (Wilson et al., 2015). The present study builds on what was previously learned using content analysis methods to examine unexplored data regarding participants' perspectives. Specific aims are to provide insight on program benefits and challenges in order to maximize the usefulness of online pain self-management.

BACKGROUND

An estimated 25 million (11%) United States (U.S.) adults experience chronic pain, which may be defined as any pain lasting at least 3 months that does not respond to treatment (Nahin, 2015). More than half of those with chronic pain describe it as "unbearable" or "excruciating" (Kennedy et al., 2014). Behavioral and cognitive therapies have been well-established in research literature as effective components that can improve pain treatment outcomes (Macea et al., 2010; Eccleston, 2011). Yet, biopsychosocial multidimensional models of pain care are less commonly delivered, at least in some nations where pharmacological options are the predominant pain treatments (National Academies Press, 2011). Unfortunately, a reliance on a biomedical approach to pain care in the U.S. has resulted in a 600% rise in opioid prescriptions over the past decade (National Academies Press, 2011). Concurrently, deaths caused by opioid overdose increased 300% (CDC, 2014). The majority of deaths occur as an unintended consequence of legitimate prescribing practices (Manchikanti et al., 2012). Respiratory depression is the main hazard of opioid use (Dumas and Pollack, 2008). It can occur as a result of opioid tolerance that develops over time as more opioids are required to receive the same pain-relieving results (Dumas and Pollack, 2008). As scrutiny increases towards prescribing physicians and patients who receive opioids, a critical need exists to offer effective, affordable multidisciplinary treatment approaches that can be widely disseminated.

The U.S. Department of Health and Human Services' National Pain Strategy calls for better access to quality pain care that does not rely solely on medication (DHHS, 2016). Non-opioid and non-pharmacologic treatments are now recommended as the preferred treatment for chronic pain (Chou et al., 2009; Manchikanit et al., 2011). It has been proposed that the call to reduce opioid prescriptions may be achieved by increasing emphasis on non-pharmacologic treatments (Hallinan et al., 2011). The Internet offers opportunities to provide accessible, affordable options, yet program developments are necessary to expand their utility in pain management. Ultimately, online programs may provide the support and education necessary to mitigate risks associated with opioid use among people with chronic pain.

Self-Management Interventions

Self-management programs are intended to assist people in mastering the tasks needed to live with a chronic condition. Such programs aim to increase confidence, or self-efficacy in one's ability to manage health symptoms (Lorig et al., 2008). Pain self-management interventions have been recommended as an essential component of evidence-based clinical practice guidelines for chronic pain (ICSI, 2011). Online and face-to-face self-management interventions have demonstrated improved outcomes in small, specific populations of patients who suffer with a variety of painful conditions, such as patients with fibromyalgia, headaches, and arthritis (Lorig et al., 2008; Macea et al., 2010). However, no such interventions have been accepted for widespread use in the general population of patients with chronic pain, and the optimal means to engage patients in pain self-management strategies remains unclear. Specifically, for those people who require opioid medicines for pain relief, more information is needed about how best to engage them in self-management programs and maximize desired effects (Wilson et al., 2015).

E-health delivers health resources or health care via electronic means. E-health offers one possible means of access to self-management for people with chronic pain, who are increasingly using the Internet for information and support (Ziebland et al., 2015). The E-health program used in the present study, the Chronic Pain Management Program (CPMP), was created by psychologists who are pain researchers. The CPMP is available to the public online with a paid subscription (approximately $25 U.S.

dollars per month). The CPMP is a self-directed, self-paced Internet-based self-management program intended for a general population of people with persistent non-cancer pain. The program targets cognitive, emotional, behavioral and social pain determinants. The main lessons provided map onto four modules that can generally be completed across 8-weeks and include: *Thinking Better, Feeling Better, Doing More,* and *Relating Better.* More description is provided on the program website https://pain.goalistics.com (Ruehlman et al., 2011).

Learning modules include didactic materials and interactive activities. For example, the *Thinking Better* module asks participants to recognize, stop, evaluate, and redirect their self-defeating thoughts, using the same techniques a cognitive behavioral therapist might teach clients as highlighted in Figure 1.

Feeling Better guides participants through relaxation exercises and builds awareness of emotional triggers as seen in Figure 2.

Figure 1. Chronic Pain Management Program Screenshot: Learning Module for Cognitions

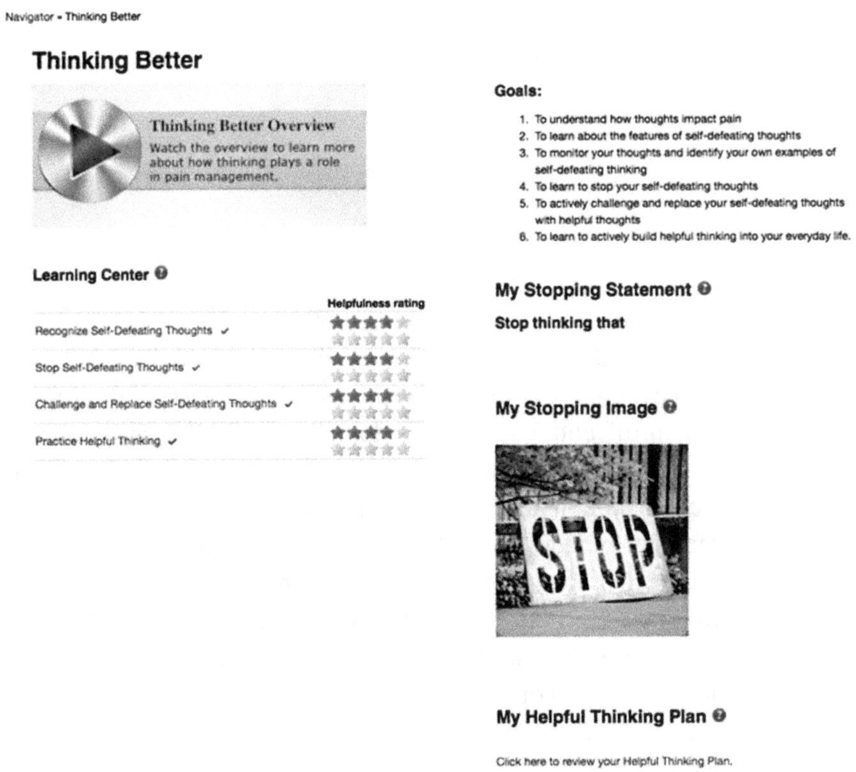

Figure 2. Chronic Pain Management Program Screenshot: Learning Module for Emotions

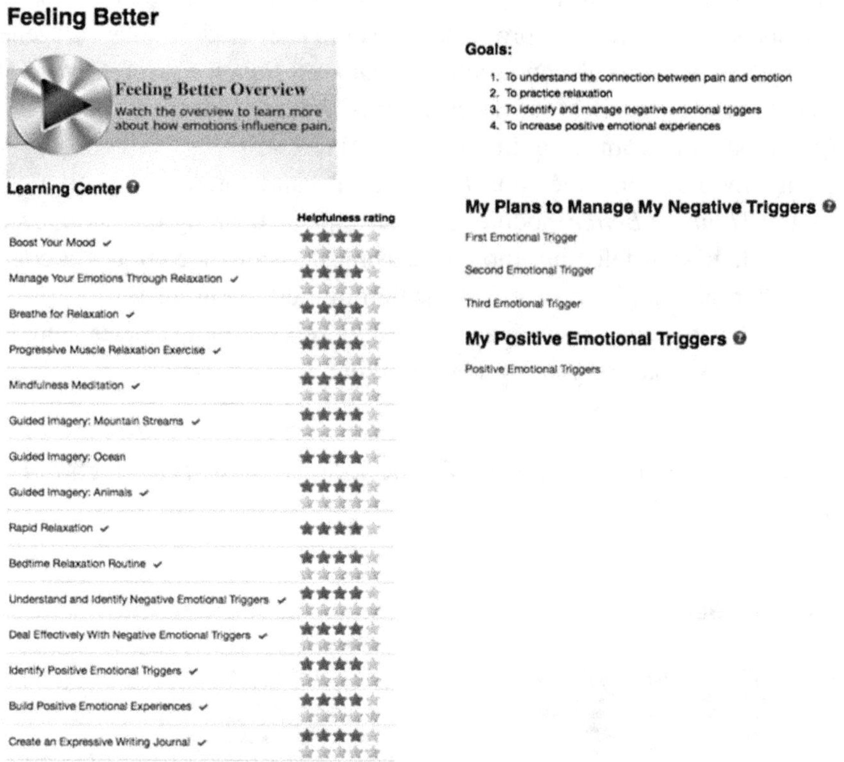

Doing More teaches pacing and fitness activities. *Relating Better* assists in building a helpful support system and scheduling social activities. At the end of each activity, participants are asked to assign a helpfulness rating using a 1-to-5- star rating where 1 star = "not at all helpful" and 5 stars = "extremely helpful." Some activities are to be completed off-line, such as physical exercises, relaxation, or self-monitoring behaviors. Prior research demonstrated the CPMP's ability to decrease pain severity, pain-related interference, perceived disability, depression, and pain-induced fear among participants recruited from the Internet (Ruehlman et al., 2011). Of note, the original RCT testing the CPMP by Ruehlman, Karoly, and Enders (2011) did not specifically recruit people using opioid medicines. Therefore, our RCT was designed to target a population prescribed opioids and determine whether they would engage in non-pharmacological pain management strategies and find benefit.

At the time of recruitment for our RCT in 2012, the CPMP was the only online self-management program specifically developed for chronic pain that was found to be publicly available. Our trial randomized 114 people with chronic non-cancer pain who had a current opioid prescription into treatment and control groups. The main published findings were that 20.9% of CPMP users compared to 6.8% of control group participants reported decreasing or discontinuing their opioid medication (Wilson et al., 2015). Moreover, in the CPMP, relative to control, participants reported significantly greater decreases in opioid misuse, increases in pain self-efficacy, and a significantly greater proportion had a clinically significant decrease (i.e. $\geq$ 2 points) in pain intensity (18% vs. 6%) (Wilson et al., 2015). Thus, the E-health program was found to improve several outcomes valued by providers and patients. However, the improvements were modest and a large number of participants engaged minimally with the program activities. Those who engaged the most had the greatest reductions in symptoms of pain intensity and pain interference, and the largest gains in pain self-efficacy (Wilson et al., 2015). One systematic review of online pain self-management programs found study withdrawal rates ranging from to 6% to 59% (Bender et al., 2011). Limited information is available to explain why those drop-outs occur, although programs with some human prompting tend to have less attrition (Bender et al., 2011). Therefore, the qualitative descriptive study presented here was designed to provide insights from participants about benefits and limitations of using the CPMP. Deeper analysis into the participant experience can generate ideas that improve the human-technology interaction and inform program enhancements for lasting, desired effects.

METHODS

Qualitative descriptive methodology and qualitative content analysis methods were selected in order to describe participants' experiences with the online pain management program and to identify common themes (Sandelowski, 2010; 2000). Our previously published RCT did not include qualitative analysis. Qualitative description is used when the goal of the research is to summarize descriptions of events or experiences in a way that depicts the unique perspectives of the participants (Sandelowski, 2010; 2000). Common themes are identified to provide details of the most prominent ideas provided by the participants' responses (Sandelowski, 2010; 2000). The methodology compliments the purpose of the present study by allowing the participants of the CPMP to give subjective input about the programs' usefulness.

Data for this study were previously collected from U.S. adult participants (n=47) prescribed opioid therapy for chronic pain who were enrolled in the RCT and who engaged in the selected online self-management program, the CPMP. Results of that trial are reported elsewhere (Wilson et al., 2015). A total of 236 potential participants were screened for the original study, and 24 were found to be ineligible, primarily due to no Internet access (33% of those ineligible) or planned surgery (29% of those ineligible). Of those eligible, 62 did not follow through with consenting procedures and 36 declined to participate, leaving a total of 114 participants who consented to join the original RCT. Of those consenting, 92 completed all study procedures (19.3% attrition). Sixty (53%) were referred from their health care provider and 54 (47%) were self-referred from Internet advertising on web pages for pain (e.g., Facebook). The present study sample of 47 is composed of those who answered the open-ended qualitative questions at the post-treatment time point. These 47 include 30 participants who responded from the original treatment group and 17 who chose to trial the CPMP after serving in the control group.

Notably, our original RCT exclusively recruited people prescribed opioids, unlike all other known Internet-based pain self-management studies at that time. The participant follow-up was, therefore, limited in duration to 8 weeks to allow participants sufficient time to engage fully in the CPMP, and also to address questions related to study feasibility, participant engagement, and retention prior to investing resources in a longer trial. Eligibility criteria included individuals 18 years of age or older who: (1) self-identified as having had a non-cancer chronic pain lasting for greater than 3 months; (2) had current prescription(s) for opioid medicine; (3) had Internet access with email capability either at home or at a public setting; and (4) had ability to read, speak and write in the English language. Exclusion criteria were chosen to limit confounding treatment effects and included: (1) planned surgical treatment in the next 2 months; (2) pregnancy; and/or (3) currently enrolled in therapy or support group with counselor, psychologist or psychiatrist for chronic pain or substance abuse. All procedures were reviewed and approved by the Institutional Review Board of the university sponsoring the study. Surveys were collected online using a secure survey site.

Pertinent to the qualitative descriptive study presented here were the open-ended survey questions included at the end of the study to evaluate participants' experiences with using the online pain self-management program. The three questions used for our present analysis were: 1) "Did you find anything about this program especially useful? What would that be?" 2) "Is there anything you would change about this program if you could? What would that be?" and 3) "What else can you share about your experience participating in this program?"

Ryan and Sawin's Individual and Family Self-Management Theory (IFSMT) (2009) provided theoretical background to our study (Ryan and Sawin, 2009). It is a descriptive, mid-level theory that allows researchers to incorporate the complexity of the human experience and build on what is known about self-management (Ryan and Sawin, 2009). In the IFSMT, the individual or family assumes responsibility for self-management, and may include health care providers as collaborators. Using the IFSMT as a guide, we can explore participants' experiences and consider unique physical, social and individual variables that may enhance or deter from achieving desired self-management program outcomes (Ryan and Sawin, 2009).

Data Analysis

Qualitative content analysis as described by Schreier was used to analyze the data (Schreer, 2012) and is the method of choice in qualitative descriptive research (Sandelowski, 2010). Conventional content analysis is appropriate when existing theory or research literature on a phenomenon is limited (Hsieh and Shannon, 2005). Print text data (responses to the three open-ended survey questions) were de-identified and transferred into a word document table for analysis. In order to meet the purpose of the present study, throughout the content analysis the researchers focused on identifying common themes in the text that were associated with participants' descriptions of the benefits and challenges of completing the online program (Schreer, 2012). Qualitative content analysis included combing concept-driven and data-driven analysis approaches to the text to summarize information (Sandelowski, 2010; Schreer, 2012). This means that the research team used their content expertise, qualitative expertise, prior experiences, and commonalities within the data and allowed themes to emerge from the data (Schreer, 2012; Hsieh and Shannon, 2005). Interpretation remains close to participants own words and is relatively free of inference (Sandelowski, 2010).

The authors initially read through the participants' responses separately to achieve immersion and made notes describing potential themes based on commonly identified statements throughout the data (Hsieh and Shannon, 2005). The researchers then met in person to discuss and compare initial findings. This meeting included reviewing initial summaries of overall impressions of the data, identifying agreed upon themes, comparing supporting quotes, and then naming and describing each theme (Schreer, 2012). During this initial meeting, a coding frame was developed, generated directly from the text data, that included the agreed upon themes (Sandelowski, 2010; Schreer, 2012). The researchers returned back to the data and using the coding frame as a reference, continued coding of data, along with contrasting similarities and differences among themes (Schreer, 2012). The researchers met several more times throughout this process to compare individual analyses, revise themes and definitions, and compare identified quotes supporting the themes (Schreer, 2012). Quantitative content analysis methods were included to represent the distribution and frequency of similar responses (Hsieh and Shannon, 2005). Reliability and credibility were addressed by the process of having each researcher initially review and analyze the data prior to each meeting and then compare consistency of agreement between the coders (Schreer, 2012; Hsieh and Shannon, 2005). Consistency was high among the commonly identified themes and supporting quotes. Validity was also addressed by considering the applicability of the themes when compared to the participants' responses, self-management theories, and the overall purpose of the study (Schreer, 2012; Hsieh and Shannon, 2005). An audit trail was kept throughout the analysis process to document decisions and next steps. Quotations from the respondents were used to support the claims made.

FINDINGS

Participants were predominantly women (80%), average age 47 years (SD 10.4) and 78% reported having education levels higher than a high school diploma. Most participants (73%) had more than one medical diagnosis related to their painful condition with the most common being back or spine pain conditions (45%), fibromyalgia (29%), arthritis (26%), or migraine headache (22%).

Five common themes were identified that provide description of the participants' perspectives about the online program. Themes were grouped into two main categories to reflect benefits and challenges of the program use. Perceived program benefits included: (1) positive reframing, (2) improved accountability, and (3) feeling supported. Perceived program challenges included: (4) ease of use and (5) desire for personalizing.

Program Benefits

Positive Reframing

The participants commonly (n=15; 32%) reported that the online pain program provided new information and techniques that could be used to make positive shifts in the way they perceive pain. Many discussed how new coping skills were gained by program enrollment and that this helped them change their negative responses and thoughts into a more positive perspective. Positive reframing as a benefit of the program can be illustrated by the following quotes:

It was extremely helpful for me to shift my mind and spirit to focus on the good and wellness instead of sickness! Huge change in me personally!

I thought that changing thinking patterns is a very important component, since chronic pain can entrench negative thought patterns.

Participants shared comments about how the program provided them with new tools to be able to change the way they approached dealing with their chronic pain. They were better able to alter their responses to pain and attempted to see their situations in a different light, as illustrated by the following comments:

This program really helped me to realize that chronic pain and a diagnosis of a condition that has no cure...doesn't mean it's hopeless. I've come to realize that a lot of how I need to deal with the pain is my attitude.

It's good for keeping myself feeling better about my pain because I have more tools for dealing with it.

Participants shared comments about noticing improvements in their coping skills when living with their chronic pain and this allowed them to "reframe" the way they thought about pain. They acknowledged that the pain was still there but they were better able to live with it:

The most helpful part of the program for me was the attitude adjustment such as not being so hard on myself.

My actual pain is about the same, but it seems to cause me less stress. I feel I have better coping mechanisms in place now.

Improved Accountability

The online program provided reminders which helped participants improve accountability of their actions. Participants were able to identify unique needs and take responsibility for meeting them. The program's built-in reminders cued participants to check in with their thoughts and actions. The theme of improved accountability was evident in 7 (15%) participants' responses and included comments regarding continuous self-evaluation of progress and steps taken to reach goals. Participants shared these examples:

It was almost like having someone ask me not to think so negatively several times a day. That alone was very helpful, at least to me.

I've found that being more self-aware is very helpful, focusing on what your body and mental state is doing to your overall pain.

Receiving reminders was described as a benefit of the program that prompted participants to continue to use the new skills they were learning. The organization that the online program provided was helpful to participants in that they found having a set plan improved coping with their pain. Benefits of improved accountability are described by the following two participants:

It created structure for my days/weeks which really helped me deal with the exhaustion and stress that goes along with the chronic pain.

I loved the idea of getting reminders on my cell phone every two hours to check my thoughts, and have texts include positive affirmations.

The program activities encouraged participants to evaluate their thoughts and their overall health status. Improved accountability led to improvements in living with chronic pain, in one participant's words:

I am back on track. Getting regular newsletters, reminders, encouragement is a necessity for me.

Feeling Supported

The theme of feeling supported was described by 5 (11%) participants in terms of decreased feelings of isolation and being misunderstood. Participants of the online program reported gaining support and understanding from their peers who shared similar stories of living with chronic pain as illustrated in the following examples:

I liked the chat groups - it really makes you aware you're not alone and other people understand.

I really enjoy being able to share my pain and experiences with others, it really helps knowing you're not alone.

Before, I felt so alone that no one understood me.

The benefit of feeling like a part of a group was often described as a reward of the program. Participants reported a realization that there are many others who are also living with chronic pain. This sense of sharing others' experiences was an expressed benefit of the support received as part of the program.

Program Challenges

Ease of Use

Ease of use of the online program was the most commonly identified challenge. Participants (n=26; 55%) desired more clarity with the directions, reduced effort of navigation, and more orientation early on explaining how to best use the online program. Experiencing technical difficulties while using the online program was reported by some. Ease of use issues are expressed by the following participants, along with specific improvement suggestions:

A fuller, detailed explanation would have had me fully engaged right from the start. For people who aren't especially computer savvy, like me, it took a while to figure things out.

I think I need a tutorial. I did want to do the program and sort of failed at it.

Frustration at not being able to fully utilize all aspects of the online program was shared by several participants. Others found the online program complicated to navigate and/or requiring too much effort as seen in these examples:

I found it very hard to go back every day and check in and keep up with check ins and to mark the activities as completed...I didn't know how to go in and mark the check-in as completed so it looked like I didn't show up that day.

Unfortunately, I was unable to access and navigate through the program as I use an iPad.

...it was difficult for me to complete all the tasks. It took a lot of time & energy which I don't seem to have. If the program could be scaled back some so the tasks didn't seem so daunting.

Participants overall seemed to desire an improved ease of use in order to successfully complete their assignments and fully engage in the online program.

Desire for Personalizing

The desire for more personalizing of the online program was commonly described in the data. Participants (n=14; 30%) expressed the need to be able to provide further explanation or more of their personal story than what the online program allowed them to do. Participants shared ideas for how to improve the online program as illustrated in the following:

Sometimes the answer is not always yes or no without explanation. I realize that's not necessarily a part of the "program" but at times I would like to explain how I feel.

To better serve others like myself who have already been exposed to many of these concepts, it would help to have a way to personalize things.

Participants wanted more options in the program to meet individual needs and to be able to provide more in-depth information. One participant's quote illustrates this clearly:

I'm open to making changes, but felt the way the program was set up, that there was no way to start from where I was at for modifications. The program seemed to assume I was starting from nothing. In reality, I have a solid pain management routine in place that includes all components the program is introducing.

Taking into account the context of each participant's unique background and experiences was voiced as a perceived challenge of the online pain management program. Improving the amount of personalization was a suggested way to improve involvement.

DISCUSSION AND CONCLUSION

Study Contributions

Participant perspectives (Figure 3) provide an essential lens through which to evaluate E-health interventions. Five major themes emerged through our analysis. Participants expressed both benefits and challenges after program use. Benefits were most often categorized as positive reframing, improved accountability, and feeling supported. Program challenges were described as a need for improving ease of use and a desire for personalizing. Ease of use was the most common category of remark, therefore, may prove to be the best starting point for increasing participant engagement and improving program usefulness.

Similar to other studies, the participants in the present study commonly reported that the online self-management intervention taught them skills that enabled them to put a positive spin on their reaction to pain. Improving coping skills or decreasing "pain catastrophizing" have been noted as benefits of other online pain self-management programs (Kristjansdottir et al., 2011; Kruijssen et al., 2015; Trudea et al., 2015). Similarly, "gaining insights" was a category endorsed by small group of six women piloting a pain program using mobile phone technology (Kristjansdottir

Figure 3. Participant Perceptions of Online Program Benefits and Challenges Weighted by Frequency of Responses

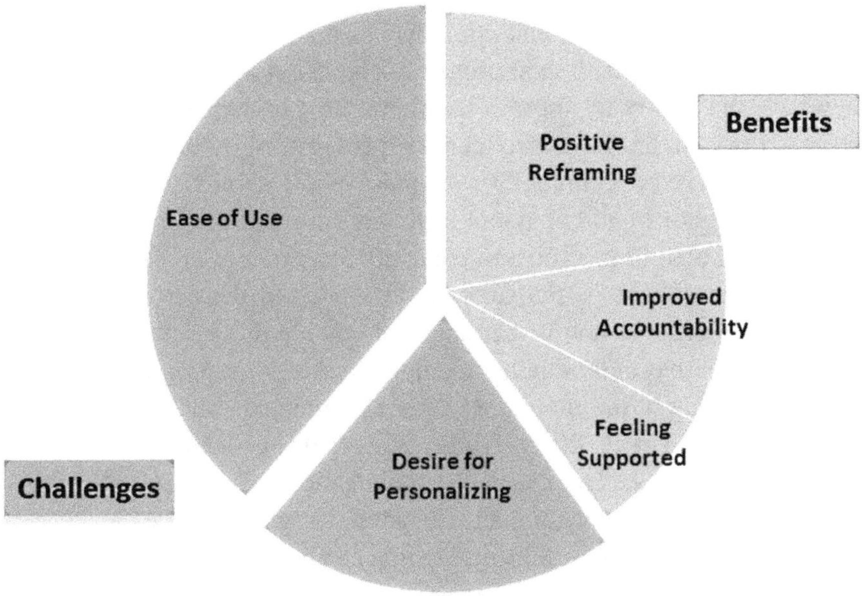

et al., 2011). Throughout the data, our participants described now having the tools to reframe negative thought patterns associated with pain. Such coping skills have been endorsed in previous studies as well. For example, "How do I cope with the pain" received high marks from 28 adults with arthritis who were asked what people want from online pain self-management programs (Trudeau et al., 2010).

Akin to prior qualitative studies of people with chronic pain, the theme of feeling supported by others or not "being alone" in their suffering was important to our participants (Andersen et al., 2014). Shared experiences, emotional support, and mutual understanding have been credited as key to success of similar interventions for people with chronic disease in group settings (Andersen et al., 2014; Barlow et al., 2009). Fewer studies have reported this from online pain self-management, so it is worth noting that social support or feeling supported can be felt within online environments. It has been suggested that online forums offer a kind of support that cannot be achieved in face-to-face sessions, therefore, they offer novel types of support that may have unique benefits (Broom, 2005). The ability to take control of one's disease and reduce inhibitions are two advantages afforded by online interactions (Broom, 2005). Emotional and informational support are the types of support seen most commonly within online communities, and self-disclosure is more frequently seen online than within face-to-face support groups (Griffiths et al., 2009).

People with chronic pain desire online programs that include information, activities and tools that will help them feel equipped to gain back control (Trudea et al., 2015; Nielsen et al., 2014). Our study participants often described that they appreciated receiving positive affirmations and reminders as part of the program and that this allowed them to check in with their progress. These actions served to remind them that they have the ability to improve their chronic pain experience through their own actions. Prior studies have also identified benefits of online self-management programs as improved accountability or improved awareness of ones' ability to choose positive actions and behaviors in living with and managing chronic pain (Kristjansdottir et al., 2011; Kruijssen et al., 2015; Trudea et al., 2015). Increasing accountability meant that participants either increased their positive actions or paused activity in order to not further aggravate their pain.

Including subjective, individualized components to online programs is a common thread noted throughout the literature to meet participants' needs (Kristjansdottir et al., 2011; Kruijssen et al., 2015; Trudea et al., 2015; Griffiths et al., 2009). Our study participants suggested increasing personalization and improving ease of use in order for them to successfully complete the online program. While the CPMP does offer daily tracking and activity scheduling that can be personalized (see Figure 4), these features were also ones that seemed to cause the most technical difficulties for some participants.

It was noted after our analysis that the emerging themes matched the CPMP's four learning modules. *Thinking Clearly* aims to reframe to more positive thought patterns, and *Feeling Better* assists in identifying and removing negative emotional triggers. *Doing More* encourages accountability with goal-setting for activities. *Relating Better* addresses the need to feel supported within healthy relationships. That these themes emerged independently of any knowledge by one of the researchers on the program modules provides compelling evidence that the program was on target in achieving what it had intended.

Study Limitations and Strengths

Because our data were collected previously, limitations of the study include the inability to question or clarify participant remarks further. The data provided were collected online and those who prefer to use verbal rather than written communications may not have fully participated. Focus groups, interviews, or online chat sessions might have allowed for more detailed input from participants. The sample was restricted to U.S. residents so may not apply to other cultures or settings. While some participants were recruited from clinical settings, many self-referred from the Internet so may not be representative of all people with chronic pain. Respondents were predominantly Caucasian and educated, like most other studies of online pain

Figure 4. Chronic Pain Management Program Daily Check-in Tool and Activity Tracker

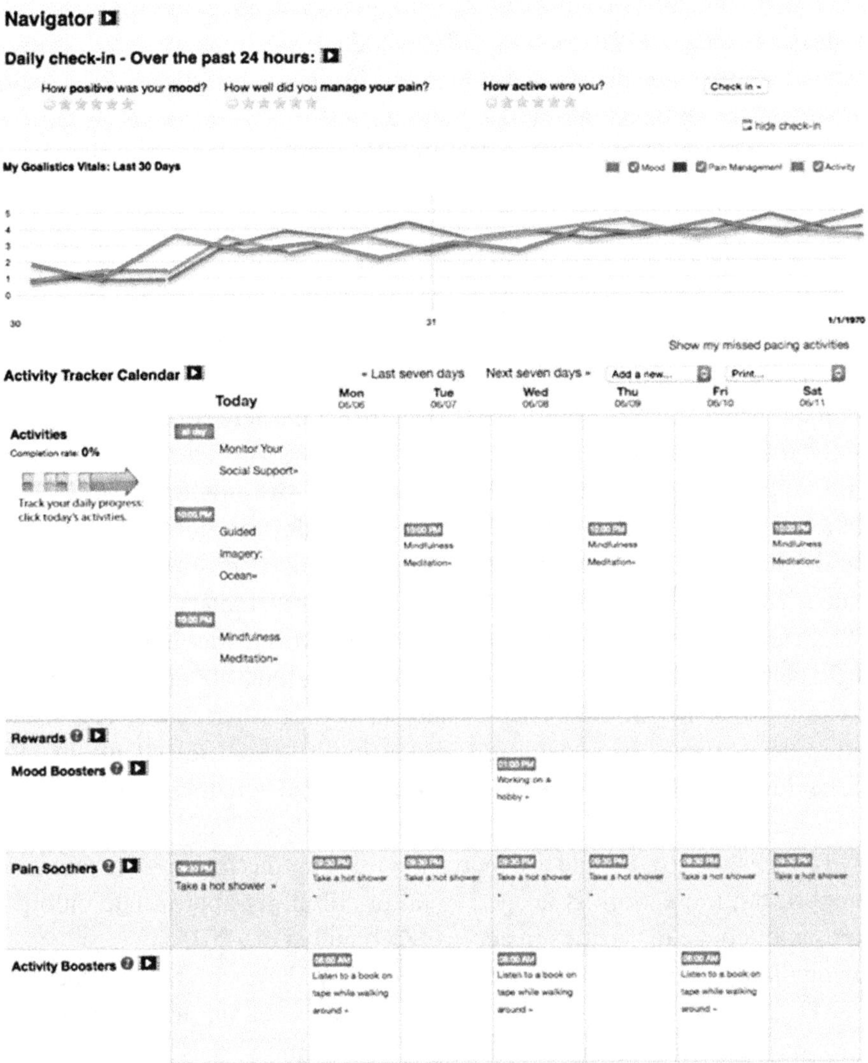

management (Bender et al., 2011), limiting generalizability. Yet, strengths of the study included the number and depth of participants' responses, and that participants were able to maintain anonymity, which has been found to be an advantage of online research (Hamitlon and Bowers, 2006). The privacy provided may have allowed more honest disclosures and freedom of expression.

Implications to Research and Practice

Our previously published RCT provided quantitative evidence of both the efficacy and the limits of the CPMP (Wilson et al., 2015), and the participants' words presented here extend, amplify, and clarify that evidence. The original published RCT included a summative program evaluation using an adapted version of the IBM Computer Usability Satisfaction Questionnaire. Seven Likert-style scale items were presented to rate satisfaction with the program's usability and usefulness, and the mean value of the combined evaluation items was interpreted to be high (Wilson et al., 2015). Yet from those data, we gleaned little insight about what participants might need to maximize the programs' usefulness and engage more vigorously, nor could we fully appreciate individual benefits. It is apparent from the deeper inquiry presented here that gains can be made using E-health for chronic pain, and also that more development is needed to fully support participants in their efforts to self-manage symptoms using technology.

Improving ease of use might be accomplished by providing more detailed orientation to the online program and offering other delivery methods such as iPad or hybrid learning options that include more personal contact along with virtual assistance. The CPMP can be accessed from computers, tablets, and smartphones, and, thus, can be accessed in a variety of ways. However, training may be needed for participants to utilize all of the functions. At present, about two-thirds of the world use the Internet at least occasionally or own a smartphone, and the most dramatic rate increases have occurred in developing countries (Poushter, 2016). Mobile health technologies are believed to hold promise to reduce accessibility gaps in mental health services, yet, it is also recognized that efficacy research is in its infancy (Anthes, 2016). People are increasingly using the Internet for information and support, but more work is needed to tailor culturally-appropriate online pain resources and reduce disparities in access (Ziebland et al., 2015).

Our qualitative descriptive approach guided by the theoretical framework of the IFSMT allowed us to identify specific variables unique to our participants' perspectives that can be explored in future intervention trials. For example, we recommend that a variety of accountability and support strategies be developed and tested for efficacy within online self-management interventions. Health care providers can serve as collaborators, as the IFSMT dictates (Ryan and Sawin, 2009). Providers can provide tangible support such as through in-person prompts, phone calls or text messages that encourage participants' progress towards goals. Family members can be enlisted to provide additional support to improve accountability. Online programs could be personalized by adding remedial training sessions for those who find computer programs daunting. Each new strategy can be tested for effects on proximal and distal outcomes as the IFSMT recommends. For example, adding family support might increase the short-term outcome of increasing physical exercise, which then might increase the desired long-term outcome of reduced health care utilization.

E-health innovations and their translation into clinical practice are worthy efforts towards expanding non-pharmacological pain care strategies, and reducing the potential harms of opioid use. Our participants' insights regarding online pain self-management can assist clinicians and researchers alike in better understanding how such programs may help people suffering with chronic pain. The knowledge generated can guide development and refinement of programs and assist in creative, technological solutions to address a multitude of health problems.

ACKNOWLEDGMENT

The data collection for this research was supported in part by the Washington State Life Sciences Discovery Fund (grant LSDF 08–02, John Roll, PI). The authors acknowledge Dr. Linda Ruehlman and Dr. Paul Karoly, creators of the Chronic Pain Management Program, for assistance in enrolling participants and sharing program activity data. Content from this paper was previously presented at Hawaii International Conference on System Science HICSS 2017 and published online at ScholarSpace doi: http://hdl.handle.net/10125/41566.

REFERENCES

Andersen, L. N., Kohberg, M., Herborg, L. G., Søgaard, K., & Roessler, K. K. (2014). Here We're All in the Same Boat: A Qualitative Study of Group Based Rehabilitation for Sick-listed Citizens with Chronic Pain. *Scandinavian Journal of Psychology*, *55*(4), 333–342. doi:10.1111jop.12121 PMID:24730653

Anthes, E. (2016, April 6). Mental Health – There's an App for That. *Nature: International Weekly Journal of Science*. Retrieved from http://www.nature.com/news/mental-health-there-s-an-app-for-that-1.19694

Barlow, J., Edwards, R., & Turner, A. (2009). The Experience of Attending a Lay-led, Chronic Disease Self-management Programme from the Perspective of Participants with Multiple Sclerosis. *Psychology & Health*, *24*(10), 1167–1180. doi:10.1080/08870440802040277 PMID:20204986

Bender, J. L., Radhakrishnan, A., Diorio, C., Englesakis, M., & Jadad, A. R. (2011). Can Pain be Managed through the Internet? A Systematic Review of Randomized Controlled Trials. *Pain*, *152*(8), 1740–1750. doi:10.1016/j.pain.2011.02.012 PMID:21565446

Broom, A. (2005). Virtually He@lthy: The Impact of Internet Use on Disease Experience and the Doctor-Patient Relationship. *Qualitative Health Research*, *15*(3), 325–345. doi:10.1177/1049732304272916 PMID:15761103

Centers for Disease Control and Prevention (CDC). (2014). Prescription Drug Overdose in the United States: Fact sheet July 3, 2014. Retrieved from http://www.cdc.gov/drugoverdose /data/prescribing.html

Chou, R., Fanciullo, G., Fine, P., Adler, J., Ballantyne, J., Davies, P., ... Miaskowski, C. (2009). Clinical Guidelines for the Use of Chronic Opioid Therapy in Chronic Noncancer Pain. *The Journal of Pain*, *10*(2), 113–130. doi:10.1016/j.jpain.2008.10.008 PMID:19187889

Department of Health and Human Services (DHHS). (2016, March 18). National Pain Strategy. Retrieved from https://iprcc.nih.gov/National_Pain_Strategy/NPS_Main.ht m

Dumas, E. O., & Pollack, G. M. (2008). Opioid Tolerance Development: A Pharmacokinetic/Pharmacodynamic Perspective. *The AAPS Journal*, *10*(4), 537–551. doi:10.120812248-008-9056-1 PMID:18989788

Eccleston, C. (2011). Can Ehealth Technology Deliver on its Promise of Pain Management for All? *Pain*, *152*(8), 1701–1702. doi:10.1016/j.pain.2011.05.004 PMID:21612868

Griffiths, K. M., Calear, A. L., Banfield, M., & Tam, A. (2009). Systematic Review on Internet Support Groups (ISGs) and Depression (2): What Is Known About Depression ISGs? *Journal of Medical Internet Research*, *11*(3), e41. doi:10.2196/jmir.1303 PMID:19793718

Hallinan, R., Osborn, M., Cohen, M., Dobbin, M., & Wodak, A. (2011). Increasing the Benefits and Reducing the Harms of Prescription Opioid Analgesics. *Drug and Alcohol Review*, *30*(3), 315–323. doi:10.1111/j.1465-3362.2011.00294.x PMID:21545563

Hamilton, R.J., & Bowers, B.J. (2006). Internet recruitment and e-mail interviews in qualitative studies. *Qualitative Health Research*. doi:10.1177/1049732306287599

Hsieh, H.-F., & Shannon, S. E. (2005). Three Approaches to Qualitative Content Analysis. *Qualitative Health Research, 15*(9), 1277–1288. doi:10.1177/1049732305276687 PMID:16204405

Institute for Clinical Systems Improvement (ICSI). (2011). Pain, Chronic; Assessment and Management of (Guideline). Retrieved from http://www.icsi.org/guidelines

Institute of Medicine Committee on Advancing Pain. (2011). *Research, Care, and Education, "Relieving Pain in America: A Blueprint for Transforming Prevention, Care, Education, and Research."* Washington, D.C.: National Academies Press.

Kennedy, J., Roll, J. M., Schraudner, T., Murphy, S., & McPherson, S. (2014). Prevalence of Persistent Pain in the U.S. Adult Population: New Data from the 2010 National Health Interview Survey. *The Journal of Pain, 15*(10), 979984. doi:10.1016/j.jpain.2014.05.009 PMID:25267013

Knoerl, R., Lavoie Smith, E. M., & Weisberg, J. (2016). Chronic Pain and Cognitive Behavioral Therapy: An Integrative Review. *Western Journal of Nursing Research, 38*(5), 596–628. doi:10.1177/0193945915615869 PMID:26604219

Kristjansdottir, O. B., Fors, E. A., Finset, A., Dulmen, S., Wigers, S. H., & Eide, H. (2011). Written Online Situational Feedback via Mobile Phone to Support Self-management of Chronic Widespread Pain: A Usability Study of a Web-based Intervention. *BioMed Central Musculoskeletal Disorders, 12*(51). Retrieved from http://www. biomedcentral.com/ 1471-2474/12/51

Kruijssen, V., Staa, A., Dwarswaard, J., Veen, J., Mennema, B., & Adams, S. (2015). Use of Online Self-Management Diaries in Asthma and COPD: A Qualitative Study of Subjects and Professionals Perceptions and Behaviors. *Respiratory Care, 60*(8), 1146–1156. doi:10.4187/respcare.03795 PMID:25922542

Lorig, K., Ritter, P., Laurent, D., & Plant, K. (2008). The Internet-based Arthritis Self-management Program: A One-year Randomized Trial for Patients with Arthritis or Fibromyalgia. *Arthritis and Rheumatism, 59*(7), 1009–1017. doi:10.1002/art.23817 PMID:18576310

Macea, D. D., Gajos, K., Calil, Y. A., & Fregni, F. (2010). The Efficacy of Web-based Cognitive Behavioral Interventions for Chronic Pain: A Systematic and Meta-analysis. *The Journal of Pain, 11*(10), 917–929. doi:10.1016/j.jpain.2010.06.005 PMID:20650691

Manchikanti, L., Abdi, S., Atluri, S., Balog, C. C., Benyamin, R. M., & Boswell, M. V. (2012). American Society of Interventional Pain Physicians (ASIPP) Guidelines for Responsible Opioid Prescribing in Chronic Non-cancer Pain: Part I--Evidence Assessment. *Pain Physician, 15*(Suppl. 3), S1–S65. PMID:22786448

Manchikanti, L., Ailinani, H., Koyyalagunta, D., Datta, S., Singh, V., & Eriator, I. (2011). A Systematic Review of Randomized Trials of Long-term Opioid Management for Chronic Non-cancer Pain. *Pain Physician, 14*, 91–121. PMID:21412367

Nahin, R. L. (2015). Estimates of Pain Prevalence and Severity in Adults: United States, 2012. *The Journal of Pain, 16*(8), 769–780. doi:10.1016/j.jpain.2015.05.002 PMID:26028573

Nielsen, M., Jull, G., & Hodges, P. W. (2014). Information Needs of People with Low Back Pain for an Online Resource: A Qualitative Study of Consumer Views. *Disability and Rehabilitation, 36*(13), 1085–1091. doi:10.3109/09638288.2013.829532 PMID:24001260

Poushter, J. (n. d.). Smartphone Ownership and Internet Usage Continues to Climb in Emerging Economies. *Pew Research Center*. Retrieved from http://www.pewglobal.org/2016/02/22/smart/phone-ownership-and-internet-usage-continues-to-climb-in-emerging-economies/

Ruehlman, L., Karoly, P., & Enders, C. (2011). A Randomized Controlled Evaluation of an Online Chronic Pain Self-Management Program. *Pain*. doi:10.1016/j.jpain.2011.02.298 PMID:22133450

Ryan, P., & Sawin, K. (2009). The Individual and Family Self-Management Theory: Background and Perspectives on Context, Process, and Outcomes. *Nursing Outlook, 57*(4), 217–225. doi:10.1016/j.outlook.2008.10.004 PMID:19631064

Sandelowski, M. (2000). Focus on Research Methods Whatever Happened to Qualitative Description? *Research in Nursing & Health, 23*(4), 334–340. doi:10.1002/1098-240X(200008)23:4<334::AID-NUR9>3.0.CO;2-G PMID:10940958

Sandelowski, M. (2010). What's in a Name? Qualitative Description Revisited. *Research in Nursing & Health, 33*, 77–84. PMID:20014004

Schreier, M. (2012). *Qualitative Content Analysis in Practice*. Thousand Oaks, CA: Sage.

Trudea, K. J., Pujol, L., DasMahapatra, P., Wall, R., Black, R., & Zacharoff, K. (2015). A Randomized Controlled Trial of an Online Self-management Program for Adults with Arthritis Pain. *Journal of Behavioral Medicine*, *38*(3), 483–496. doi:10.100710865-015-9622-9 PMID:25686538

Trudeau, K. J., Ainscough, J., Pujol, L. A., & Charity, S. (2010). What Arthritis Pain Practitioners and Patients Want in an Online Self Management Program. *Musculoskeletal Care*, *8*(4), 189–196. doi:10.1002/msc.183 PMID:21108492

Wilson, M., Roll, J. M., Corbett, C., & Barbosa-Leiker, C. (2015). Empowering Patients with Persistent Pain using an Internet-based Self-Management Program. *Pain Management Nursing*, *16*(4), 503–514. doi:10.1016/j.pmn.2014.09.009 PMID:26088940

Ziebland, S., Lavie-Ajayi, M., & Lucius-Hoene, G. (2015). The Role of the Internet for People with Chronic Pain: Examples from the DIPEx International Project. *British Journal of Pain*, *9*(1), 62–64. doi:10.1177/2049463714555438 PMID:26516557

This research was previously published in the International Journal of Healthcare Information Systems and Informatics (IJHISI), 12(4); edited by Qiang (Shawn) Cheng and Joseph Tan, pages 52-67, copyright year 2017 by IGI Publishing (an imprint of IGI Global).

Chapter 8
Systematic Review and Evaluation of Pain-Related Mobile Applications

Anabela G. Silva
University of Aveiro, Portugal

Hilma Caravau
University of Aveiro, Portugal

Alexandra Queirós
University of Aveiro, Portugal

Alina Ferreira
University of Aveiro, Portugal

Nelson P. Rocha
University of Aveiro, Portugal

INTRODUCTION

Pain and in particular chronic pain is highly prevalent in the general population across all age groups. A survey including 15 European countries and Israel and 46,394 adults (>18 years), found that chronic pain prevalence varies between 12% in Spain to 30% in Norway (Breivik, Collett, Ventafridda, Cohen, & Gallacher, 2006). Of these, 46% reported pain for 10 years or longer that interfered with daily activities such as maintaining relationships with family and friends, performing household activities, walking or exercising. When asked how many times they had seen their doctor because of the condition that causes their pain, 60% of respondents reported to have seen their doctor two to nine times and 11% had seen their doctor at least 10 times. The high prevalence, high disability and high costs associated with pain that were reported in this study are supported by findings of other authors in other countries and for specific pain conditions (Jakobsson, 2010; Leadley, Armstrong, Lee, Allen, & Kleijnen, 2012; Manchikanti, Singh, Datta, Cohen, & Hirsch, 2009; Parsons et al., 2007).

DOI: 10.4018/978-1-7998-1680-5.ch008

The World Health Organization (WHO) defines mobile health (mHealth) technologies as a component of eHealth. mHealth covers medical and public health practice supported by mobile devices, such as mobile phones, patient monitoring devices, personal digital assistants, and other wireless devices (WHO, 2011). It is an emerging and rapidly developing field that can contribute to the transformation of healthcare and increase its quality and efficiency while simultaneously containing costs (de la Vega & Miro, 2014). The International association for the Study of Pain has published in December 2013 a clinical update recognizing the importance of mobile technology in managing chronic pain as a means to improve access to healthcare, contain costs and improve clinical outcomes (Vardeh, Edwards, & Jamison, 2013). However, this publication also highlights the need to evaluate existing solutions.

Electronic applications can cover a wide range of purposes including easy access to information related to patient's health conditions or treatments, provide patients with simple applications to organize and track their health information, help patients self-manage their disease or conditions, help patients to document, show or communicate potential conditions to health care providers and enable patients or health care providers to interact with health care record systems (US Food and Drug Administration, 2013). In terms of pain related applications, the most common include:

1. Electronic diaries which are used to monitor aspects of pain such as pain intensity, location, aggravating factors and/or intake of medication,
2. Internet-based interventions which usually consist of structured self-administered therapy programs and
3. Text messaging, for communication between patients and healthcare professionals (Vardeh et al., 2013).

Electronic applications are virtually available to everyone in the general population independently of their ability to critically assess its content and without being necessarily indicated by a health professional. In addition, there is no one to recur to if anything unexpected occurs (Rocio de la Vega & Miro, 2014) and the available guidance for health care applications developers is still in its early steps (US Food and Drug Administration, 2013). Taken together these aspects suggest that it is particularly important that electronic applications in general and, pain-related applications in particular, are carefully designed and evaluated before being made available to the general public. There is a need to guarantee that applications are both suitable for users and based on the best available evidence in order to promote its potential (Moore, 2012). The aim of this systematic review is to review and evaluate mobile applications in terms of user involvement, healthcare professionals' involvement, usability, reliability, validity and clinical usefulness for pain-related mobile applications available both at a commercial store and in scientific databases.

It is considered that if applications involve users and healthcare professionals during their development and/or testing they are more likely to meet the users' needs both in terms of content and usability and be based on up to date scientific evidence. If the application is used to measure any pain characteristic such as pain intensity, pain duration, location or pain associated disability it has to fulfil the requirements of any measurement device: measure what it is intended to measure (validity) in a consistent manner (reliability). Furthermore, to be of clinical value, the use of the application has to result in any health benefit for its users (clinical usefulness), for example improved adherence to pain medication.

METHODS

This section describes the methods of this systematic review.

Data Sources and Searches

This systematic review employed a two-phase search.

In the first phase, a search for pain applications in the Android platform was performed using the terms pain and ache. This platform was used because it is the number one in the ranking of Smartphone operating systems worldwide (Singla & Mendiratta, 2014). The search was conducted on the 7th of October 2014. This search aimed to identify applications related to pain.

In the second phase, we performed a search on pain-related applications in five databases (Pubmed, Web of Science, Science Direct, Academic Search Complete and IEEE). Databases were searched since 1st January 2000. The following search terms were used: (pain OR *ache) AND i) (smartphone OR "personal digital assistant" OR PDA); ii) ("mobile application" OR APP), iii) (pain OR *ache) AND ("electronic application" OR "electronic APP") PubMed was searched using MeSH terms. This search was performed on the 9th of October and aimed to identify articles describing the development of pain-related applications and/or the assessment of usability, reliability, validity and clinical usefulness of pain-related applications.

Selection of Applications

To be included in this review, an application had to have the following characteristics:

- Have the patient has the intended primary user;
- Claim some informational, assessment, management facilitating or curative capacity relating to pain;

- Be written in English or Portuguese;
- Pain featured within the keywords or text description.

Applications were excluded if:

- They could be applied to pain but were not advertise for that;
- They are for use in a clinical context only (e.g. hospitals or other health care centers).

Selection of Publications

To be included in this review, publications must characterize the development of a pain-related application (including the characterization of users' needs) or assess usability, reliability, validity and/or clinical usefulness of those applications. For the terms of this review, the following definitions were used:

- **Usability:** Relates to user interfaces ease of use (Carrol, 2009);
- **Reliability:** Refers to the consistency of the measurements taken over time (Streiner & Norman, 2003);
- **Validity:** Refers to the accuracy of measurements when compared to a golden standard (Streiner & Norman, 2003);
- **Clinical Usefulness:** Refers to as whether using the application results in any benefit for the patient as for example more accurate diagnosis or more appropriate care.

Data Extraction and Synthesis: Applications

Relevant information regarding the general characteristics of the applications were collected using customized forms specifying: release date, download cost, file size, source of application contents, documentation of a healthcare professional's involvement in the development of the application, primary purpose of the application and targeted pain-related condition(s). In addition applications were classified into at least one of the following categories:

1. **Education and Awareness:** One way communication applications mainly intended to provide information or advice on a pain condition;
2. **Monitoring and Assessment:** One or two way communication applications mainly intended to monitor pain characteristics;
3. **Diagnosis or Intervention:** Applications designed to provide support for diagnosis and/or to deliver pain-related interventions.

These categories were adapted from (Källander et al., 2013).

Data Extraction and Synthesis: Studies

Those studies that were eligible to enter this systematic review were read, and the following information retrieved using customized forms: authors, application name/description, pathology and target population, users and health professionals' involvement in the development of the application, and category:

1. Education and awareness,
2. Monitoring and assessment, and
3. Diagnosis or intervention.

Additionally, for studies reporting on pain-related applications usability, reliability, validity and/or clinical usefulness, the procedure of assessment and results were retrieved.

RESULTS

The search performed in the Android platform resulted in 250 applications of which 108 did not meet the inclusion criteria and were excluded from this review. The search performed in the 5 databases resulted in 2997 references, of which 331 were duplicates. Therefore, 2666 titles and/or abstracts were screened for inclusion and 2583 did not meet the inclusion criteria. The full text of 80 articles was retrieved (it was not possible to find the full papers of 3 references) and after being read another 53 articles were excluded because they did not report on applications, applications were not related to pain or the intended primary user was not the patient. Therefore, a total of 142 applications retrieved from the Android platform and 26 papers retrieved from databases were analyzed and included in this review (Figure 1).

Pain-Related Applications

A total of 142 applications entered this analysis. Different versions of an application were counted as different applications because they have different features. For example, the free version of an application is usually different from the paid version and the first does not include all the features of the latter.

The number of applications available increased from 9 in 2011 to 86 in 2014. Most applications (n=93/142) were available for free. Those that were not free had prices between 0.59 to 30.14 euros (mean$\pm$sd=3.05$\pm$2.95 euros). Most applications

Figure 1. Flowchart of search and results

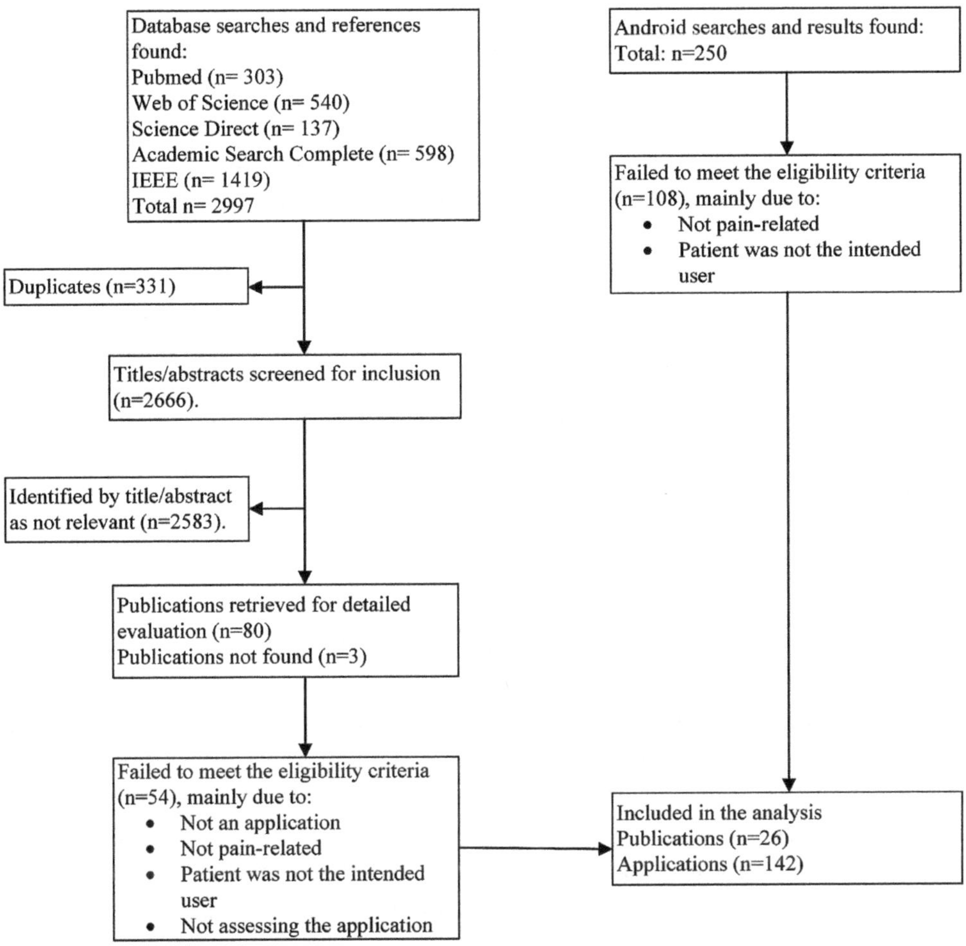

were included in the education and awareness category (n=114/142), because they were primarily 1-way communication applications providing information on the characteristics of a pain condition or giving advice on what to do. The remaining applications were categorized as monitoring and assessment (n=28/142) as they were primarily intended for registering pain related information. Of the 142, only 26 mentioned that a health professional had been involved in the development of the application or the source from where the information displayed in the application was retrieved. Most applications were intended for pain associated with musculoskeletal pathology (n=69/142), including conditions such as neck pain, back pain, arthritis or fibromyalgia or for pain in general (56/142).

Papers Characterizing Pain-Related Applications

Of the 26 papers included for analysis at this stage, 19 described applications primarily intended for pain assessment and monitoring and 7 described applications aiming to deliver pain-related interventions and were, therefore, included in the diagnostic and intervention category. Some applications were for pain/chronic pain in general (n=13) while others target specific pain conditions, such as migraine (n=4), cancer pain (n=4), pain associated with sickle cell disease (n=2), fibromyalgia (n=1), rheumatoid arthritis (n=1) and vulvar pain (n=1). The intended primary user was a child or an adolescent in 8 of the applications described and the remaining were described as for adults in general. A detailed characterization of the papers included in this systematic review is presented in Table 1. Of the 26 papers, 15 described aspects of usability (57.7%), 2 assessed reliability (7.7%), 7 assessed validity (26.9%) and 3 investigated clinical usefulness (11.5%) of pain-related applications. This adds up to more than 26 papers as some papers reported on more than one aspect. The following sections present a detailed description of both the applications and the articles retrieved.

User and Healthcare Professionals involvement

All papers described applications in which there was the involvement of healthcare professionals. This judgment was based on the fact that at least one of the authors of the paper was a healthcare professional (e.g. doctor, physiotherapist, nurse or psychologist). However, only two studies explicitly stated the involvement of healthcare professionals other than the paper authors in the development or assessment of the application (Ghinea, Spyridonis, Serif, & Frank, 2008; Jibb et al., 2014). Similarly, only four articles reported on user's involvement to inform the development of the applications on aspects other than usability (for example, overall concept, content, target needs) (Liu, Holroyd, Zhu, Shen, & Zhou, 2010; Stinson et al., 2013, 2014; Zhu, Liu, & Holroyd, 2012).

Usability

Usability assessment was described in 15 studies (Alfvén, 2010; Anatchkova, Saris-Baglama, Kosinski, & Bjorner, 2009; Baggott et al., 2012; Rocío de la Vega et al., 2014; Garcia-Palacios et al., 2014; Ghinea et al., 2008; Hachizuka et al., 2010; Jacob et al., 2012; Kleiboer, Sorbi, Merelle, Passchier, & van Doornen, 2009; Kristjansdottir et al., 2011; Marceau, Link, Jamison, & Carolan, 2007; Moloney et al., 2009; Nguyen et al., 2014; Shah, Jonassaint, & De Castro, 2014; Stinson et al., 2013; Wood et al., 2011). Methods of usability assessment included interviews

Table 1. General characteristics of articles retrieved from academic databases

Authors	APP Aim/Description	Patology/Target Population	Category	User Involvement	Health Professionals Involvement
(Alfvén, 2010)	SMS to capture recurrent pain intensity and disability	Children aged 9–15 with pain	Monitoring & assessment		Yes
(Anatchkova et al., 2009)	A computerized adaptive test of chronic pain (CHRONIC PAIN-CAT)	Adults with pain	Monitoring & assessment		Yes
(Baggott et al., 2012)	eDiary designed to assess severity of pain, nausea, vomiting, fatigue, and sleep quality	Adolescents with cancer pain	Monitoring & assessment		Yes
(Boormans et al., 2009)	A Continuous Pain Score Meter that measures pain score in a continuous, instead of a single, manner	Adults with pain	Monitoring & assessment		Yes
(Rocío de la Vega et al., 2014)	Painometer that includes 4 pain intensity scales: the Faces Pain Scale-Revised, the numerical rating scale-11, the Coloured Analogue Scale, and the visual analog scale	Pain in general in children and adults	Monitoring & assessment		Yes
(Garcia-Palacios et al., 2014)	An eletronic diary to assess pain intensity, fatigue intensity and mood	Women with fibromyalgia	Monitoring & assessment		yes
(Ghinea et al., 2008)	A 3-D representation of the human body, which can be marked in color to visualize and record the pain data	Pain in general	Monitoring & assessment		Conducted in collaboration with a team of clinicians from the Rheumatology Department of the Northwick Park Hospital, London
(Hachizuka et al., 2010)	A PDA system to collect information on symptoms such as pain and mood	Adults with cancer	Monitoring & assessment		Yes
(Heiberg et al., 2007)	A PDA to collect information on pain, fatigue, and global disease	Rheumatoid Arthritis	Monitoring & assessment		Yes
(Jacob et al., 2012)	Web based eDiary that included items from paper-based measures of pain and symptoms	Children and adolescents with sickle cell disease	Monitoring & assessment		Yes
(Jamison et al., 2002)	Eletronic visual analogue scale(eVAS) to assess pain intensity	Adults with pain in general	Monitoring & assessment		Yes

continued on following page

Table 1. Continued

Authors	APP Aim/Description	Patology/Target Population	Category	User Involvement	Health Professionals Involvement
(Jibb et al., 2014)	Smartphone-based pain management app capable of providing adolescents with pain management support	Children with cancer	Diagnostic or intervention	Iterative qualitative testing was conducted with adolescents with cancer to vet and refine the developed algorithm and system requirements for the real-time smartphone app	15 international experts (clinicians, scientists, and a consumer) in pediatric pain, pediatric oncology and mHealth design, who participated in a 2-day consensus conference to develop consensus on important pain inputs, pain management advice, and system design requirements.
(Junker et al., 2008)	A pain questionnaire on a hand-held computer	Adults with pain in general	Monitoring & assessment		Yes
(Kleiboer et al., 2009)	A generic software-based method designed to support behavioral training	Migraine	Diagnostic or intervention		Yes
(Kristjánsdóttir et al., 2013)	Smartphone-delivered intervention with written diaries and therapist feedback	Adults with chronic widespread pain	Diagnostic or intervention		Yes
(Kristjansdottir et al., 2011)	Four-week Internet intervention delivered by a Web-enabled mobile phone	Adults with chronic widespread pain	Diagnostic or intervention		Yes
(Liu et al., 2010)	iPhone application was developed to help manage migraine	Adolescents with migraine	Diagnostic or intervention	Yes, adolescents with migraine pinpointed aspects that need to be considered in the application	Yes
(Marceau et al., 2007)	A software program designed for use on a personal digital assistant incorporating pain questionnaires to fill in	Adults with chronic pain	Monitoring & assessment		Yes
(Marceau et al., 2010)	A software program designed for use on a personal digital assistant incorporating pain questionnaires to fill in	Adults with chronic pain	Monitoring & assessment		Yes

continued on following page

Table 1. Continued

Authors	APP Aim/Description	Patology/Target Population	Category	User Involvement	Health Professionals Involvement
(Moloney et al., 2009)	An Internet-based headache diary containing pain scales and open-ended questions	Adults with migraine	Monitoring & assessment		Yes
(Nguyen et al., 2014)	A smartphone application to collect data on vulvar pain and factors that may influence vulvar pain level	Adult women with vulvar pain	Monitoring & assessment		Yes
(Shah et al., 2014)	A mobile application designed for sickle cell disease	Sickle cell disease	Monitoring & assessment		Yes
(Stinson et al., 2013)	The app functions as an electronic pain diary and is unique in its ability to collect data on pain intensity, duration, location, and the impact pain has on an adolescent's life (ie, relationships, school work, sleep, mood).	adolescents with cancer	Monitoring & assessment	The overarching concept for the app and the app's design elements were developed in consultation with adolescents	Yes
(Stinson et al., 2014)	An online chronic pain self-management program	Adolescents with chronic pain	Diagnostic or intervention	Yes; authors conducted a needs assessment to inform the development of the application	Yes
(Wood et al., 2011)	Electronic versions of pain scales fill in using a PDA	Children with pain	Monitoring & assessment		Yes
(Zhu et al., 2012)	iBMM is a behavioral intervention mobile application	Adults with migraine	Diagnostic or intervention	Yes; 15 participants used iBMM to relax by following a relaxation exercise were asked to describe any issues they encountered; the authors observed all user interaction with the app	Yes

or questionnaires designed by the paper authors for the application of interest. No study reported on the use of a validated usability questionnaire. In general, authors assessed ease of use, errors, suggested changes and users' acceptability.

Reliability

Reliability assessment was reported in 2 papers. Both papers assessed test-retest reliability (measurement consistency between two measurement occasions) and one found acceptable to good reliability for an application aiming to assess pain intensity and disability (Alfvén, 2010) and the other reported good reliability for a continuous pain intensity meter (Boormans, van Kesteren, Perez, Brölmann, & Zuurmond, 2009).

Validity

Validity assessment was reported in 7 papers (Garcia-Palacios et al., 2014; Heiberg et al., 2007; Jacob et al., 2012; Jamison et al., 2002; Junker et al., 2008; Marceau et al., 2007; Wood et al., 2011). All papers assessed criterion validity by comparing scores obtained with the applications against paper-based methods. In general, results of the 7 studies indicate that there are no relevant differences between the two methods and, therefore, that the electronic applications are valid.

Clinical Usefulness

Clinical usefulness was assessed in 3 papers (Kleiboer et al., 2009; Kristjánsdóttir et al., 2013; Marceau, Link, Smith, Carolan, & Jamison, 2010). In two of these studies, authors compared whether a treatment intervention partially delivered using an electronic application resulted in better patient outcomes than a traditional intervention (without the use of an application) (Kleiboer et al., 2009; Kristjánsdóttir et al., 2013). One paper reported no significant differences between the two methods of intervention delivery in migraine patients (Kleiboer et al., 2009) and the other using the same type of patients, reported that a Smartphone based intervention can reduce catastrophizing and prevent functional decline and increases in symptoms (Kristjánsdóttir et al., 2013). Another paper assessed clinical utility, by asking the patients whether they believed that using the application resulted in any improvement in care delivery. Results indicated that 23% of patients reported healthcare improvement resulting from the use of the application (Marceau et al., 2010). A detailed characterization of reliability, validity, usability and clinical usefulness is presented in Table 2.

Table 2. Reliability, validity, usability, and clinical usefulness

Authors	Reliability	Validity	Usability	Clinical Usefulness
(Alfvén, 2010)	Test-retest reliability; Acceptable to good reliability - verbal scale - K= between 0.50 and 0.73		The easiness of giving numerical answers was indicated on a Likert scale with five verbal options	
(Anatchkova et al., 2009)			Time needed to completion	
(Baggott et al., 2012)			10 to 15 minute interviews to assess adherence to daily reports, perception about using the application and technical problems	
(Boormans et al., 2009)	Test–retest reliability; Good reliability (ICC between 0.79 and 0.86)			
(Rocío de la Vega et al., 2014)			Semi structured interview; the domains measured were ease of use, errors in usage, most popular characteristics, suggested changes, and acceptability	
(Garcia-Palacios et al., 2014)		47 participants used paper diary and ED diary for one week; positive and significant correlation between both assessments ($r = 0.79$, $p < 0.001$)	Acceptability and preference questionnaires	
(Ghinea et al., 2008)			A questionnaire in which opinions over a range of statements were recorded on a 5-point Likert scale	
(Hachizuka et al., 2010)			Interviews	
(Heiberg et al., 2007)		Compare results between PDA and paper-pencil; Average scores did not differ between PDA and paper-pencil		
(Jacob et al., 2012)		80% of concordance between pre-completed paper-based measures and the web-based e-Diary	Asked to rate their ability to use the smartphone and how much of a bother it was on a scale from 0 to 5	
(Jamison et al., 2002)		Correlation for ratings between eVAS and paper VAS; r=0.91		

continued on following page

Table 2. Continued

Authors	Reliability	Validity	Usability	Clinical Usefulness
(Junker et al., 2008)		200 chronic pain patients were given two pain questionnaires, one on paper and one on a hand-held computer; overall results from the two questionnaire types were highly consistent		
(Kleiboer et al., 2009)			Acceptability was assessed by a structured interview and confirmed by positive participant responses concerning usefulness, supportiveness, and low burden	31 patients with migraine who received ODA during BT and at 6 months' follow-up were compared with a matched group of 31 participants who received BT only. ODA participants did not mark better improvements considering migraine attack frequency, internal control, and migraine-specific quality of life compared to those that underwent BT only.
(Kristjánsdóttir et al., 2013)				140 women with chronic widespread pain participated in a 4-week inpatient rehabilitation program were randomized into 2 groups: with or without a smartphone; the results suggest that a SP based intervention can reduce catastrophizing and prevent functional decline and increases in symptoms
(Kristjansdottir et al., 2011)			Rated as supportive, meaningful and user-friendly by the majority of the women; the response rate to the daily registration entries was high and technical problems were few	
(Marceau et al., 2007)		36 chronic pain patients were asked to monitor their pain, mood, activity interference, medication use, and pain location on either a paper or electronic diary for 2 weeks; No differences were found between paper and electronic tracking on pain	Patients found the electronic diary easier to use and would continue using it over paper if given the choice	

continued on following page

Table 2. Continued

Authors	Reliability	Validity	Usability	Clinical Usefulness
(Marceau et al., 2010)				134 chronic pain patients were asked to monitor their pain, mood, activity interference, medication use, and pain location on either a paper or electronic diary immediately before each monthly clinic visit for 10 months; 23% of patients in the experimental condition felt that the data from the electronic diaries improved their care and less than 15% believed that their doctor made a change in their treatment based on the summary diary information
(Moloney et al., 2009)			77 interviews; the Internet-based headache diary is a feasible, acceptable data collection tool	
(Nguyen et al., 2014)			24 women were asked to complete a survey regarding their opinions and experiences of the application; the women believed that the technology was easy to use and would prefer using the smartphone over a computer or paper and pencil method	
(Shah et al., 2014)			94% of 17 participants reported that the app was easy to use	
(Stinson et al., 2013)			A qualitative usability testing approach was used with iterative cycles of semi-structured audiotaped interviews	
(Wood et al., 2011)		202 children provided self reports of their pain on a PDA and on a paper version; The overall weighted Kappa was 0.85; Spearman correlation was 0.91 ($p < 0.0001$)		

K – Cohen's K; ICC – intraclass correlation coefficient; PDA - personal digital assistant; VAS – visual analogue scale; p – level o significance; r – correlation coefficient; ODA - ; BT - behavioral therapy.

DISCUSSION

This review aimed to characterize existing pain-related applications in a commercial store versus scientific data on the assessment of pain-related applications in scientific databases. Results showed that there is a lot more applications (n=142) than papers assessing its characteristics in terms of usability, reliability, validity and clinical usefulness (n=26), suggesting a discrepancy between what is commercially available to consumers and what has been published in scientific and peer-reviewed databases.

While applications described in papers found in academic databases usually report the involvement of a healthcare professional, the involvement of healthcare professionals in the applications available in the store or the specification of the source of the information displayed in the application is reported for 18% of applications only. No information was found on the involvement of the users for applications available in the Android store. The enrollment of patients and health professionals in the application development process could take place as earlier as the stage of defining the requisites and characteristics of the application (Jibb et al., 2014; Liu et al., 2010; Stinson et al., 2013, 2014; Zhu et al., 2012). This will improve the likelihood of the application to meet the needs of both patients and clinicians by assessing/doing what is relevant for them. Consequently, this is likely to increase the odds of the application being used. The involvement of healthcare professionals also contributes to an application that is scientifically grounded, i.e., based on information that is both scientifically sound, appropriate to the target patient population and based on the best available evidence while decreasing the odds of doing harm or deceiving the patient. For example, one of the applications found in the Android store claimed to help patients to easily and effectively get rid of their back pain. However, research shows that at 12 months follow up 20% of patients with low back pain are not improved or are worse (Verkerk et al., 2014). Therefore, it is likely that a considerable number of patients with low back pain using the application do not get better. This is of particular concern, considering that patients with pain might be desperately seeking a solution to their problems and lacking the appropriate knowledge to make a critical assessment of the available applications. Further critical analysis of the available applications is warranted.

Usability was assessed most of the times through interviews. Although this is an appropriate method to assess usability, it makes it difficult to compare results between studies and applications and it does not guarantee that all relevant aspects of usability are being assessed in all studies. Therefore, we suggest that in addition to interviews, validated questionnaires and frameworks should be used. For example, Brown et al. (2013) proposed an evaluation framework for assessing the usability of mHealth applications. This framework includes the concepts of error prevention, completeness, memorability, information needs, flexibility/customizability, learnability, performance speed, competency and other outcomes. Appropriately assessing usability is crucial for the success of an application as it seems either to potentiate or hinder the use an application. Lack of attention to the usability of applications may result in less satisfied users, decreased effectiveness, and/or increased error costs (Kaufman, Roberts, Merrill, Lai, & Bakken, 2006).

If an application is intended to collect data on a set of variables it needs to fulfill two important requisites of any measurement device, be both reliable and valid. It is reliable if it gives similar results in similar circumstances at repeated points in time. It is valid if it measures what it is intended to. The first is assessed by comparing data collected at different points in time, providing that the patient conditions did not change. The second is usually assessed by comparing data collected with one device with data collected using a gold standard. In the case of mobile pain-related applications, the gold standards are likely to be paper-based questionnaires which have been previously shown to be valid measures. This systematic review found 2 studies that reported on the reliability of pain applications (Alfvén, 2010; Boormans et al., 2009) and another 7 that reported on their validity (Garcia-Palacios et al., 2014; Heiberg et al., 2007; Jacob et al., 2012; Jamison et al., 2002; Junker et al., 2008; Marceau et al., 2007; Wood et al., 2011). Although these papers show promising results in terms of applications' reliability and validity, they also show that these important characteristics of measurement devices are not being routinely evaluated before applications intended to assess pain are made available to the general public. However, the validity and reliability of an application intended to assess pain cannot be assumed only because the paper version is reliable and valid. For example, the wording of questions, its presentation or order, are factors that can affect reliability and validity (Streiner & Norman, 2003). In a mobile application, the number of questions presented at the same time might change, the answer to previous questions might not be displayed, the ability to go back and review/change answers may need to be considered and all these factors can both influence how the questions and instructions are interpreted and, consequently, the responses given. The use of bolding, italics, colors, fonts, and capitalization can affect the readability of items and draw attention to or from different key parts of the instruction (Wantland, Portillo, Holzemer, Slaughter, & McGhee, 2004).

Even if the application is reliable and valid, it does not guarantee that its use either results in any benefit for the patient or, at least, is as effective as the traditional way of performing pain-related assessments or delivering pain-related interventions. Furthermore, it does not guarantee that using the application results in no harm for the patient. Therefore, when developing an application, developers must assess the impact of their use on patients' conditions. For example, does using the application helps the patients to better manage their condition or improve the care provided by the healthcare professionals? This could be assessed by comparing the use of the application against the traditional way of doing things. In this systematic review only 3 studies assessed the clinical usefulness of the mobile application by comparing pain characteristics and improvement of a group of participants receiving an intervention in which a mobile application was used against the traditional way of care delivery (Kleiboer et al., 2009; Kristjánsdóttir et al., 2013) or by asking patients whether the use of a mobile application affected care delivery (Marceau et al., 2007). Comparing applications with the traditional way should be favored in relation to studies on patients' opinions as they are less prone to bias, in particular, using randomized clinical trials.

SOLUTIONS AND RECOMMENDATIONS

From the overall analysis of the pain-related applications available in the commercial store and the papers retrieved from the databases search, it seems crucial that pain-related applications are carefully assessed for their content, usability, reliability, validity and clinical usefulness before made available to the general public. Each of these aspects should be assessed in studies with methodologically sound designs and using participants who are representative of intended users. We believe that this is crucial to a responsible and wider use of electronic applications. It is unlikely that patients and health professionals would engage in routine use of electronic applications if they are not convinced that these are as valid and reliable as the traditional way of performing patients' assessment and intervention and result in at least equal benefit without harming the patients in any way. This is also of concern to the American Food and Drug Administration agency (US Food and Drug Administration, 2013).

FUTURE RESEARCH DIRECTIONS

Research in the health-related mobile applications area would benefit from interdisciplinary teams as questions that need to be answered also come from different areas and in particular from the fields of technology and health. This interdisciplinary work between who knows the health conditions and the data needed to provide a better care (the healthcare professionals) as well as patients' needs (the patients and the healthcare professionals) and who knows the technology (such as engineers, graphic designers) is likely to result in an end product more adjusted to patients/healthcare professionals needs that is also more likely to be used by its intended users. A detailed analysis of the content of available electronic applications should also be performed in order to determine whether they meet users' requirements and whether its content is scientifically sound. More studies aiming to assess the reliability, validity and clinical usefulness of electronic applications are also needed. Future work can also expand on our review by including other electronic platforms (such as iPhone) and electronic applications available in other languages.

CONCLUSION

Pain-related mobile applications have the potential to improve healthcare outcomes. However, its potential is hindered by lack of routine consideration of users' needs, health professionals' involvement and standardized assessment of its usability, reliability, validity and clinical usefulness, in particular for those applications available in commercial stores. These aspects should be considered for both existing and new pain-related applications.

REFERENCES

Alfvén, G. (2010). SMS pain diary: a method for real-time data capture of recurrent pain in childhood. *Acta Paediatrica, 99*(7), 1047–1053. Retrieved from doi:10.1111/j.1651-2227.2010.01735.x

Anatchkova, M. D., Saris-Baglama, R. N., Kosinski, M., & Bjorner, J. B. (2009). Development and Preliminary Testing of a Computerized Adaptive Assessment of Chronic Pain. *The Journal of Pain, 10*(9), 932–943. doi:10.1016/j.jpain.2009.03.007 PMID:19595636

Baggott, C., Gibson, F., Coll, B., Kletter, R., Zeltzer, P., & Miaskowski, C. (2012). Initial Evaluation of an Electronic Symptom Diary for Adolescents with Cancer. *JMIR Res Protoc., 1*(2), e23. doi:10.2196/resprot.2175 PMID:23612521

Boormans, E. M., van Kesteren, P. J., Perez, R. S., Brölmann, H. A., & Zuurmond, W. W. (2009). Reliability of a Continuous Pain Score Meter: Real Time Pain Measurement. *Pain Practice, 9*(2), 100–104. doi:10.1111/j.1533-2500.2009.00260.x

Breivik, H., Collett, B., Ventafridda, V., Cohen, R., & Gallacher, D. (2006). Survey of chronic pain in Europe: Prevalence, impact on daily life, and treatment. *European Journal of Pain (London, England), 10*(4), 287–333. doi:10.1016/j.ejpain.2005.06.009 PMID:16095934

Brown, W. III, Yen, P.-Y., Rojas, M., & Schnall, R. (2013). Assessment of the Health IT Usability Evaluation Model (Health-ITUEM) for evaluating mobile health (mHealth) technology. *Journal of Biomedical Informatics*, *46*(6), 1080–1087. doi:10.1016/j.jbi.2013.08.001 PMID:23973872

Carrol, J. (2009). Human Computer Interaction (HCI). In M. Soegaard & R. Dam (Eds.), *Encyclopedia of Human-Computer Interaction*. Aarhus: The Interaction Design Foundation.

De la Vega, R., & Miro, J. (2014). mHealth: A Strategic Field without a Solid Scientific Soul. A Systematic Review of Pain-Related Apps. *PLoS ONE*, *9*(7). doi:10.1371/journal.pone.0101312 PMID:24999983

De la Vega, R., Roset, R., Castarlenas, E., Sánchez-Rodríguez, E., Solé, E., & Miró, J. (2014). Development and Testing of Painometer: A Smartphone App to Assess Pain Intensity. *The Journal of Pain*, *15*(10), 1001–1007. doi:10.1016/j.jpain.2014.04.009 PMID:24854065

Garcia-Palacios, A., Herrero, R., Belmonte, M. A., Castilla, D., Guixeres, J., Molinari, G., ... Botella, C. (2014). Ecological momentary assessment for chronic pain in fibromyalgia using a smartphone: A randomized crossover study. *European Journal of Pain (London, England)*, *18*(6), 862–872. doi:10.1002/j.1532-2149.2013.00425.x PMID:24921074

Ghinea, G., Spyridonis, F., Serif, T., & Frank, A. O. (2008). 3-D pain drawings - Mobile data collection using a PDA. *IEEE Transactions on Information Technology in Biomedicine*, *12*(1), 27–33. doi:10.1109/TITB.2007.903266 PMID:18270034

Hachizuka, M., Yoshiuchi, K., Yamamoto, Y., Iwase, S., Nakagawa, K., Kawagoe, K., & Akabayashi, A. (2010). Development of a personal digital assistant (PDA) system to collect symptom information from home hospice patients. *Journal of Palliative Medicine*, *13*(6), 647–651. doi:10.1089/jpm.2009.0350 PMID:20509795

Heiberg, T., Kvien, T. K., Dale, O., Mowinckel, P., Aanerud, G. J., Songe-Moller, A. B., ... Hagen, K. B. (2007). Daily health status registration (patient diary) in patients with rheumatoid arthritis: A comparison between personal digital assistant and paper-pencil format. *Arthritis & Rheumatism-Arthritis Care & Research*, *57*(3), 454–460. doi:10.1002/art.22613 PMID:17394232

Jacob, E., Stinson, J., Duran, J., Gupta, A., Gerla, M., Lewis, M. A., & Zeltzer, L. (2012). Usability Testing of a Smartphone for Accessing a Web-based e-Diary for Self-monitoring of Pain and Symptoms in Sickle Cell Disease. *Journal of Pediatric Hematology/Oncology*, *34*(5), 326–335. doi:10.1097/MPH.0b013e318257a13c PMID:22627570

Jakobsson, U. (2010). The epidemiology of chronic pain in a general population: Results of a survey in southern Sweden. *Scandinavian Journal of Rheumatology, 39*(5), 421–429. doi:10.3109/03009741003685616 PMID:20476853

Jamison, R. N., Gracely, R. H., Raymond, S. A., Levine, J. G., Marino, B., Herrmann, T. J., ... Katz, N. P. (2002). Comparative study of electronic vs. paper VAS ratings: A randomized, crossover trial using healthy volunteers. *Pain, 99*(1/2), 341–347. doi:10.1016/S0304-3959(02)00178-1 PMID:12237213

Jibb, L., Stevens, B., Nathan, P., Seto, E., Cafazzo, J., & Stinson, J. (2014). A Smartphone-Based Pain Management App for Adolescents With Cancer: Establishing System Requirements and a Pain Care Algorithm Based on Literature Review, Interviews, and Consensus. *JMIR Res Protoc., 3*(1), e15. doi:10.2196/resprot.3041 PMID:24646454

Junker, U., Freynhagen, R., Laengler, K., Gockel, U., Schmidt, U., Toelle, T. R., ... Kohlmann, T. (2008). Paper versus electronic rating scales for pain assessment: A prospective, randomised, cross-over validation study with 200 chronic pain patients. *Current Medical Research and Opinion, 24*(6), 1797–1806. doi:10.1185/03007990802121059 PMID:18485269

Källander, K., Tibenderana, J. K., Akpogheneta, O. J., Strachan, D., Hill, Z., ten Asbroek, A., ... Meek, S. (2013). Mobile health (mHealth) approaches and lessons for increased performance and retention of community health workers in low-and middle-income countries: A review. *Journal of Medical Internet Research, 15*(1), e17. doi:10.2196/jmir.2130 PMID:23353680

Kaufman, D., Roberts, W., Merrill, J., Lai, T., & Bakken, S. (2006). an evaluation framework for health information system design, development, and implementation. *Nursing Research, 55*(2Supplement 1), S37–S42. doi:10.1097/00006199-200603001-00007 PMID:16601633

Kleiboer, A., Sorbi, M., Merelle, S., Passchier, J., & van Doornen, L. (2009). Utility and Preliminary Effects of Online Digital Assistance (ODA) for Behavioral Attack Prevention in Migraine. *Telemedicine Journal and e-Health, 15*(7), 682–690. doi:10.1089/tmj.2009.0014 PMID:19694591

Kristjánsdóttir, O., Fors, E., Eide, E., Finset, A., Stensrud, T., van Dulmen, S., ... Eide, H. (2013). A Smartphone-Based Intervention With Diaries and Therapist-Feedback to Reduce Catastrophizing and Increase Functioning in Women With Chronic Widespread Pain: Randomized Controlled Trial. *Journal of Medical Internet Research, 15*(1), e5. doi:10.2196/jmir.2249 PMID:23291270

Kristjansdottir, O. B., Fors, E. A., Eide, E., Finset, A., van Dulmen, S., Wigers, S. H., & Eide, H. (2011). Written online situational feedback via mobile phone to support self-management of chronic widespread pain: A usability study of a Web-based intervention. *BMC Musculoskeletal Disorders, 12*(1), 51. doi:10.1186/1471-2474-12-51 PMID:21352516

Leadley, R., Armstrong, N., Lee, Y., Allen, A., & Kleijnen, J. (2012). Chronic diseases in the European Union: The prevalence and health cost implications of chronic pain. *Journal of Pain & Palliative Care Pharmacotherapy, 26*(4), 310–325. doi:10.3109/15360288.2012.736933 PMID:23216170

Liu, C., Holroyd, K. A., Zhu, Q., Shen, K., & Zhou, W. (2010). *Design and implementation of a behavioral migraine management iPhone app for adolescents with migraine*. World of Wireless Mobile and Multimedia Networks (WoWMoM), 2010 IEEE International Symposium on a. 10.1109/WOWMOM.2010.5534985

Manchikanti, L., Singh, V., Datta, S., Cohen, S. P., & Hirsch, J. A. (2009). *Comprehensive Review of Epidemiology, Scope, and Impact of Spinal Pain*. Academic Press.

Marceau, L., Link, C., Jamison, R., & Carolan, S. (2007). Electronic diaries as a tool to improve pain management: Is there any evidence? *Pain Medicine, 8*(Suppl 3), S101–S109. doi:10.1111/j.1526-4637.2007.00374.x PMID:17877520

Marceau, L., Link, C. L., Smith, L. D., Carolan, S. J., & Jamison, R. N. (2010). In-Clinic Use of Electronic Pain Diaries: Barriers of Implementation Among Pain Physicians. *Journal of Pain and Symptom Management, 40*(3), 391–404. doi:10.1016/j.jpainsymman.2009.12.021 PMID:20580526

Moloney, M. F., Aycock, D. M., Cotsonis, G. A., Myerburg, S., Farino, C., & Lentz, M. (2009). An Internet-Based Migraine Headache Diary: Issues in Internet-Based Research. *Headache: The Journal of Head & Face Pain, 49*(5), 673–686. Retrieved from doi:10.1111/j.1526-4610.2009.01399.x

Moore, J. (2012). The benefits of mobile apps for patients and providers. *Br J Healthc Manag, 18*(9), 465–467. doi:10.12968/bjhc.2012.18.9.465

Nguyen, R., Turner, R., Sieling, J., Williams, D., Hodges, J., & Harlow, B. (2014). Feasibility of Collecting Vulvar Pain Variability and Its Correlates Using Prospective Collection with Smartphones. *Pain Research and Treatment, 2014*, 1–7. doi:10.1155/2014/659863 PMID:25006458

Parsons, S., Breen, A., Foster, N., Letley, L., Pincus, T., Vogel, S., & Underwood, M. (2007). Prevalence and comparative troublesomeness by age of musculoskeletal pain in different body locations. *Family Practice*, *24*(4), 308–316. doi:10.1093/fampra/cmm027 PMID:17602173

Shah, N., Jonassaint, J., & De Castro, L. (2014). Patients Welcome the Sickle Cell Disease Mobile Application to Record Symptoms via Technology (SMART). *Hemoglobin*, *38*(2), 99–103. doi:10.3109/03630269.2014.880716 PMID:24512633

Singla, D., & Mendiratta, L. (2014). Android VS IOS. *IJIRT*, *1*(5), 592–596.

Stinson, J. N., Jibb, L. A., Nguyen, C., Nathan, P. C., Maloney, A. M., Dupuis, L. L., ... Orr, M. (2013). Development and Testing of a Multidimensional iPhone Pain Assessment Application for Adolescents with Cancer. *Journal of Medical Internet Research*, *15*(3), 137–151. doi:10.2196/jmir.2350 PMID:23475457

Stinson, J. N., Lalloo, C., Harris, L., Isaac, L., Campbell, F., Brown, S., ... Kaarim, A. (2014). iCanCope with Pain™: User-centred design of a web- and mobile-based self-management program for youth with chronic pain based on identified health care needs. *Pain Research & Management*, *19*(5), 257–265. doi:10.1155/2014/935278 PMID:25000507

Streiner, D., & Norman, G. (2003). *Health measurement scales: a practical guide to their development and use (3rd ed.)*. Oxford, UK: Oxford University Press.

US Food and Drug Administration. (2013). *Medical Device Development Tools - Draft Guidance for Industry, Tool Developers, and Food and Drug Administration Staff* (pp. 1–26). Retrieved from Available at: http://www.fda.gov/MedicalDevices/DeviceRegulationandGuidance/GuidanceDocuments/ ucm374427.htm

Vardeh, D., Edwards, R., & Jamison, R. (2013). *There's an App for That: Mobile Technology, Pain Clinical Updates*. IASP.

Verkerk, K., & Luijsterburg, P. J., Heymans, M. W., Ronchetti, I., Miedema, H. S., Koes, B. W., & Pool-Goudzwaard, A. (2014). Prognostic factors and course for successful clinical outcome quality of life and patients' perceived effect after a cognitive behavior therapy for chronic non-specific low back pain: A 12-months prospective study. *Manual Therapy*, 1–7. doi:10.1016/j.math.2014.07.003 PMID:25107827

Wantland, D., Portillo, C., Holzemer, W., Slaughter, R., & McGhee, E. (2004). The Effectiveness of Web-Based vs. Non-Web-Based Interventions: A Meta-Analysis of Behavioral Change Outcomes. *Journal of Medical Internet Research*, *6*(4), e40. doi:10.2196/jmir.6.4.e40 PMID:15631964

WHO. (2011). *Based on the findings of the second global survey on eHealth*. Global Obs.

Wood, C., von Baeyer, C. L., Falinower, S., Moyse, D., Annequin, D., & Legout, V. (2011). Electronic and paper versions of a faces pain intensity scale: Concordance and preference in hospitalized children. *BMC Pediatrics*, *11*(1), 87. doi:10.1186/1471-2431-11-87 PMID:21989306

Zhu, Q., Liu, C., & Holroyd, K. A. (2012). From a traditional behavioral management program to an m-health app: Lessons learned in developing m-health apps for existing health care programs. *Software Engineering in Health Care (SEHC), Proceedings of the 4th International Workshop on Software Engineering in Health Care*, (pp. 69-72). doi:10.1109/SEHC.2012.6227006

KEY TERMS AND DEFINITIONS

Application: A type of software designed to run on a mobile device.

Clinical Usefulness: Refers as to whether using the application results in any benefit for the patient as for example more accurate diagnosis or more appropriate care.

M-Health: A component of eHealth, that covers medical and public health practice supported by mobile devices.

Pain: According to the International Association for the study of pain, pain is defined as unpleasant sensory and emotional experience associated with actual or potential tissue damage, or described in terms of such damage.

Reliability: Relates to the consistency of repeated measurements.

Usability: Relates to user interfaces ease of use.

Validity: Relates to whether the measurement device is measuring what it is intended to.

This research was previously published in the Encyclopedia of E-Health and Telemedicine edited by Maria Manuela Cruz-Cunha, Isabel Maria Miranda, Ricardo Martinho, and Rui Rijo, pages 383-400, copyright year 2016 by Medical Information Science Reference (an imprint of IGI Global).

Chapter 9
Headache App:
Usability Assessment and Criterion Validity

Tânia Dantas
University of Aveiro, Portugal

Milton Rodrigues dos Santos
University of Aveiro, Portugal

Alexandra Queirós
University of Aveiro, Portugal

Anabela G. Silva
University of Aveiro, Portugal

ABSTRACT

Mobile applications show great potential for the assessment and registration of information regarding headaches. However, data on the content and usability of mobile applications for headache that are accessible to the public in European Portuguese are scarce, as well the criterion validity. Therefore, this article aims to search for and characterize the mobile applications related to headache in terms of content, usability and criterion validity. A search in the Android app store of applications was conducted. Four mobile applications were found in European Portuguese that matched a set of predefined criteria. These were characterized in terms of general characteristics, content, usability and criterion validity. Three of the applications were specific for headaches and one could be used for any type of pain, including headache. All applications allowed recording of pain characteristics and its extraction in a form of a report. In the discussion section several challenges related to the use of mobile applications in the assessment and management of headache are discussed.

DOI: 10.4018/978-1-7998-1680-5.ch009

INTRODUCTION

The World Health Organization (WHO) defines mobile health (mHealth) technologies as a component of eHealth. mHealth covers medical and public health practice supported by mobile devices, such as mobile phones, patient monitoring devices, personal digital assistants, and other wireless devices (WHO, 2011). It is an emerging and rapidly developing field that can contribute to the transformation of healthcare and increase its quality and efficiency while simultaneously containing costs (de la Vega & Miró, 2014).

According to the Food and Drug Administration (FDA), the mobile applications for health should: i) help people (which means the users of the app) monitoring their health conditions without providing treatment suggestions; ii) provide simple tools to organize and control health information; provide easy access to information related with health; iii) help to document the health conditions, making this easier to share information with the health providers; iv) automate simple tasks for health care providers; and v) be intended to transfer, store and display medical data (FDA, 2013).

The adoption of mobile applications on a continuous basis can be affected by some barriers like the lack of confidence among patients, healthcare professionals and citizens regarding their reliability and their ability to accurately measure what is intended. Therefore, special attention should be given to them, before making them available to the general public and/or health professionals, especially if they have the potential to be a source of harm in normal use or have the potential to be misused (Queirós et al., 2016).

Regulations should effectively address issues such as certification of devices as well as applications. In addition, clinical usefulness is also an important issue for patients, citizens and healthcare professional's acceptance (EC, 2014). Clinical usefulness can be defined as to whether using the application results in any benefit for the patient such as more accurate diagnosis or more appropriate care (Silva, Queirós, Caravau, Ferreira, & Rocha, 2016). It depends on other aspects such as whether the application is measuring what it is intended to measure (validity), whether measurements taken with the application are consistent across repeated measurements in similar conditions (reliability) (Streiner & Norman 2003). In addition, the experience of the end user when using the application and its ease of use (usability) can also be a barrier or a facilitator when considering the use of mobile applications. This means that before the use of an application can be considered and results trusted a broaden assessment of this application, from different but complementary perspectives, should be undertaken. It is assumed that this assessment performed as an interactive process should be performed by interdisciplinary teams constituted by professionals from different areas (e.g. informatics, health) and end users to improve the likelihood of the applications to be used.

RELATED WORK

According to the International Headache Society (IHS, 2013), headaches are classified as primary headaches (Migraine, Tension-type headache, Trigeminal autonomic cephalalgias and other primary headache disorders) and secondary headaches (headaches attributed to trauma, injury, disorder or other condition). The prevalence of headache disorders among adults defined as symptomatic at least once within the last year is about 50% and about one third of adults aged 18–65 years have reported at least one episode of migraine (WHO, 2016). The Global Burden of Disease Survey 2010 (Vos et al., 2013) estimated that tension-type headache and migraine have a global prevalence of 20.1% and 14.7%, respectively, and are ranked as second and third most common diseases in the world. Migraine was recognized as the seventh highest among specific causes of disability.

A study on the impact of headache in Europe (Steiner et al., 2014) conducted across 15 different countries and a total of 8,271 participants revealed that the one-year prevalence of any headache was 79.6%, being slightly higher in females (86.0%) when compared to males (71.1%). Personal headache impact was assessed using a set of seven questions (encompassing areas such as the impact of headache on education, career prospects, earnings, relationships, work). Results showed that headaches negatively impact all these areas of life and are associated with a significant loss of useful time (17.7% of males and 28.0% of females with migraine lost >10% of days), which have implications for health policy and a high socioeconomic burden.

Wöber-Bingöl et al. (2014) in their study also refer to the impact of headache in children and adolescents. Their study results showed that 20.7% of the participants with headache reported to have lost at least one day of school and 48.8% reported that there was at least one day that they were unable to do the activities they had wanted to due to headache. Also, participants who reported headache also reported lower quality of life when compared to participants that did not report headaches.

The International association for the Study of Pain has published in December 2013 a clinical update recognizing the importance of mobile technology in managing chronic pain as a means to improve access to healthcare, contain costs and improve clinical outcomes (Vardeh, 2013). However, this publication also highlights the need to evaluate existing solutions.

Several authors suggest that mobile applications will have a crucial role in the future in maintaining social relationships, health and well-being (Mikkonen, Va, Ikonen, & Heikkila, 2002). However, mobile applications for health should go through a process of assessment in order to guarantee the quality and accuracy of its content as well as its usability (Boulos, Brewer, Karimkhani, Buller, & Dellavalle, 2014).

The usability of applications is a quality attribute related to the ease of use, more specifically, refers to the degree of ease of use, efficiency, errors and the number of users that like to use the applications (Nielsen & Loranger, 2006).

The objectives of this study were to characterize in terms of content and assess in terms of usability and criterion validity mobile applications related to headache.

METHODS

In order to facilitate the description of all procedures involved in this study, it was divided in three different phases. Phase A, included the selection and analysis of mobile applications and evaluation of its content. Phase B corresponded to the evaluation of their usability. Phase C corresponded to the assessment of criterion validity for one mobile application.

Phase A: Selection and Assessment of Mobile Applications

Pain related applications available in the Android platform between the 7th of October 2014 and the 15th of March 2015 were systematically searched (Silva et al., 2016). The search was conducted in this platform because it is the most used in terms of applications (Singla & Mendirata, 2014). In brief, this systematic review employed a two-phase search. In the first phase, we performed a search for pain applications in the Android platform using the terms pain and ache. In the second phase, we performed a search for publications on pain-related applications in five databases (Pubmed, Web of Science, Science Direct, Academic Search Complete and IEEE). The following search terms were used: (pain OR *ache) AND i) (smartphone OR "personal digital assistant" OR PDA); ii) ("mobile application" OR APP), iii) (pain OR *ache) AND ("electronic application" OR "electronic APP").

Retrieved applications were subcategorized according to several criteria, including the pathology for which they designed. The analysis in this paper refers to applications related to headache.

To be included in the present study the applications had to meet the following criteria:

- Allow the registration of information about headache
- Have the individual as primary user
- Have a version in European Portuguese language
- Be free of charge

The search resulted in four applications that met the inclusion criteria: i) Headache App; ii) Pain Diary; iii) Migraine Diary; and iv) Simple Record.

The general characterization of each of the four applications consisted of: description of the application; size; number of downloads, version; date last updated, number of evaluations made by users and average score (in stars – from 0 to 5).

A content analysis of each application was also performed, using a set of criteria adapted from Reynoldson et al. (2014) to assess pain related mobile applications. There were a total of 19 criteria, including aspects of: pain location (e.g., frontal, temporal); onset of pain (day and time); characteristics of the pain (how the pain is defined); associated symptoms (e.g. nausea, dizziness): duration of pain (duration of the pain episode); aggravating factors or relief factors (e.g. worsens with increasing brightness, improves with rest); environment (where the pain began, for example, work or home); pain intensity (existence of a pain intensity scale – for example, from 0 to 10); medication or treatment (details of the drugs and pain treatment); additional notes (ability to enter additional information); modification of existing options and results (existence of a results section). Each criterion was scored as 1 (if present) or 0 (if not) for a maximum score of 19 points.

The content analysis of each application was performed independently by two researchers.

Phase B: Usability Assessment

Only 3 applications enter the usability assessment phase because the applications Simple Record, was not available in the Play Store (platform for downloads belonging to Android) at this stage.

A convenience sample of 22 older adults recruited at Universidade Sénior de Cacia (USIDEC), Universidade Sénior de Estarreja (USR) and from the general community were asked to assess the usability of the mobile applications. Those who agreed to participate had to give their written consent. Participants were eligible if they were able to use an electronic device.

The sample was characterized in terms of: gender, age, level of education and computer literacy through a questionnaire developed for the purpose of this study.

For the application's usability evaluation, participants answered a questionnaire of usability, the International Classification of Functioning - Usability Scale I (ICF-US I), which is based on the International Classification of Functioning, Disability and Health (Martins et al., 2013). This instrument consists of 10 items covering aspects of ease of use, satisfaction and learning process; expected results and clarity of information. To answer each of the 10 items, the respondent has to report on whether the aspect being considered is a barrier or a facilitator and graduate the magnitude of the barrier or facilitator in a Likert scale of three points (barrier: -3: complete;

-2: large and -1: small; facilitator: 1:small; 2:large and 3: complete). The maximum score is 30 points. The ICF-US I was completed after using all three applications according to a written script of tasks aimed to ensure that all participants used each application in a similar way and explored its different functionalities in the same way.

In parallel to the usability evaluation, a performance evaluation was also performed. For this evaluation a script was given to participants in order for them to complete a series of tasks using the application (for example, register pain intensity or medication intake). For each task, the researcher assessed the following aspects: i) number of attempts that each participant needed to successfully complete each task; ii) whether participants were able to complete the tasks without any support, with verbal support or needed physical assistance and iii) the time that each participant took to complete all tasks. These procedures were piloted in 2 individuals not belonging to the final sample.

Phase C: Criterion Validity Assessment of Headache App

Only one application was used at this phase – the Headache App. Participants in this phase were students of the 1st year of the Bachelor in Physiotherapy at Health Sciences School, University of Aveiro. The sample was characterized in terms of gender and age.

Students were asked to install the application in their smartphones and to register headache episodes during two weeks. In parallel, they were also asked to register headache episodes on a paper-based pain diary. This paper-based pain diary included the following information: date (day/month/year), time of the day, factors relieving the headache and a 10 cm visual analogue scale anchored with "no pain" and "worst pain imaginable". This scale has been found to be valid (Ferreira-Valente, Pais-Ribeiro, & Jensen, 2011). At the end of the two weeks period, students exported the headache pain report from the Headache Application and delivered the paper-based pain diary for comparison.

DATA ANALYSIS

Data was analyzed using the Statistical Package for the Social Sciences, version 22.0 for Windows. The characterization of the sample, usability and performance of applications was made descriptive statistics (mean, standard deviation, frequencies, minimum and maximum). An ANOVA was used to compare the total score of the ICF-US I and performance (time to complete the task script) among the three applications. In addition, a spearman correlation coefficient was used to compare pain intensity ratings as measured in the application and using the VAS in the paper-based pain diary. Percentage of agreement was used to compare date, time of day and medication intake. The significance level was set at $p<0.05$.

RESULTS

The results will be presented according to the phases described previously.

Phase A: Selection and Analysis of Mobile Applications

All applications enabled the recording of episodes of headache by users, and the possibility to insert various characteristics of the headache. In terms of size, the larger application was Pain Diary with 9.5 MB, the application presenting a greater number of downloads (between 1000 and 50000) was Headache App; the application last updated (2/2/2014) was Simple Record; the application with the highest number of evaluations made by users was the Headache App; and the applications better assessed by users (a mean score of 4.1 out of 5) were the Pain Diary and Simple Record.

The content assessment of various applications, as mentioned above, was performed independently by two reviewers. The percentage of agreement ranged between 84.21% (Pain Diary) and 100% (Migraine Diary). However, after discussion, reviewers reached 100% agreement for all applications.

Table 1 presents the result of content assessment adapted from (Reynoldson et al., 2014).

Only the application Pain Diary refers to headache duration and allows for the modification of existing options. In contrast, all the applications evaluated allow the imputation of the date; the time of day pain first appeared and intensity of pain. All applications are faithful to the information given by the programmer in the description; all have a results section, and these can be filtered and formatted in a final report. The application with the highest final score (15 points out of a maximum of 19 points) was Pain Diary and the application with the lowest final score (8 points) was the Simple Record.

Phase B: Usability Assessment

The sample consisted of 22 participants, 54.5% (n=12) female and 45.5% (n=10) of males, with a mean (±SD) age of 72.3 (±8.2) years old. Regarding level of education, 31.8% (n=7) had an university degree. As regards the level of computer literacy, all participants (n=22) had at least one mobile device and 59.1% (n=13) used mobile devices every day.

Table 1. Content assessment of applications

Onset of pain	Pain Diary	Headache App	Migraine Diary	Simple Record
Day the pain appeared	1	1	1	1
Time of day the pain appeared	1	1	1	1
Characteristics – pain definition and pattern	1	1	0	0
Location	0	1	1	0
Associated symptoms (another symptom beyond the pain, like nausea, blurred vision, dizziness)	1	1	0	0
Duration (how long has this pain episode)	1	0	0	0
Factors of worsening or relief				
Factors influencing pain worsening	1	1	1	0
Factors influencing pain relief	0	0	0	0
Environment (place where the pain occurred, for example home, work, external environment)	0	0	0	0
Intensity (existence of scale of evaluation, for example numerical - from 1 to 10)	1	1	1	1
Section of treatment and medication	1	1	0	0
Drug dose section, treatment details	1	1	0	0
Section about changes after treatment or medication	0	0	0	0
Notes (possibility to add extra notes relating to the pain episode)	1	1	0	1
Possibility to change options (for example, options can be added or removed in order to make the application more relevant to the user)	1	0	0	0
The application remains true to the claims made by the programmer in the market description	1	1	1	1
Results				
Presence of a results section	1	1	1	1
Possibility to filter the results	1	1	1	1
Presence of a final report	1	1	1	1
Total	**15**	**14**	**9**	**2**

The application with the highest score in terms of usability (ICF-US I) was the Headache Application (Mean±sd ICF_US I=25.4 ±0.4), followed by the Pain Diary (Mean±sd ICF_US I=24.7±3.9) and the application Migraine Diary (Mean±sd ICF_US I= 13.6±3.7). There were no statistically significant differences in the final score of the ICF-US I between the three applications (p=0.21), suggesting that they have similar usability levels.

Table 2. Mean (±SD) of attempts to complete tasks and number (±SD) of participants needing verbal and/or physical support to complete the tasks

	No. of tasks	Number of attempts to complete tasks			Type of support needed	
		1ª	2ª	3º	Physical	Verbal
Migraine Diary	12	14,9 (±2,3)	4,3 (±2,1)	1,5 (±0,9)	0,85 (±0,9)	1,0 (0,9)
Headache Application	11	15,4 (1,6)	3,6 (±1,0)	1,5 (±1,8)	0,8 (±1,1)	0,8 (±1,1)
Pain Diary	12	14,4 (±2,8)	3,2 (1,7)	2,4 (±0,9)	1,0 (±0,9)	1,1 (±1,0)

Table 2 presents the number attempts to finish the tasks, as well as the type of support needed. The support needed to finish the tasks was physical, the evaluator could help the participant showing how to complete the task, or verbal, the evaluator explains orally how to perform the task.

The application for which participants took longer to complete the task script was the Migraine Diary (mean ±sd=7.1±3.3min.), followed by Headache Application (mean ±sd=6.2 ±2.9 min.) and Pain Diary (mean ±sd=5.1 ±2.7 min). No significant differences were found between applications ($p<0.05$).

Phase C: Criterion Validity Assessment of Headache Application

A total of eight students (5 males and 3 females) aged between 18 and 20 years old, participated in the study and made a total of 26 registries referring to 26 episodes of headache in different days that were registered in the application. Each student reported on one to four different episodes of headache and a similar number of episodes was registered both in the application (n=26) and in the pain diary (n=24). Therefore, comparisons were carried out for the 24 episodes of headache registered in both the application and the paper-based diary. Figure 1 shows a screenshot taken from the application.

Mean pain intensity as reported in the application was 4.10±2.02 and 3.90±2.31 when measured using the VAS and correlation between pain intensity measured in the application and in the pain, diary was r=0.91.

When comparing dates and time of day at which participants reported headache episodes, there was 100% agreement between data provided by the application and data provided in the pain diary. For medication intake, there was 90% agreement between data registered in the application and in the pain diary.

Figure 1. Screenshot of the Headache Application filled in by one participant

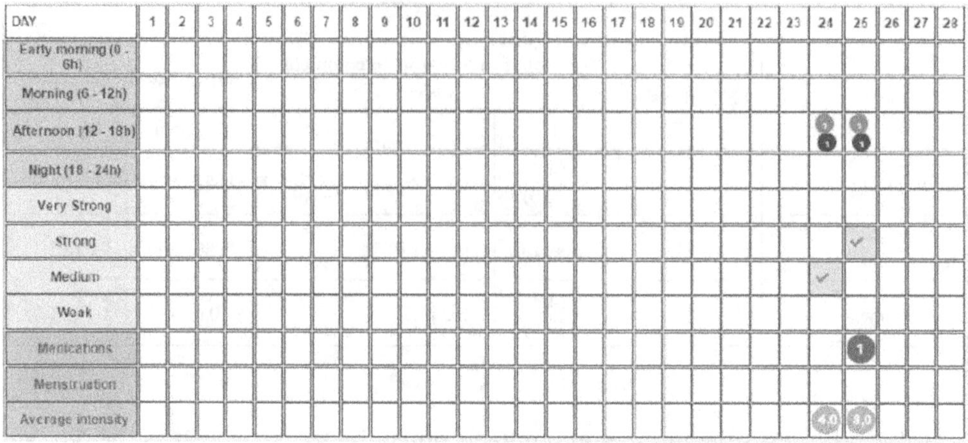

DISCUSSION

The present study characterized three mobile applications related to (i) Migraine Diary; ii) Pain Diary and iii) Headache App) in terms of general characteristics, content, usability and validity.

In terms of content, all applications allowed the insertion of information regarding the characteristics of the headache and all applications included a final report that could be exported or sent by email. These contents are in line with the European principles of management of common headache disorders in primary care developed by WHO, the World Headache Alliance, International Headache Society and European Headache Federation (Steiner, 2005). One of the recommendations was related to the importance of diaries to record symptoms and temporal patterns that contribute to the correct diagnosis; assessment of medication use and overuse; or other associations with the pain episode. In addition, keeping a calendar is also recommended to remember the medication intake, record the treatment effects or monitor acute medication use or overuse during follow-up. The majority of the applications analyzed have these functionalities.

Concerning the usability of the applications assessed in this study, the high mean score of ICF-US (minimum of 24.7 out of 30) suggests that applications were relatively easy to use. Nevertheless, this could have been influenced by the high literacy levels of our sample. This is also shown by the fact that most participants were able to perform the tasks requested in the task script at a first attempt. According to several studies (Hachizuka et al., 2010; Kristjánsdóttir et al., 2011; Marceau, Link, Jamison, & Carolan, 2007), pain related mobile applications tend to be considered easy to use by end users. Mobile applications can help reduce the burden associated to chronic conditions and the disability due to pain, ensuring the continuous recovery of a particular pathology, and to alert informal caregivers to any changes in medication or access to information (CTA, 2011). Considering these, it is important that usability questions are considered in the development of mobile applications for management of headache, in what concerns design, functionalities and interaction.

Mobile applications for the management of headache may be of high importance for older people, as they cover the most important clinical aspects of headache and allow communication with health professionals, for example, by sending an email with the data collected using the application. They might be relevant in terms of assessment and monitoring of symptoms before and after an intervention, allowing health professionals to have a more accurate feedback on the impact of interventions (Alban, De Marchi, Scortegagna, & Leguisamo, 2012; CTA, 2011; McDowell, 2006; Scanaill, Ahearne, & Lyons, 2006). Also, Mosadeghi-Nik et al. (2016) refer the importance of involving patients and clinicians in the development of applications in order to create effective tools to identify trigger factors of migraine, improving self-management of headache disorders, and mediating the interactions between headache sufferers and their treating doctors. Despite the availability of numerous mobile applications for headache the evidence base to support their effectiveness and clinical safety is still very weak. Nevertheless, there is a need to ensure that its content is accurate and its mode of use appropriate to end users. Furthermore, this study results show that the information collected using the application and traditional methods (such as paper-based diaries) give comparable results, suggesting that data collected using the application is valid. These findings suggest that the headache application can be used to collect real time data on headache characteristics. The results of the present study are in line with the results of Pombo et al. (2016), that refers that electronic diaries produce reliable data; however training is critical to improve the adherence. Special attention should be given to technological safety in mobile applications to avoid system failures and missing values. Another issue considered relevant is related to the loss of mobile devices, their use to store health records implies the risk of losing data and personal information or applications discontinuity.

One of the characteristics of mobile applications is related to the integration of data in Electronic Health Record (EHR). Effectively, several studies demonstrated that the main characteristic present in mobile applications are related to monitoring and management of a specific health condition (Queirós et al., 2016). Recent studies related to remote care emphasize the need of interoperability between systems (Jin & Chen, 2015; Mohammadzadeh & Safdari, 2014). Mohammadzadeh et al. (2014) identified several challenges in the use of mobile heath applications, some already referred in this section like the privacy and confidentiality of data and usability assessment and, in particular, challenges related to the interoperability with other EHR or other health systems. Interoperability and information share is necessary to facilitate the health decision making, reduce medical errors is reduced and increase quality of remote health care. In the applications analyzed, a final report was referred, but some participants reported difficulties when attempting to export data. Furthermore, the document that was exported was a pdf file what makes difficult to share information and it is a barrier to semantic interoperability, the ability to exchange the content of the data among mobile applications, EHR, or other health systems. However, it is not explicit if the data collected can be shared with health professionals or EHR, or other health systems. This seem to mean that even technological interoperability may be missing.

CONCLUSION

This study results suggest that 3 mobile applications related to headache and which are available in European Portuguese are adequate in terms of content and usability and one of them collects valid data. It also explores some challenges related to the use of mobile applications, namely the privacy and confidentiality of data, the usability assessment and the interoperability with other EHR or other health systems.

The present study has some limitations in what concerns the number of applications tested. In fact, there were only three applications available in European Portuguese in the Android platform. Another limitation is related to the sample used. It would have been interesting to have usability and validity data on both samples (older adults and young adults), which would have allowed for comparison of results.

Future studies may test more applications, including those available at different platforms like Microsoft or IOS and with participants with different levels of digital literacy and across age groups. Future studies could also look at the interoperability of mobile applications with EHR, or other health systems and investigate whether using mobile applications to assess headache and share the information with health professionals results in better health care when compared to the traditional methods of assessment.

ACKNOWLEDGMENT

Special thanks to all the people who agreed to participate in this study, as well as the Universidade Sénior de Cacia (USIDEC) and Universidade Sénior de Estarreja (USR) and 1st year BSc students of Physiotherapy (2016/2017).

REFERENCES

Alban, A., De Marchi, A. C. B., Scortegagna, S. A., & Leguisamo, C. P. (2012). Ampliando a usabilidade de interfaces web para idosos em dispositivos móveis: uma proposta utilizando design responsivo. *RENOTE*, *10*(3).

Boulos, M. N. K., Brewer, A. C., Karimkhani, C., Buller, D. B., & Dellavalle, R. P. (2014). Mobile medical and health apps: State of the art, concerns, regulatory control and certification. *Online Journal of Public Health Informatics*, *5*(3). PMID:24683442

CTA. (2011). mHealth Technologies: Applications to Benefit Older Adults: Center for Technology and Aging.

de la Vega, R., & Miró, J. (2014). mHealth: A strategic field without a solid scientific soul. a systematic review of pain-related apps. *PLoS One*, *9*(7), e101312. doi:10.1371/journal.pone.0101312 PMID:24999983

EC. (2014). *GREEN PAPER on mobile Health ("mHealth")*. Brussels: European Commission.

FDA. (2013). *Mobile medical applications: guidance for industry and Food and Drug Administration staff*. USA: Food and Drug Administration.

Ferreira-Valente, M. A., Pais-Ribeiro, J. L., & Jensen, M. P. (2011). Validity of four pain intensity rating scales. *Pain*, *152*(10), 2399–2404. doi:10.1016/j.pain.2011.07.005 PMID:21856077

Hachizuka, M., Yoshiuchi, K., Yamamoto, Y., Iwase, S., Nakagawa, K., Kawagoe, K., & Akabayashi, A. (2010). Development of a personal digital assistant (PDA) system to collect symptom information from home hospice patients. *Journal of Palliative Medicine*, *13*(6), 647–651. doi:10.1089/jpm.2009.0350 PMID:20509795

IHS. (2013). The international classification of headache disorders, (beta version). *Cephalalgia*, *33*(9), 629–808. doi:10.1177/0333102413485658 PMID:23771276

Jin, Z., & Chen, Y. (2015). Telemedicine in the cloud era: Prospects and challenges. *IEEE Pervasive Computing*, *14*(1), 54–61. doi:10.1109/MPRV.2015.19

Kristjánsdóttir, Ó. B., Fors, E. A., Eide, E., Finset, A., van Dulmen, S., Wigers, S. H., & Eide, H. (2011). Written online situational feedback via mobile phone to support self-management of chronic widespread pain: A usability study of a Web-based intervention. *BMC Musculoskeletal Disorders*, *12*(1), 51. doi:10.1186/1471-2474-12-51 PMID:21352516

Marceau, L. D., Link, C., Jamison, R. N., & Carolan, S. (2007). *Electronic diaries as a tool to improve pain management: is there any evidence?* The Oxford University Press.

Martins, A., Queirós, A., Cerqueira, M., Silva, A., Francesco, S., & Rocha, N. (2013). *AAL Living Lab Methodologies based on ICF*. In Assist. Technol. From Res. to Pract.

McDowell, I. (2006). *Measuring health: a guide to rating scales and questionnaires*. Oxford university press. doi:10.1093/acprof:oso/9780195165678.001.0001

Mikkonen, M., Va, S., Ikonen, V., & Heikkila, M. (2002). User and concept studies as tools in developing mobile communication services for the elderly. *Personal and Ubiquitous Computing*, *6*(2), 113–124. doi:10.1007007790200010

Mohammadzadeh, N., & Safdari, R. (2014). Patient monitoring in mobile health: Opportunities and challenges. *Medicinski Arhiv*, *68*(1), 57. doi:10.5455/medarh.2014.68.57-60 PMID:24783916

Mosadeghi-Nik, M., Askari, M. S., & Fatehi, F. (2016). Mobile health (mHealth) for headache disorders: A review of the evidence base. *Journal of Telemedicine and Telecare*, *22*(8), 472–477. doi:10.1177/1357633X16673275 PMID:27799450

Nielsen, J., & Loranger, H. (2006). *Prioritizing web usability*. Pearson Education.

Pombo, N., Garcia, N., Bousson, K., Spinsante, S., & Chorbev, I. (2016). Pain Assessment–Can it be Done with a Computerised System? A Systematic Review and Meta-Analysis. *International Journal of Environmental Research and Public Health, 13*(4), 415. doi:10.3390/ijerph13040415 PMID:27089351

Queirós, A., Silva, A. G., Ferreira, A., Caravau, H., Cerqueira, M., & Rocha, N. P. (2016). Assessing Mobile Applications Considered Medical Devices. In Encyclopedia of E-Health and Telemedicine (pp. 111–127). Hershey, PA: IGI Global. doi:10.4018/978-1-4666-9978-6.ch010

Reynoldson, C., Stones, C., Allsop, M., Gardner, P., Bennett, M. I., Closs, S. J., & Knapp, P. (2014). Assessing the Quality and Usability of Smartphone Apps for Pain Self-Management. *Pain Medicine*, *15*(6), 898–909. doi:10.1111/pme.12327 PMID:24422990

Scanaill, C. N., Ahearne, B., & Lyons, G. M. (2006). Long-term telemonitoring of mobility trends of elderly people using SMS messaging. *IEEE Transactions on Information Technology in Biomedicine*, *10*(2), 412–413. doi:10.1109/TITB.2005.859890 PMID:16617630

Silva, A. G., Queirós, A., Caravau, H., Ferreira, A., & Rocha, N. P. (2016). Systematic Review and Evaluation of Pain-Related Mobile Applications. In Encyclopedia of E-Health and Telemedicine (pp. 383–400). Hershey, PA: IGI Global.

Singla, D., & Mendirata, L. (2014). Android VS IOS. *IJIRT*, *1*(5), 592–596.

Steiner, T. J. (2005). Lifting The Burden: The global campaign to reduce the burden of headache worldwide. *The Journal of Headache and Pain*, *6*(5), 373–377. doi:10.100710194-005-0241-7 PMID:16362709

Steiner, T. J., Stovner, L. J., Katsarava, Z., Lainez, J. M., Lampl, C., Lantéri-Minet, M., & Barré, J. (2014). The impact of headache in Europe: Principal results of the Eurolight project. *The Journal of Headache and Pain*, *15*(1), 31. doi:10.1186/1129-2377-15-31 PMID:24884549

Vardeh, D. E. R., Jamison, R., & Eccleston, C. (2013). There's an App for That: Mobile Technology Is a New Advantage in Managing Chronic Pain. *ISAP Pain Clinical*, *21*(6).

Vos, T., Flaxman, A. D., Naghavi, M., Lozano, R., Michaud, C., Ezzati, M., & Aboyans, V. (2013). Years lived with disability (YLDs) for 1160 sequelae of 289 diseases and injuries 1990–2010: A systematic analysis for the Global Burden of Disease Study 2010. *Lancet*, *380*(9859), 2163–2196. doi:10.1016/S0140-6736(12)61729-2 PMID:23245607

World Health Organization (WHO). (2011). *Atlas eHealth country profiles: based on the findings of the second global survey on eHealth.*

WHO. (2016). Headache Disorders Fact Sheet No 277 (2007). Retrieved from http://www.who.int/mediacentre/factsheets/fs277/en/

Wöber-Bingöl, Ç., Wöber, C., Uluduz, D., Uygunoğlu, U., Aslan, T. S., Kernmayer, M., & Siva, A. (2014). The global burden of headache in children and adolescents–developing a questionnaire and methodology for a global study. *The Journal of Headache and Pain*, *15*(1), 86. doi:10.1186/1129-2377-15-86 PMID:25496532

This research was previously published in the International Journal of Mobile Computing and Multimedia Communications (IJMCMC), 9(2); edited by Agustinus Waluyo, pages 1-11, copyright year 2018 by IGI Publishing (an imprint of IGI Global).

Section 4
Self-Management and Therapy

Chapter 10
The Role of Self-Efficacy and Aging in Managing Disease

Debra Weiss-Randall
Florida Atlantic University, USA

ABSTRACT

In 1900, life expectancy in the U.S. was 47 years and infectious diseases were the leading cause of mortality; today, life expectancy in the U.S. is almost 80 years and chronic diseases are the leading causes of mortality. Eighty percent of adults 65 and older have multiple chronic health conditions, which are costly to treat. Offering older adults an evidence-based self-management program can reduce medical costs and improve patient outcomes and quality of life. Research has shown that self-efficacy is a key factor in effective self-management programs. The Chronic Disease Self-Management Program (CDSMP) is an evidence-based program that helps patients to boost their self-efficacy and improve their disease self-management, under the supervision of a physician. In addition, the use of evidence-based complementary modalities is recommended as part of an integrative approach to self-management to help patients manage the daily anger, fear, and depression that frequently accompany living with an incurable disease.

INTRODUCTION

Gone are the days when the doctor (usually a male) told the patient what to do and the patient accepted it without reservation. Today patients are consumers, and they select healthcare providers from a roster of names accepted by their health plan. Thanks to the Internet, which has widely disseminated health information through websites such as WebMD, patients are much better informed today than they were

DOI: 10.4018/978-1-7998-1680-5.ch010

25 years ago. They are also prey to "infomercials" and a host of advertisers selling products that will "cure" them of obesity, cancer, depression, and more, if they pay a monthly fee to receive certain supplements, potions, and balms. *Caveat emptor*—buyer beware.

In the U.S., chronic diseases cause 7 of 10 deaths each year, and treating chronic diseases accounts for 86% of the nation's healthcare costs (Centers for Disease Control and Prevention, 2013). In 2012, about half of all U.S. adults—117 million people—had at least one chronic health condition; 25% of adults had two or more chronic health conditions (Ward et al., 2014). The healthcare provider's aim in dealing with patients who have chronic diseases such as diabetes and asthma is adequate self-management in order to maintain good quality of life. Control over risk factors such as diet, exercise, and smoking make an enormous difference in outcome.

Today patients are partners in their own healthcare. This chapters posits that, for patients to be able to achieve adequate self-management of chronic diseases, they need a chronic disease self-management program that provides education about disease management and helps patients to apply what they have learned at home. Furthermore, in order to feel empowered to act, patients need to develop self-efficacy, i.e., belief in their capacity to exercise control over their lives and effect behavior change. A diagnosis of a serious illness such as cancer can lead to fear, depression, and feelings of powerlessness, which must be treated in order for the patient to be an effective partner in his or her care. Evidence-based non-pharmacologic complementary therapies can be a great help in this regard, providing emotional and psychological support.

This chapter describes the contributions of self-efficacy theory and positive psychology to disease self-management. Next, the chapter provides a review of the literature on chronic disease self-management programs, with a discussion of the Chronic Disease Self-Management Program (CDSMP), an evidence-based program developed in the mid-1990s that has been found to boost patients' self-efficacy and improve outcome measures. The chapter also examines the effectiveness of individual components of chronic disease self-management programs. The chapter then provides a detailed discussion of evidence-based non-pharmacologic complementary therapies, which are a useful adjunctive treatment that should be used under the supervision of a physician. These complementary therapies provide symptom relief, reduce stress, improve patients' ability to perform daily tasks, and facilitate adoption of healthy lifestyle habits.

Next, the chapter looks at the U.S. statistics on aging and disease, and the implications for healthy aging. Aging places an additional burden on patients. Seniors with chronic diseases may feel hopeless about recovery and need supportive services aimed at their age group to encourage self-efficacy and to keep them motivated to participate in rehabilitation. Elderly patients may need adaptive physical activities to accommodate age-related physical limitations. Access to appropriate facilities, and transportation to get there, are two additional challenges seniors face.

The chapter concludes by summing up the recommendations for chronic disease self-management, including the use of an evidence-based self-management plan such as CDSMP, and the use of complementary therapies to provide symptom relief and promote adoption of healthy behaviors. Treatment should be tailored to the patient's specific age cohort and be culturally sensitive as well, respecting the patient's ethnic, racial, and religious background.

SELF-EFFICACY THEORY

Albert Bandura's groundbreaking work in self-efficacy posited that "expectations of personal efficacy determine whether coping behavior will be initiated, how much effort will be expended, and how long it will be sustained in the face of obstacles and aversive experiences" (Bandura, 1977, p. 191).

An outcome expectancy is a person's belief that a particular course of action will produce certain outcomes. Bandura (1977) differentiates it from self-efficacy, which is a person's belief that he or she can successfully execute the behavior required to produce the outcomes. Bandura notes that individuals can believe that a particular course of action will produce certain outcomes, but if they entertain serious doubts about whether they can perform the necessary activities such information does not influence their behavior (Bandura, 1977, p. 193).

Perceived self-efficacy is based on four principal sources of information (Bandura, 1982):

- Performance attainments
- Vicarious experiences observing others
- Verbal persuasion and social influence, and
- Physiological states.

Performance attainments refer to success the person has experienced; these successes build confidence in the person's ability to succeed again in the future. Observing someone who is perceived to be of similar competence succeed can give the observer confidence that she, too, can succeed. Conversely, watching a peer fail can put a damper on one's enthusiasm for tackling a similar task. Pep talks (verbal persuasion) have the greatest effect on those who believe they can produce effects through their actions. Experiencing negative physiological states such as high arousal with tension and agitation (e.g., nerves before a speech), or fatigue with aches and pains (e.g., aching back before a race) may deter a person from continuing toward his goal (Bandura, 1982). The higher the perceived self-efficacy, the more likely the person is to persevere and overcome obstacles to attain the desired goal. Bandura (1982) emphasizes the centrality of the self-efficacy mechanism in human agency. Perceived self-efficacy influences a person's thought patterns, actions, and emotional arousal. The higher the level of self-efficacy, the higher the performance accomplishments will be.

There is an inverse relationship between level of self-efficacy and emotional arousal; the higher the former, the lower the latter. Why is this the case? Emotional arousal is debilitating and, hence, reduces a person's confidence that he or she can complete the desired task. Confidence, in turn, is influenced by one's outlook in life. An optimistic outlook promotes confidence in one's ability to overcome obstacles and achieve a desired outcome. Self-efficacy theory is closely related to positive psychology, which promotes an optimistic outlook on life.

POSITIVE PSYCHOLOGY

Martin Seligman, founder of the positive psychology movement, defines it as "the scientific study of the strengths that enable individuals and communities to thrive" (Seligman, 2015). In contrast to the traditional disease model, which focuses on weaknesses and dysfunction, the positive psychology model focuses on authentic happiness and flourishing (Seligman, 2011). Seligman's PERMA model of well-being has five components:

- Positive Emotions
- Engagement
- Relationships
- Meaning
- Accomplishment

When life is frustrating and a person's efforts to attain desired goals are thwarted, is the glass half full or half empty? From a positive pschology point of view, it is always half full.

Given challenging circumstances, the optimist feels that he or she can persevere and attain a desired goal. The pessimist, on the other hand, doesn't even want to try because it seems like a hopeless cause. Can a person's outlook on life be changed? Positive psychologists believe the answer is "Yes!" Positive psychology posits that a person's thoughts profoundly affect his or her actions. Therefore, thinking positive thoughts will engender positive actions. If you believe in your ability to attain a goal, you are likely to do it!

Positive psychology builds on strength and resilience, with the patient no longer viewed as "a passive vessel," but rather as a decision maker (Bandura, 1989; Seligman, 2011). Rather than emphasizing disease and dysfunction, positive psychology focuses on well-being, optimal experience, happiness, and self-determination. It posits that a positive personality can be *developed* because human beings are adaptive entities. Furthermore, because people and experiences are embedded in a social context, it is vital to take positive communities and institutions into account (Seligman & Csikszentmihalyi, 2000).

How can people change their mindset to a more positive one? In Seligman's view, people can become more optimistic by cultivating kindness, developing friendships, exercising, using their strengths, finding their flow, finding meaning through spirituality, and by expressing gratitude, mindfulness, and hope (Seligman, 2015). Mroczek (2014) argues for the plasticity of the personality, for the possibility that personality traits such as conscientiousness—an important element of self-management—can be cultivated. Some authors (Chapman et al., 2014; Magidson et al., 2014) advocate interventions that cultivate the trait of conscientiousness, which, in turn, leads to improved health behaviors.

When people have a life-threatening chronic disease (such as heart disease or cancer), the coping mechanisms they use, in part, determine their emotional well-being (Carver et al., 1993; Hart et al., 1987; Stanton et al., 2007). When problems are controllable, the most effective strategy, and the one most closely related to emotional well-being, is active coping (problem-solving and seeking information and social support). When problems are uncontrollable, the most effective coping strategies are acceptance of the problem, positive reappraisal of the situation (e.g., considering it an opportunity to adopt a healthier lifestyle, to appreciate the truly important things in life), and the use of a sense of humor (Angeles Ruiz, 2011). A positive attitude toward the illness has a beneficial effect on recovery. Research has found that positive expectations predicted patients' recovery from a myocardial infarction (Agarwal et al., 1995). Dispositional optimism is also an important predictor of recovery from a cardiovascular episode or surgery (Scheier et al., 1989).

REVIEW OF THE LITERATURE

Forty years ago, most patients went to their primary doctor and took whatever medication was prescribed; doctors were in charge of disease management, and patients followed their advice. With the founding of the World Wide Web in 1989, the flow of information on medical diseases and conditions increased exponentially. Patients became health consumers who searched medical websites for information about their health conditions. Today, patients can optimize their quality of life by taking an active role in self-management of their chronic diseases and conditions, under the supervision of a healthcare provider.

Overview of Chronic Disease Self-Management

Lorig and Holman (2003) give an overview of the history of disease self-management. The term "self-management" as applied to chronic disease indicates that the patient is an active participant in treatment. One of its early proponents was Thomas Creer, who used it in his work with chronically ill children at the Children's Asthma Research Institute and Hospital (Creer et al., 1976). For someone with a chronic disease, self-management is generally a lifelong task. The burden of day-to-day disease management falls largely on the patient.

Self-management of chronic disease comprises three tasks—medical management, role management, and emotional management (Lorig & Holman, 2003). The medical management of the disease or condition includes taking medications and monitoring vital signs such as blood pressure and heart rate; it also may necessitate adhering to a special diet and/or using medical devices such as an inhaler for asthma. The role management of the chronic disease or condition involves maintaining, changing, and creating new behaviors or life roles to accommodate the limitations imposed by the disease. For example, people with chronic back pain may need to modify how they participate in a sport (Lorig & Holman, 2003). Emotional management involves dealing with the anger, fear, frustration, and depression that are often experienced by an individual with a chronic, incurable disease; dealing with the disease requires daily management of symptoms and adaptation to the limitations imposed by the disease (Lorig & Holman, 2003). Corbin and Strauss's (1988) research on individuals with chronic diseases and conditions yielded the finding that self-management programs must be problem based, i.e., they need to solve the underlying problem that is perceived by the patient to be the core issue. They cite the example of arthritis: traditional arthritis programs focused on preventing or limiting disability; however, for the patients, pain management was the underlying problem. Therefore, disability prevention should be taught in the context of pain management (Corbin & Strauss, 1988). The first step in self-management program should be a detailed needs assessment to ascertain what the most important issues are for the patient.

In order to execute these tasks successfully, one must master five core self-management skills—1) problem solving, 2) decision making, 3) resource utilization, 4) forming a patient-provider partnership, and 5) taking action (Lorig & Holman, 2003). In solving a problem, one must first define it, then generate ideas for possible solutions, implement a plan to resolve the problem, and then evaluate the results. The Americans with Disabilities Act (ADA), passed by Congress in 1990, prohibited discrimination in employment, public services, public accommodations, and telecommunications. It led to the requirement that public buildings have access ramps for wheelchairs that buses accommodate wheelchairs, and that public services and facilities (including theatres and museums) offer accommodations for individuals with disabilities. Therefore, when a person with a chronic condition or disease has a problem regarding transportation (a frequent concern), it is now easier than it was before ADA to problem solve and get them where they need to go using public transportation. Decision making might revolve around being able to understand when a symptom is serious enough to require a visit to the doctor or hospital, to know how much exercise is "enough," or to know how to read food labels to make sure the item does not contain anything not on the individual's special diet.

The third skill, resource utilization, requires getting the consumer to the resource. It may involve acquiring new skills, such as learning to surf the Web to locate a desired resource. In addition, Lorig and Holman (2003) suggest casting a wide net by contacting several sources of information at once rather than calling only one and waiting for someone to get back to you. The fourth skill, forming a partnership with the physician or other healthcare provider, requires re-thinking the traditional approach to the patient-provider relationship, which was predicated on diagnosing and treating acute, infectious diseases. In the U.S. today, chronic diseases such as heart disease, cancer, and stroke are the major killers, and people live with chronic diseases for decades. When dealing with chronic diseases, the provider-patient relationship has to be a partnership, with the physician supervising and teaching the patient about self-management.

Finally, taking action involves skill mastery and confidence in one's ability to carry out an action plan in the next week or two. The objective should be quite specific and measurable; for example, "This week I will walk to the corner store and back (2 blocks in all) before dinner on Monday, Wednesday, and Saturday." (Lorig & Holman, 2003). In addition, the plan should be realistic and "doable," and the person should be confident that he or she can achieve the objective. On a scale of 1 (totally unconfident) to 10 (totally confident), the person planning to take action should have a confidence score of 7 or above. If it is below 7, more problem solving may be needed (Lorig & Holman, 2003). To improve compliance with an action plan and to make sure that it is appropriate, self-tailoring is needed; this requires that the individual has learned the principles behind behavior change, decision making, and problem solving. In addition, the individual must believe in his or her capacity to effect behavior change, as self-efficacy (Bandura, 1977, 1982, 1989, 1991) is the mechanism driving the success of self-management interventions (Lorig & Holman, 2003). (For a discussion of self-efficacy, see Theoretical Framework.)

Chronic Disease Self-Management Program (CDSMP)

CDSMP is a self-management education program for individuals with chronic illnesses or health conditions. Lorig and colleagues (Lorig et al., 1999) developed it in a longitudinal study at the School of Medicine at Stanford University. The aim of CDSMP is to improve self-management of chronic disease by improving self-efficacy through the use of goal setting, performance mastery, modeling, and social persuasion techniques (Melchior et al., 2014). The Centers for Disease Control and Prevention (CDC) recommends CDSMP as an effective evidence-based tool for chronic disease self-management (CDC, 2016).

The CDSMP randomized controlled trial (RCT) at Stanford University had more than 1,000 participants with heart disease, lung disease, stroke, or arthritis. The outcome measures the researchers studied were changes in the participants' health status (self-rated general health, disability, social limitations, pain/physical discomfort, energy level, shortness of breath, psychological well-being, depression), health care usage (visits to physicians and emergency department, hospitalizations), self-efficacy (to perform self-management behaviors, manage disease in general, achieve outcomes), and self-management behaviors (exercise, manage cognitive symptoms and stress, use community resources, and communicate with physician).

Lorig et al. (1996) state that four factors motivated them to undertake the CDSMP study, namely, 1) an aging population, 2) increases in both chronic disease and comorbidity, 3) new concepts about healthy aging, and 4) a lack of health education programs for those with multiple chronic diseases or conditions (Lorig et al., 1996). The aims of developing such a self-management program were to improve quality of life for an aging population suffering from chronic diseases, and to reduce healthcare costs (Lorig et al., 1996).

The researchers had previous experience with an Arthritis Self-Management Program (ASMP), and developed their theoretical framework for CDSMP based on the results of ASMP Lorig et al., 1989).. They found that participants in ASMP who experienced positive changes in pain reported an increased sense of control over their symptoms, whereas those who did not were more likely to report that nothing could be done for their symptoms. Feelings of control were operationalized as perceived self-efficacy to feel confident that they could manage arthritis symptoms (Lenker et al., 1984). This hypothesis that ASMP increased self-efficacy and that this increase was associated with improvements in pain was tested and demonstrated in subsequent research (Lorig et al., 1999).

The CDSMP RCT offered weekly workshops that taught skills useful for managing chronic diseases and conditions. The workshops were held in community settings such as senior centers, churches, libraries, and hospitals; participants met 2 1/2 hours per week for 6 weeks. The workshops were facilitated by two trained leaders, one or both of whom were non-health professionals with a chronic disease (Lorig et al., 1999). The topics covered in the workshops included: 1) techniques to deal with problems such as frustration, fatigue, pain and isolation, 2) appropriate exercises for strength, flexibility, and endurance, 3) appropriate use of medications, 4) communicating effectively with family, friends, and health professionals, 5) nutrition, 6) decision making, and, 7) how to evaluate new treatments (Lorig et al., 1999).

The Stanford study (Lorig et al., 1999) found that participants who took CDSMP, when compared to those who did not, demonstrated significant improvements in exercise, ability to do social and household activities, communication with physicians, self-reported general health, health distress, fatigue, and disabilities. They also spent fewer days in the hospital. There was a cost to savings ration of approximately 1:4 (Lorig et al., 1999).

From 2008 to 2010, the Healthy Aging Regional Collaborative in South Florida (Melchior et al., 2014) evaluated the effectiveness of CDSMP in a study at multiple agencies in community settings over a six-week period. Seven agencies delivered 108 CDSMP workshops at 81 sites in Broward, Miami-Dade, and Palm Beach Counties. Each weekly 2½-hour workshop was led by two trained instructors; there were a total of 94 instructors. The study comprised a total of 811 participants, who filled out surveys at baseline and at the end of the six-week intervention (Melchior et al., 2014). Topics covered during the 6-week CDSMP intervention included managing fear, anger, and depression; problem solving and decision making; exercise techniques; communication skills; and nutrition. At the end of each workshop, participants created an action plan with a specific weekly goal to be accomplished before the next workshop. Outcome measures included health behavior outcomes (exercise frequency and perceived level of interference in social and daily activities by chronic disease symptoms) and self-efficacy outcomes (self-confidence in ability to manage chronic disease adequately). The outcomes that showed statistically significant improvement included self-efficacy to manage disease ($p =.001$), self-efficacy to manage emotions ($p = .026$), time spent walking ($p = .008$), and perceived social/role activities limitations ($p = .001$). In sum, the intervention found that CDSMP was effective at improving self-efficacy, increasing physical activity, and decreasing perceived limitations in social and daily activities (Melchior et al., 2014).

In addition to improving health outcomes and lifestyle behaviors, CDSMP also has been shown to reduce medical costs (Anh et al., 2013; Ory et al., 2013). In a study of 1,170 community-dwelling CDSMP patients in 17 states, participants showed significant reductions in ER visits (5%) at the 6-month and 12-month follow up assessments, and in hospitalizations (3%) at 6 months (Anh et al., 2013). The researchers calculated that the potential net savings would be $364 per CDSMP participant (Anh et al., 2013). That equates to a national savings of $3.3 billion if 5% of adults with chronic conditions were offered the intervention (Anh et al., 2013).

The median age of the study participants was 65.4 years, a geriatric population (Ory et al., 2013). CDSMP has been replicated across the United States and is considered a state-of-the-art intervention for disease self-management (CDC, 2016).

The CDSMP model of chronic disease self-management has been adapted for use with consumers who suffer from chronic mental illnesses and disorders. The Health and Recovery Program (HARP) is a six-session intervention delivered by mental health peer leaders; its aim is to help participant become more effective managers of their chronic illnesses (Druss et al., 2010). The use of peer leaders is growing rapidly in the U.S. as an avenue to address concerns about elevated morbidity and premature mortality among those with chronic mental illnesses (Parks & Svedsen, 2006). Individuals with serious mental illness are at risk of developing a number of chronic medical conditions (Sokal, 2004; Carney et al., 2006; Carney & Jones, 2006).

Effectiveness of Specific Components of Disease Management Programs

Rather than advocating a specific disease management program, Pimouguet et al. (2011) sought to identify the effective components of disease management programs. Their rationale was as follows: "Because disease-management programs are heterogeneous, the effective components need to be identified to improve program implementation" (Pimouguet et al., 2011, E115). They further noted that there was no "consensual definition" of disease management. Pimouguet et al. (2011, p. E116) defined disease management as follows:

the ongoing and proactive follow-up of patients that includes at least two of the following five components: patient education (dietary and exercise counselling, self-monitoring, and knowledge of disease and medication); coaching (the disease manager encourages the patient to overcome psychological or social barriers that impede autonomy or improvement in medication compliance); treatment adjustment (the disease manager is able to start or modify treatment with or without prior approval from the primary care physician); monitoring (the disease manager gets medical data from the patient); and care coordination (the disease manager reminds the patient about upcoming appointments or important aspects of self-care and informs the primary care physician about complications, treatment adjustment or therapeutic recommendations).

Pimouguet et al.'s meta-analysis (2011) focused on disease management in patients with Type 1 and 2 diabetes mellitus. Only RCTs were included in the meta-analysis. The outcome measure evaluated was the impact of specific components of disease management programs on hemoglobin (A.sub.1C) levels. Forty-four studies met the inclusion criteria, but three had missing data on hemoglobin (A.sub.1C) at baseline and so were excluded, leaving a total of 41 RCTs in the meta-analysis. The trials were conducted between 1990 and 2009 and enrolled a total of 7013 participants. The RCTs were international; 26 trials were conducted in the U.S., five in Canada, three in Europe, and seven in Asia. The results showed that diabetes management programs had a clinically moderate but significant impact on hemoglobin (A.sub.1C) levels; effective components of the programs were a high frequency of patient contact and the ability for disease managers to adjust treatment with or without prior physician approval (Pimouguet et al., 2011). Further study might be useful in determining the effectiveness of specific disease management components with different diseases and for various subpopulations, in order to provide self-tailoring of CDSMP and other evidence-based self-management programs.

The following section discusses adjunctive non-pharmacologic therapies that can be used as part of an integrative approach to treatment. All of the modalities described below are evidence-based; it should be noted that they are not alternative, but rather, complementary treatments to be used under a physician's supervision.

Evidence-Based Non-Pharmacologic Complementary Therapies

Evidence-based integrative medicine includes non-pharmacologic complementary therapies that provide symptom relief. Memorial Sloan Kettering Cancer Center, a pioneer in complementary treatments, recommends the following safe, effective, evidence-based complementary modalities: 1) mind-body techniques (yoga, meditation, qi gong, tai chi, and relaxation techniques), 2) music therapy, 3) acupuncture, 4) diet and nutrition, including herbs, 5) physical activity, and 6) massage therapy (Bao, 2014). The six complementary modalities are displayed in Figure 1.

Complementary modalities can be used with older adults, but they need to be tailored to their specific needs; for example, the Integrative Medicine Institute of Memorial Sloan Kettering Cancer Center has a program, *65+*, for older adults with cancer. It is staffed by experts in geriatric medicine, rehab, nutrition, social work, pain, and palliative care. Five mind-body techniques are discussed in the following section.

Complementary modalities should not be confused with alternative therapies, which eschew traditional medical practices. Complementary, or integrative, therapies are rational and noninvasive and have demonstrated safety, value, and benefits (Deng & Cassileth, 2014).

A discussion of the six recommended complementary non-pharmacologic therapies follows. Increasingly, major medical centers are offering these therapies under the umbrella of an Integrative Institute, with all care supervised by a physician, who is part of a healthcare team.

Figure 1. Six evidence-based complementary modalities
Recommended by Memorial Sloan Kettering Cancer Center for disease management (Bao, 2014).

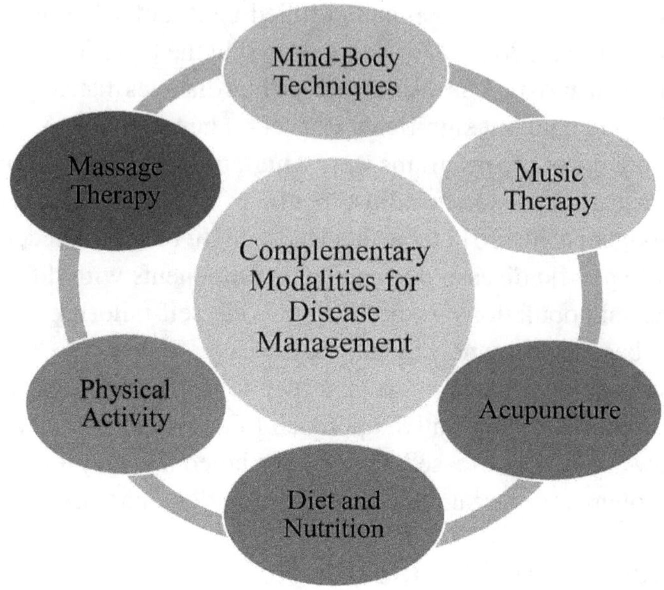

Mind-Body Techniques

Mind-body techniques reflect an integrative approach to health; the body influences the mind, and the mind, in turn, affects the functioning of the body. The evidence-based mind-body techniques used as complementary therapies in the treatment of chronic diseases such as cancer and heart disease are depicted in Figure 2.

Yoga

At Albert Einstein College of Medicine, a longitudinal research study on the effects of mind-body studies on cancer has focused on yoga. This randomized wait-list controlled study began in 2001. The yoga intervention in the Einstein study was developed for use with breast, lung and colorectal cancer patients by Dr. Chirag Shah, a U.S.-board certified oncologist and certified yoga instructor, in consultation with Integral Yoga expert Richard Sisco. The Yoga-based Cancer Rehabilitation Program served 240 patients between 2001 and 2009 (Moadel et. al., 2009). It comprised four components—warm up, yoga asanas (poses), pranayama (yogic breathing), and meditation. To avoid falls, all components were done either seated or laying down, with rests between each pose, and modifications added as needed for lymphedema, abdominal pain, fatigue, and anxiety. Props (mats, blankets, and

Figure 2. Evidence-based mind-body techniques used in disease management

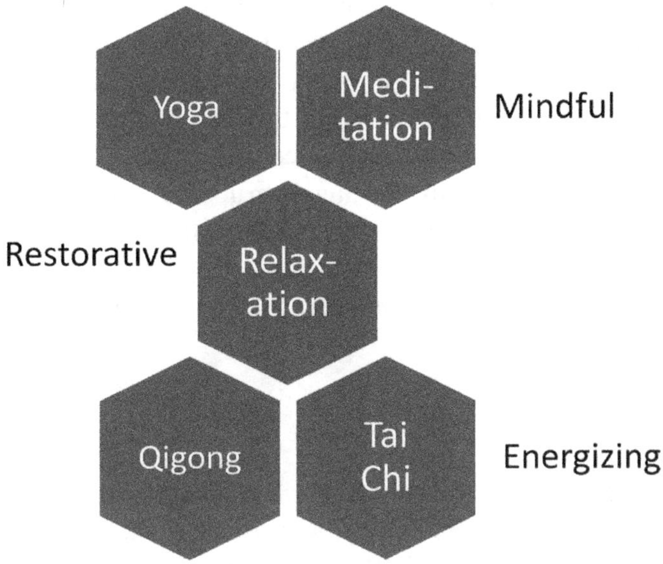

blocks) were used for support and to minimize pain (Moadel et al., 2009). Improved mood and decreased distress were found in the intervention group compared to the wait group; the intervention helped them to cope better (Moadel, 2010).

Lin et al. (2011) conducted a meta-analysis of RCTs evaluating the effects of yoga on psychological health, quality of life, and physical health of patients with cancer. Compared to the waitlist control groups, the yoga groups showed significantly greater improvements in psychological health: anxiety (P = .009), depression (P = .002), distress (P = .003), and stress (P = .006). However, due to the quality and small number of studies conducted, the findings have to be considered preliminary. More high-quality research using RCTs is needed.

Meditation

Mindfulness meditation is one of the most studied body-mind therapies. Mindfulness is defined as "a state of being attentive to and aware of what is taking place in the present" (Brown & Ryan 2003, p. 822). Mindfulness-based techniques enable an individual to be a detached observer of his or her thoughts, perceptions, and emotions; this detachment allows the person to respond to stressful events in an accepting, nonjudgmental manner (Michel et al., 2014). Mindfulness meditation is frequently offered as part of Mindfulness-Based Stress Reduction (MBSR), an eight-week program that includes mindfulness meditation, body scan, and yoga. Mindfulness-

Based Stress Reduction has been found to reduce anxiety and stress, and improve sleep and overall quality of life (Shennen et al., 2011; Ledesma & Kumano, 2009; Cramer et al., 2012b; Zainal et al., 2013; Piet et al., 2012).

Meditation that uses visualization is another complementary technique that is closely tied to the self-efficacy theory of Bandura and positive psychology. A cancer patient may visualize macrophages--cells that attack cancer cells--as blue elephants stomping on cancer cells, sucking them up into their trunks, and squirting them out and eliminating them from the body. Patients may spend up to two hours a day affirming that they can recover, visualizing the cancer being eliminated, and meditating to control the emotional arousal of the mind and create a state of calm equanimity (Barasch, 1994).

Qigong and Tai Chi

Qigong (also spelled ch'i kung) comprises two Chinese words: Qi, which means "life force" or "vital energy," and Gong, which means "accomplishment or skill cultivated through steady practice." The intention of qigong practice is "to restore, circulate, balance and/or enhance personal life energy" (Dunbar, 2015). When qigong is practiced by individuals to improve their own health and well-being, it is referred to as "internal qigong." When a certified qigong practitioner uses the principles of Traditional Chinese Medicine (TCM) to heal others, it is referred to as "external qigong" (Dunbar, 2015). Qigong is considered a form of moving meditation. Qigong developed in China about 5,000 years ago. It enhances healing of the body by improving the flow of energy, or qi (ch'i), along energy pathways known as meridians throughout the body. Acupuncture and acupressure also work on the meridians. In Chinese medicine, good health is believed to be the result of a free-flowing, well-balanced energy system; when vital energy flow is blocked, a systemic dysfunction occurs, and illnesses and disorders result. T'ai-chi ch'üan is a Chinese internal style martial art and exercise for relaxation, energy, and overall well-being. Tai chi, which is a flowing series of poses, grew out of qigong more recently—about 200 years ago.

Kelley and Kelley (2015) completed a systematic review of meta-analyses on meditative movement therapy (MMT) (yoga, tai chi, and qigong) and its effects on Health-Related Quality of Life (HRQOL) in adults. (For more about HRQOL, see Centers for Disease Control & Prevention, 2000). The Kelley and Kelley (2015) review included only randomized controlled trials for adults age 18 and over, and those in which the difference in HRQOL between the intervention group and control group was a primary outcome reported as the standardized mean difference (SMD) effect size. The studies that met the inclusion criteria included the following diseases and conditions: cancer, schizophrenia, low back pain, heart failure, and diabetes.

The percentile improvement in HRQOL between the intervention group and the control group by type of modality ranged from 9.9 to 48.9 for yoga (Buffart et al., 2012; Cramer et al., 2012a; Cramer et al., 2013a; Cramer et al., 2013b, Shneerson et al., 2013; Zhang et al., 2012), 25.8 to 42.1 for tai chi only (Pan et al., 2013), 21.9 and 46.3 for qigong only (Wang et al., 2013; Zeng et al., 2014), and 47.4 for tai chi and qigong combined (Zeng et al., 2014). The researchers believe this is the first such study examining the effects of MMT on HRQOL for RCTs. The researchers recommend that, based on their review findings, "it would appear both prudent and safe at this time to suggest that HRQOL may be improved by participating in MMT at least 3 times per week for about 71 minutes per session" (Kelley & Kelley, 2015). They recommend that further research be conducted, and that future studies include cost-effectiveness of the interventions as well as dose-response of the MMT and description of the specific type of MMT (e.g., specify form of yoga used).

Relaxation Techniques

One of the most commonly used complementary modalities for patients with chronic disease and disorders is relaxation techniques. They are used to improve well-being, relieve stress, and elevate mood. The term "relaxation response" was coined by Herbert Benson (Benson & Klipper, 1975/2001), a cardiologist at Harvard Medical School, to describe a physiological and psychological state that was evoked through meditative practices and that was the opposite of the fight or flight response elicited by a stressor. The relaxation response is characterized by

- Decreased metabolism, heart rate, blood pressure, and rate of breathing
- A "calming" in brain activity
- An increase in attention and decision-making functions of the brain
- Changes in gene activity that are the opposite of those associated with stress (Benson & Proctor, 2010)

The relaxation response may be elicited by sitting quietly, focusing on slow, deep breathing, and saying a calming word or sound associated with the person's belief system on each exhale. The mind should focus only on the breath and on relaxing. Research has shown the relaxation response to be effective with hypertension (Benson et al., 1974, Peters et al., 1977) and irregular heartbeat (Benson & Proctor, 2010). It does not require the agility of yoga practice or even the muscular control of progressive muscle relaxation, and so is suitable for frail seniors.

Reig-Ferrer et al.'s (2014) randomized controlled study of seniors in a nursing home was a trial of the effectiveness of Benson's relaxation response with an elderly population. Previous research (Kiecolt-Glaser et al., 2010) had shown that a

Jacobson-type muscle relaxation technique improved cellular immune competence in the elderly. Reig-Ferrer et al. (2014) wanted to achieve a similar effect without muscular effort, to accommodate elderly individuals who have muscle and joint disorders. They selected Benson's relaxation response, which has been shown to decrease stress (Esch et al., 2003) and anxiety, and to enhance cognitive performance in healthy aging (Galvin, 2006). Reig-Ferrer et al. (2014) evaluated the effects of this relaxation technique on psychological well-being and quality of life, biomedical variables, and immune changes of participants compared to a waitlist control group.

The intervention was two weeks, with a 3-month follow up. Reig-Ferrer et al. (2014) hypothesized that the relaxation technique would elevate psychological well-being, which would enhance immune functioning and enhance quality of life. Reig-Ferrer et al.'s (2014) RCT excluded anyone with health problems directly related to immune function or on drugs with significant effects on endocrine or immune function. The following biomedical measures were taken at the beginning of the intervention, 15 days after the intervention concluded, and three months after the intervention concluded: 1) clinical history, 2) functional assessment, using Katz Index of Activities of Daily Living, 3) weight, height, BMI, blood pressure and heart rate, 4) red and white blood cell counts, CBC, hemoglobin hematocryte, MCV, platelets, ESR, and 5) glucose, creatinine, urea, uric acid, lipids, AST, ALT, GGT, total proteins, and serum albumin. Psychological well-being was measured with the Satisfaction with Life Scale (SWLS) and Bradburn's Affect Balance Scale (ABS); Health-Related Quality of Life was measured using the Nottingham Health Profile (NHP) (Reig-Ferrer et al., 2014).

The Reig-Ferrer et al. (2014) trial was the first time a relaxation technique had been used in a nursing home in Spain and in which the psychological, biomedical and immunological measures were obtained. The aim was to test the Benson relaxation method as a psycho-gerontological intervention for enhancing well-being and immune parameters. The results showed a decrease in negative affect, psychological discomfort, and symptom perception in the treatment group, and improved quality of life. There were significant differences in immune parameters after the trial between the intervention group and waitlist group in CD19, CD71, CD97, CD134, and CD137 lymphocyte subpopulations. However, the sample size was very small and further research is needed with larger samples (Reig-Ferrer et al., 2014).

Prasad et al. (2010) administered a cross-sectional, point-of-care survey to patients attending the Cardiology Outpatient Clinic at Mayo Clinic in Rochester, Minnesota to document the use of complementary and alternative (CAM) therapies among patients with cardiovascular disease; the top four modalities used for heart-related symptoms were relaxation techniques, stress management, meditation, and guided imagery. A total of 23.9% of those surveyed reported using mind-body therapies for heart-related symptoms. Improvement in heart-related symptoms after using these therapies was reported by 22.2% for palpitations, 21.8% for sleep disturbance, 20.0% for chest pain, and 19.4% for leg swelling (Prasad et al., 2010).

COPD is a progressive disease associated with an abnormal inflammatory response of the lungs to noxious particles or gases (Volpato et al., 2015). Due to continuous exposure to risk factors and increases in life expectancy, COPD is expected to move from sixth to fourth cause of mortality and morbidity worldwide (Pauwels et al., 2001; Lopez et al., 2006; Murray & Lopez, 1997). Interventions aimed at COPD patients tend to focus on the physical aspects of the disease and to ignore the considerable anxiety, depression, and feelings of helplessness and powerlessness that often accompany the disease as it progresses (Karadag et al., 2008). Volpato et al. (2015) did a systematic review of the literature on the effect of relaxation techniques on anxiety, depression, quality of life, and percentage of Forced Expiratory Volume (FEV_1) in patients with COPD. FEV_1 is the maximal amount of air a person can forcefully exhale in one second. Volpato et al.'s (2015) review included only RCTs, and they had to focus on anxiety, depression, quality of life, and/or percentage of FEV_1. Volpato et al. (2015) found that relaxation techniques can have a moderate positive impact on psychological well-being and respiratory function; they believed that the results sustain the importance of relaxation techniques as a tool for managing COPD. Various relaxation techniques were used in the RCTs, including several different breathing techniques, singing, yoga, and tai chi. Volpati et al. (2015) noted the need for more high-quality research.

Music Therapy

The power of music to improve mood and emotions has been extolled by poets for centuries. Shakespeare put it this way: "If music be the food of love, play on" (Shakespeare, 1602/1623). Music therapy is the clinical and evidence-based use of music interventions by a credentialed professional to address the physical, emotional, cognitive, and social needs of patients (American Music Therapy Association, 2015). Music therapy may be used as part of a complementary medicine program in the context of an integrative approach to disease management. It is important to note that music therapy does NOT replace medical treatment; rather, it is an adjunctive therapy that supports patients by facilitating their coping with pain, anxiety, fear, and depression (Stanczyk, 2011). It is used to promote wellness, manage stress, alleviate pain, express feelings, enhance memory, improve communication, and promote physical rehabilitation (American Music Therapy Association, 2015). With oncology patients, music therapy focuses on the physiological and psychological needs of the patient, including anxiety about the future, fear of pain, and side effects from treatments (Stanczyk, 2011). Controlled trials have found that music therapy reduces anxiety (Salamon et al., 2003), stress, (Allen et al., 2001) depression, and pain (Good et al., 2002). Music therapy was also effective in reducing pain in oncology patients (Zimmerman et al., 1989).

Some cancer treatment centers have implemented drum circles for cancer survivors. At Albert Einstein College of Medicine, the Bronx Oncology Living Daily (BOLD) program offers free mind-body workshops to those in the local community affected by cancer as part of the Psychosocial Oncology program (Moadel, 2010). The BOLD drum circle helps patients to connect, get support, and feel empowered (Bongo therapy, 2011). The BOLD Program followed the model of integrative medicine at Memorial Sloan Kettering Cancer (MSKCC). At MSKCC, music therapy is used to calm agitation and distress, to lower blood pressure, and to help patients relax during difficult tests or procedures (Bao, 2014). Music therapy may be provided pre-treatment, during treatment, and after treatment. Researchers found that providing music therapy to patients prior to receiving radiation treatment decreased State-Trait anxiety and systolic blood pressure in cancer patients (Chen et al., 2013).

Acupuncture

Acupuncture was developed in China more than 3,000 years ago. Insertion of the needles into specific pressure points on the body stimulates the parasympathetic system and calms down the sympathetic nervous system. Acupuncture needles are regulated as a medical device in the United States; they are sterile, single-use, filiform, 32 gauge to 36 gauge, and 30 mm to 40 mm in length. The needle is inserted a few millimeters to a few centimeters into the skin. A typical treatment session lasts for 20 minutes to 40 minutes (Deng & Cassileth, 2014). Acupuncture has been shown to reduce pain (Vickers et al., 2012). Meta-analyses of acupuncture trials for four chronic pain conditions-- back and neck pain, osteoarthritis, chronic headache, and shoulder pain—have found significant effect sizes; acupuncture was superior to no acupuncture control and sham acupuncture, offering greater pain relief in all comparisons ($p<0.001$) (Vickers et al., 2012; Vickers & Linde, 2014). Acupuncture has also has been found to be effective in controlling chemotherapy-induced vomiting (Ezzo et al., 2005). In the hands of a licensed acupuncturist, acupuncture is very safe. Sterile needles are used, and they are disposed of after a single use. For those who cannot tolerate needles, acupressure is a needle-less alternative to acupuncture that uses the same pressure points but without needles (Bao, 2014).

Diet and Nutrition

There is an old saying, "You are what you eat." Making healthy food choices is free and should be easy to implement. However, Americans live in an obesogenic environment where fast food franchises such as McDonalds reign supreme, and where fatty fried foods and soda are the norm. Filmmaker Morgan Spurlock raised public consciousness about the dangers of consuming sugary soda and junk food with his 2004 film, *Supersize Me.* In the film, he ate nothing but McDonalds food for one month to document the adverse health consequences of such a diet. Spurlock pointed out that those marketing healthy food choices, such as the 5 A Day Fruit and Vegetable Campaign of the American Cancer Society, spent a mere $2 million a year on promotion, while McDonald's spent $1.4 billion on direct advertising and Hershey's spent $200 million (*Supersize Me*, 2004). Nevertheless, Spurlock's film did cause McDonald's to stop making Supersize fries; it also stopped frying potatoes in saturated fat after consumers sued McDonald's.

Heart disease is the number one killer in the United States today for both men and women; approximately 610,000 people die of heart disease in the United States every year–that's 1 in every 4 deaths (Centers for Disease Control and Prevention, 2015). More than half of older adults have hyperlipidemia and more than half have hypertension (Racine et al., 2011). Hyperlipidemia is a term that means there are elevated lipids (fats) in the blood; it refers primarily to cholesterol and triglycerides. Cholesterol is found primarily in saturated fat, which comes from animal products (meat, poultry, dairy). The American Heart Association (2015) recommends that adults reduce their consumption of saturated fat to no more than 5 to 6 percent of total calories. For a person who eats 2,000 calories a day, that's about 11 to 13 grams of saturated fat. Trans fat is another source of cholesterol that should be reduced; trans fat causes double trouble, as it raises LDL (low density lipoproteins, the "bad" cholesterol, and lowers HDL (high density lipoproteins, the "good" cholesterol). A person with hyperlipidemia should consult a doctor for medical treatment of the condition. However, medication alone is not sufficient; lifestyle factors are very important. Making healthy diet choices and getting an adequate amount of exercise are important steps in lowering high cholesterol, even if a person is on a statin (American Heart Association, 2015).

Hypertension refers to high blood pressure, defined as a diastolic blood pressure of 90 or above and a systolic blood pressure of 140 or above. High systolic blood pressure is a major risk factor for cardiovascular disease for people 50+ years old. Systolic blood pressure tends to rise with age due to increasing stiffness of large arteries, long-term build-up of plaque, and increased incidence of cardiac and vascular disease (American Heart Association, 2015). The American Heart Association recommends eating a healthy diet low in sodium, exercising regularly, maintaining a healthy weight, managing stress, and avoiding tobacco smoke to prevent hypertension. Regular consumption of green tea also may reduce the risk of hypertension (Yang et al., 2004, Cassileth, 2011).

Once diagnosed with hypertension, your physician may prescribe medication; however, the recommended lifestyle factors should still be followed (American Heart Association, 2015). The National Heart, Lung, and Blood Institute (2015) recommends that adults with risk factors for heart disease, including age 50+, elevated lipids, hypertension, smoking, and a family history, follow the Dietary Approach to Stop Hypertension (DASH) diet. The Dash diet reduces intake of saturated fat, total fat, sodium, and cholesterol, increases intake of fruits and vegetables, and increases consumption of potassium, calcium, magnesium, fiber, and protein. The DASH diet has been found to be effective in reducing blood pressure in adults (Appel et al., 1997; Blumenthal et al., 2010; Dickinson et al., 2006; Elmer et al., 2006). The DASH eating plan goals for a 2,000-calorie-a-day diet are shown in Table 1.

A high-fat, low-fiber diet is a key factor in the current epidemic of Type 2 diabetes mellitus (T2DM) in the U.S. and other countries. It is estimated that 23.6 million people have diabetes (about 20% of those are undiagnosed) in the United States; T2DM represents about 90 to 95 percent of cases of diagnosed diabetes. One-quarter of American adults 65 and over have diabetes (American Diabetes Association, 2015). In other countries, the highest prevalence rates of T2DM are in indigenous peoples who have experienced rapid change in their lifestyle (Venn & Mann, 2004). In the next 20 years, the greatest number of cases of T2DM are predicted to occur

Table 1. Daily and weekly DASH eating plan goals for a 2,000-calorie-a-day diet

Food Group	Daily Servings
Grains	6–8
Meats, poultry, and fish	6 or less
Vegetables	4–5
Fruit	4–5
Low-fat or fat-free dairy products	2–3
Fats and oils	2–3
Sodium	2,300 mg*
	Weekly Servings
Nuts, seeds, dry beans, and peas	4–5
Sweets	5 or less

*1,500 milligrams (mg) sodium lowers blood pressure even further than 2,300 mg sodium daily.

Source: National Heart, Lung, and Blood Institute. National Institutes of Health, U.S. Department of Health & Human Services.

in China and India. Diabetes is a chronic disease; its effective management is "a constant juggling act" that requires careful attention to medication dosing, eating, activity, and other variables (DiMeglio, 2013). Unlike Type 1 diabetes, which appears in childhood, T2DM has an onset in adulthood.

Diabetes mellitus is a metabolic disorder characterized by hyperglycemia, insulin resistance and insulin insufficiency; living with diabetes elevates the risk of heart disease and can lead to long-term complications such as neuropathy, retinopathy, and nephropathy. A common sight in America today is middle-aged and older adults in wheelchairs missing one or both legs from amputations due to complications from diabetes. All of the health problems attendant to diabetes decrease quality of life and increase risk of mortality (American Diabetes Association, 2015; Constantino et al., 2013; Santaguida et al, 2005).

Dietary management of a case of presumed diabetes was first documented in 1500 B.C., with the recommendation that the patient consume wheat grains, grapes, honey, and berries (Leeds, 1979). Many other dietary prescriptions were tried between then and 1921, when insulin was discovered. The Food and Agriculture Organization (FAO) of the World Health Organization (WHO) recommends a diabetes-prevention diet in which the bulk of carbohydrates consumed are rich in nonstarch polysaccharides and have a low glycemic index (GI), with liberal intake of cereals, vegetables, legumes, and fruits (FAO/WHO, 1998). Diabetes organizations in many countries, including Australia, the United Kingdom, the United States, and continental Europe, have endorsed the dietary recommendations of the FAO/WHO for prevention of T2DM as well as for treatment of both types I and II diabetes mellitus (Venn & Mann, 2004).

The development of T2DM is associated with a number of risk factors (Venn & Mann, 2004):

- Excess energy intake, leading to obesity
- High intakes of saturated and trans fats
- High intakes of fiber-depleted refined grain foods
- Lack of physical exercise

Medical nutrition therapy (MNT) is an important component of management of diabetes management. A registered dietician can help set up a menu for diabetic patients. People with diabetes are advised to avoid fried and fatty foods, and processed, refined carbohydrates, which have high advanced glycation end products (AGEs); foods with high AGEs can increase chronic inflammation and contribute to heart disease and other complications from diabetes (Weisenberger, 2014). A review of the literature on nutrition management of type II diabetes mellitus (T2DM) found strong support for the high intake of whole grain foods being a protective factor against the development of type II diabetes mellitus (T2DM). Adults who consumed approximately three servings per day of whole grain foods were less likely to develop T2DM than were low consumers (<3 servings per week), with a risk reduction of 20%-30% (Venn & Mann, 2004). Mirmiran et al. (2014) recommend consuming a whole-grain diet of functional foods to manage T2DM. They note that previous studies have shown that dietary carbohydrate modification in patients with metabolic syndrome has had favorable results, including increased insulin sensitivity and decreased adipocyte cell size (Laaksonen et al., 2005; Kallio et al., 2007). Mirmiran et al. (2014) propose a novel approach to NMI, one that makes functional foods-- especially whole grains, phytochemical-rich fruits and vegetables, legumes, nuts, dairy products, green tea and some spices--a required component of a health-promoting diet for diabetic patients. Bioactive compounds in whole grain foods (e.g., rye, oatmeal, barley, brown rice) have shown promise in regulating glycemic response, increasing insulin sensitivity, improving pancreatic β-cell functions, and increasing insulin secretion (Rosén et al., 2009; Shen et al., 2011). The American Diabetes Association recommends the Mediterranean diet, which is rich in whole grains, vegetables, legumes, nuts and seeds, and fruits; it uses heart-healthy monounsaturated olive oil and polyunsaturated oil (from nuts and seeds) rather than saturated fat Neithercott, 2014).

Herb and dietary supplements are a commonly used complementary modality in the self-management of many chronic diseases and conditions. The Memorial Sloan Kettering Cancer Center (MSKCC) Integrative Medicine website provides an extensive listing of herbs, botanicals, and other supplements used as adjunctive therapy for cancer treatment (MSKCC Integrative Medicine, 2015). In addition, MSKCC's Bendheim Integrative Medicine Center offers Nutritional and Dietary-Supplement Counseling for its on patients and for those in the community (MSKCC Bendheim Integrative Medicine Center, 2015).

Caution should be used in taking herbs and other dietary supplements as an adjunctive treatment for disease management; since they are not regulated substances, their quality and strength may vary. In addition, they may interact with medications and other medical treatments. An integrative approach to treatment is recommended, with the healthcare provider supervising all dietary supplements to make sure that there are no harmful side effects or drug interactions.

Physical Activity

Physical activity is a leading health indicator for our nation (*Healthy People 2020*). Getting regular physical activity that meets the federal guidelines (*Healthy People 2020*) is critical to maintaining a healthy weight. In 2012, half of adults age 18 and over met the guidelines for aerobic physical activity (at least 150 minutes per week of moderate physical activity, or 75 minutes per week of vigorous physical activity, or an equivalent combination). The levels of aerobic physical activity varied by gender: more adult males (53.8%) than females (46.5%) met the federal guidelines. The levels also varied by race; the number of non-Hispanic white adults who met the federal guidelines for aerobic physical activity was nearly one and a half times that of both Hispanic/Latino adults and non-Hispanic black adults. For adults with activity limitations, only 30.5% met the federal guidelines for aerobic physical activity, versus 53.9% of adults without activity limitations. All of the percentages are age-adjusted. (*Healthy People, 2020*).

Encouraging Americans to get regular exercise is a key factor in the fight against obesity. We live in an obesogenic environment that has produced an epidemic of obesity: more than one-third of American adults and 17% of youth are obese, with a Body Mass Index (BMI) of 30 or greater (Ogden et al., 2014). Among non-Hispanic Blacks and Hispanics, the age-adjusted prevalence rates of obesity are 47.8% and 42.5%, respectively. Obesity rates vary with age; prevalence is 39.5% among adults aged 40-59 years old. Obesity is a risk factor for heart disease, diabetes, stroke, and cancer. The fight against obesity comprises two main components: 1) changing eating habits to include high-fiber, low-fat items; and 2) increasing the level of physical activity.

Increasing one's level of physical activity aids in weight management. In addition, meeting the federal guidelines for aerobic physical activity reduces the risk of cardiovascular disease, (Wannamethee & Shaper, 2001; Sesso et al., 2000), ischemic stroke (Hu et al., 2000; Gorelick et al., 1999; Wannamethee & Shaper, 1999), T2DM (Hu et al., 2001; Pfohl & Schatz, 2001; Fulton-Kehoe et al., 2001), colon cancer (Brownson et al., 1991; Giovannucci et al., 1995), osteoporosis (Kohrt et al., 1995), depression (Fox, 1999; Camacho et al., 1991; Weyerer, 1992), and fall-related injuries (Meyer et al., 1993; Jaglal, 1993).

The first step in physical activity participation among adults is being knowledgeable about the benefits of physical activity. Once adults are aware that getting adequate physical activity is likely to lengthen their life and to reduce their risk for heart disease, ischemic stroke, diabetes, cancer, osteoporosis, depression, and fall-related injuries, they should be motivated to exercise, right? Unfortunately, knowledge alone may not be sufficient to facilitate physical activity. In the Dallas Heart Study, a 7-year longitudinal study of cardiovascular health in a multi-ethnic adult population, participants were asked about their physical activity and health beliefs (Mathieu et al., 2012). A whopping 94% of participants felt that physical activity was effective in preventing a heart attack; yet only 46% of Hispanics, 59% of African-Americans, and 78% of Whites participated in physical activity. Whites had higher rates of participation in physical activity than did African-Americans or Hispanics. Lack of physical activity was associated with higher cardiovascular mortality overall and among African Americans in particular. The researchers concluded that there were other ethnic-specific factors that required further study (Mathieu et al., 2012).

The second step in physical activity participation among adults is health promotion, including counselling, to encourage physical activity. In the Netherlands, chronically ill patients pay regular visits to their family practitioner to monitor their disease; during the visit the practice nurse provides lifestyle counseling. The most common type of promotion is verbal advice, followed by print and computer-based interventions. It is not clear which type of exercise promotion works best in the long term (Foster et al., 2005). One method that shows great promise is computer-based patient self-management programs such as mHealth (mobile phone Apps) and other E-health applications, which facilitate patient self-management (McDermott & While, 2013).

Verwey et al. (2014a) developed a smartphone physical activity App, called *It's Life*, embedded in a Self-management Support Program (SSP). They are testing the tool and the SSP in a randomized controlled trial of participants who have been diagnosed with either COPD or T2DM. The trial has three arms: the use of a monitoring and feedback tool embedded in the SSP (group 1), the SSP without the tool (group 2), and usual care (group 3). The participants are 40-70 years old, in primary care, and do not comply with national standards of physical activity (Verwey et al., 2014a). The primary outcome measure is physical activity in daily life, and the hypothesis is that the intervention group will increase their physical activity compared to the control group. The secondary outcome measures are self-efficacy (measured by General Self-Efficacy Scale and Exercise Self-Efficacy Scale (Everett et al., 2009)), quality of life (measured by SF-36), and health status (measured by Diabetes Symptom checklist-revised for T2DM participants and Chronic Respiratory Questionnaire for COPD participants). The trial began with a pre-measurement period during which time participants got used to wearing and entering comments on their accelerometer (part of the tool). They received two sessions about barriers, facilitators, and activity planning, with the aim of modifying factors known to influence physical activity, such as social support and self-efficacy (Verwey et al., 2014a). After two weeks, patient and nurse set a goal of physical activity per day; then the patient received feedback in the form of tips, encouragement, rewards, suggestions—all written in a positive tone.

***In the pilot study, a positive trend was seen for use of the tool; the mean level of physical activity increased by more than 10 minutes per day and patients reported a higher quality of life (Verwey et al., 2014b). The results of the longitudinal RCT, when completed, should yield valuable data on how to increase physical activity for patients suffering from serious chronic illnesses.*

Massage Therapy

In the Who's rock opera, *Tommy*, the protagonist sings "See me, feel me, touch me, heal me!" Touch is healing; it may be vital to survival at an early stage in life. In the 1940s, psychoanalyst Rene A. Spitz studied child development. He observed that infants in foundling homes who were well fed and warm but not held or touched, tended to wither and die. Of 91 babies he observed, 27 died in infancy, followed by seven more in their second year of life; in some foundling homes, up to 90 percent of the babies died in early infancy (Cassileth & Vickers, 2004). Human touch was needed for proper development. Therapeutic massage relaxes muscular tension. When licensed massage therapists work with chronically ill patients, special training is recommended to enable them to work on patients safely and effectively (Miner, 2007). Therapeutic massage with oncology patients reduces pain and anxiety, and improves quality of life; it also has been shown to reduce chemo-induced nausea and vomiting (Calenda, 2006; Bao, 2014). The use of therapeutic massage in cancer centers and hospitals in increasing. Massage has a positive effect on the body's biochemistry, increasing the neurotransmitter dopamine, the lymphocytes, and the natural killer cells (Calenda, 2006).

Healing Touch is another complementary therapeutic modality used by many nurses and health providers today. It is a form of massage that involves only light touching or stroking. The Healing Touch practitioner works on the patient's energy field surrounding his or her body, rather than directly on the muscles themselves. Healing Touch is a good choice of modality for frail patients, as it is gentle but penetrating. It was first offered as a continuing education program for nurses in the 1980s. The principle behind Healing Touch is promoting well-being through work with the energy system of the body (Mentgen, 2002). It is used in the U.S. and around the world at outpatient pain centers, in private practices, and in operating rooms.

Wardell and Weymouth (2004) did a systematic review of studies using Healing Touch with chronically ill patients. In their review of the literature on Healing Touch, Wardell and Weymouth (2004) categorized studies by disease or disorder. Nine of the studies of Healing Touch used the modality for chronic pain relief; three studies used Healing Touch with cancer patients for functional status, well-being, mood, fatigue, blood pressure, and pain; four studies used Healing Touch to improve immune system functioning; three used the modality on patients who had had cardiovascular procedures or were critical ill with CV disease; five studies were with elderly dementia patients; four studies were with mentally ill patients (depression, PTSD, anxiety, chronically stressed); two were in theoretical areas, and one was in pediatrics (Wardell & Weymouth, 2004). Seven of the nine pain studies showed decreased pain with Healing Touch, and an eighth showed a decrease when reflexology and Healing Touch were used together. The cancer studies showed that both massage therapy and Healing Touch were more effective in reducing pain, fatigue, and blood pressure in chemotherapy patients than was Caring Presence or standard care alone. Among the elderly who received Healing Touch, compared to the control group, the intervention group improved significantly on all ten behavioral items (appetite, sleep, freedom from pain, orientation, compliance with daily routine, socialization, emotional stability, nonverbal responses, conversational communication, and freedom from jargon). Elderly dementia patients who were given Healing Touch three times a week for four weeks showed significant decreases in agitation. Outcomes from the studies with elderly adults were positive; the intervention groups showed enhanced appetite, improved sleep, and reduced pain; worry and outbursts were decreased. Functional ability and compliance with daily routines increased. The other areas studied had limited or inconclusive results.

In sum, Healing Touch is supported for use with older adults. Further study with larger sample sizes and rigorous methods is needed to replicate these finding, which show great promise for use of Healing Touch for pain relief, as an adjunctive therapy with cancer treatment, and with elderly patients suffering from dementia (Wardell & Weymouth, 2004).

SUMMARY: USE OF NON-PHARMACOLOGIC COMPLEMENTARY MODALITIES

In conclusion, the use of non-pharmacologic complementary modalities as an adjunctive treatment in chronic disease self-management can significantly enhance patients' quality of life, reduce symptoms, relieve stress, and give much-needed support. The main complementary modalities that have been shown to be effective with cancer and other chronic diseases are 1) mind-body techniques (yoga, meditation, relaxation techniques, qigong, and tai chi), 2) music therapy, 3) acupuncture, 4) diet and nutrition, 5) physical activity, and 6) massage therapy. Participation in complementary modalities must be done under the supervision of a physician. All complementary practitioners must have undergone special training to deal safely and effectively with a frail, sick, and aging patient population. Increasingly, complementary therapies are being offered by major medical centers through their own Integrative Medicine Institutes, which facilitates smooth coordination of care.

AGING AND CHRONIC DISEASE

In 2010, there were 40 million adults age 65 or over in the United States, accounting for 13% of the population (U.S. Census Bureau, 2010). By 2030, the adult population 65 and over is expected to grow to 72 million, or almost 20% of the total population

(Federal Interagency Forum on Aging-Related Statistics, 2012). In *Older Americans 2012: Key Indicators of Well-Being,* the Federal Interagency Forum (Forum) on Aging-Related Statistics (2012) describes the condition of U.S. adults aged 65 and over using 37 indicators in the following five broad areas:

- Population
- Economics
- Health status
- Health risks and behaviors
- Health care

Three of the five areas involve health, which reflects the national concern over the skyrocketing costs of healthcare for an aging elderly population.

The report compiles data from more than a dozen federal agencies to construct broad indicators of well-being for adults 65 and over. The report forecasts increasing numbers of older women in the workforce, declining poverty rates, increasing housing problems, increasing obesity, and increasing use of hospice. A natural consequence of aging is a decline in the immune response, which renders a person more susceptible to disease (Panda et al., 2009). Almost half of all Americans have at least one chronic disease; 31.5% of Americans suffer from multiple chronic conditions (MCC) (Gerteis et al., 2014. Prevalence of MCC increases with age; 80% of adults 65 and over suffer from MCC. The healthcare costs of MCC are staggering; 71% of all healthcare spending in the U.S. goes towards treating people with MCC (Gerteis et al., 2014). Chronic diseases/health conditions for adults 65 and over in the United States are listed in Table 2.

The leading causes of death for Americans 65 and over in 2009 were heart disease, cancer, and chronic respiratory diseases, followed by stroke and Alzheimers Disease. From 1998 until 2006, stroke was the third leading cause of death, but it was surpassed in 2008 by chronic respiratory diseases and fell to fourth place. Deaths from Alzheimers disease climbed from 1998 to 2009, surpassing deaths from influenza/pneumonia and diabetes in 2003 to become the fifth leading cause of mortality for adults 65 and over (Federal Interagency Forum on Age-Related Statistics, 2012). Almost a quarter of adults 65 and over reported being in fair or poor health, and 13.7% reported suffering from clinical depression.

Dietary adequacy was assessed using 12 components from the total Healthy Eating Index-2005 score. The total score was 67 out of 100, or poor. The lowest ratings were for dark green and orange vegetables and legumes (36), whole grains (34), and sodium (33). Given the dietary recommendations for a Mediterranean diet low in sodium and high in vegetables, legumes, and whole grains, the diet was far from adequate (Federal Interagency Forum on Age-Related Statistics, 2012). Diet quality for adults aged 65 and over is shown in Table 3.

Table 2. Chronic health conditions: Percentage of people age 65 and over who reported having selected chronic health conditions, by sex and race and Hispanic origin, 2009–2010

	Heart Disease	Hyperten-sion	Stroke	Asthma	Chronic Bronchitis or Emphysema	Any Cancer	Diabetes	Arthritis
Total	30.4	55.9	8.6	11.3	10.3	24.0	20.5	51.2
Men	36.9	54.1	9.1	9.7	9.6	27.6	23.5	44.8
Women	25.5	57.2	8.2	12.5	10.8	21.2	18.2	56.1
Non-Hispanic White	32.1	54.2	8.5	11.3	10.9	26.9	18.0	52.6
Non-Hispanic Black	25.1	69.2	11.7	11.5	8.4	13.9	31.6	51.0
Hispanic	22.2	57.2	7.2	11.1	7.1	10.4	32.5	43.8

Note: Data are based on a 2-year average from 2009-2010. See data sources for the definition of race and Hispanic origin in the National Health Interview Survey.

Source: Federal Interagency Forum on Age-Related Statistics (compiled from CDC, National Center for Health Statistics, National Health Interview Survey).

Although physical activity level for adults 65 and over increased from 1998 to 2010, it still was very low; only 5.5% of senior adults met the federal guidelines for physical activity (Federal Interagency Forum on Age-Related Statistics, 2012). Physical activity levels for adults 65 and over are shown in Table 4.

IMPLICATIONS FOR HEALTHY AGING

The population in the United States is aging. People are living longer, and many—especially women—are working longer. With most infectious diseases under control in the U.S. (STDs are an exception), disease management is largely about chronic conditions. People's expectations have changed, too. Television commercials advertise sexual aids for seniors, along with a host of products to make older adults feel, look, and act younger. Healthy Aging isn't about cosmetic surgery and botox, however; it is about adopting healthy lifestyle habits, especially making healthy dietary choices, exercising regularly, avoiding tobacco, and practicing stress management. Depression, anxiety, fear, and feelings of helplessness often follow a diagnosis of a chronic disease such as cancer or COPD. Complementary therapies such as yoga, meditation, qigong, tai chi, and relaxation techniques can be helpful in reducing negative affect and distress, and in enhancing feelings of well-being. Massage therapy (including Healing Hands), acupuncture, and qigong can provide effective non-pharmacologic pain relief.

Table 3. Diet quality: Average diet scores, population age 65 and over, by age group, 2007–2008

	Age		
	65 and Under	**65-74**	**75 and Over**
Total Healthy Eating Index-2005 Score	67	66	67
Adequacy Components			
Total fruit	90	86	94
Whole fruit	100	100	100
Total vegetables	84	86	82
Dark green and orange vegetables and legumes	36	36	35
Total grains	100	100	100
Whole grains	34	32	37
Milk	60	58	63
Meat and beans	100	100	100
Oils	75	77	73
Moderation Components			
Saturated fat	60	59	63
Sodium	33	32	35
Solid fats, alcoholic beverages, added sugar	59	59	59

Note: The Healthy Eating Index-2005 (HEI-2005) has 12 components, and a higher score indicates a higher quality diet. The moderation components (e.g., sodium) are scored in reverse; i.e., excessively high intakes get 0 percent and as intakes decrease towards the standard, scores increase up to 100 percent.

Reference population: These data refer to the resident noninstitutionalized population.

Source: Federal Interagency Forum for Age-Related Statistics (compiled from multiple agencies).

It is estimated that one-third of Americans—about 100 million people—experience chronic pain, and 5 to 8 million of them treat it with opioid drugs (National Institute on Drug Abuse, 2015). Opioids are highly addictive, and opioid abuse is rampant. In 2012, more than 259 million prescriptions were written in the U.S. for opioid painkillers such as Vicodin and OxyContin. That amounts to one bottle of pain pills for every U.S. adult. In 2011, 17,000 people died from prescription painkiller overdoses (National Institute on Drug Abuse, 2015). There is a safe, healthy alternative to opioids for pain. Research has shown that use of complementary modalities such as acupuncture, massage therapy, qigong, and music therapy aid in pain relief and should be incorporated into disease management plans for patients who experience chronic pain. Even medically fragile seniors can benefit from music therapy and Healing Hands, or learn MBSR or Benson's relaxation technique; none of these modalities requires physical strength or agility.

Table 4. Percentage of people age 45 and over who reported participating in leisure-time aerobic and muscle-strengthening activities that meet the 2008 Federal physical activity guidelines, by age group, 1998–2010.

Year	45-64	65	65-74	75-84	85 and Over
1998	11.4	5.5	7.0	3.9	2.0
1999	11.9	5.9	7.7	4.5	0.9
2000	12.8	6.9	8.4	5.7	1.9
2001	13.1	6.7	7.7	6.1	3.1
2002	14.2	7.1	8.8	5.8	2.1
2003	14.6	7.6	9.2	6.7	2.9
2004	14.0	7.8	9.7	6.4	3.5
2005	14.4	7.9	10.5	5.7	3.0
2006	13.8	7.5	9.1	6.5	3.0
2007	15.0	7.9	9.5	6.6	4.1
2008	16.3	9.5	11.3	9.3	2.3
2009	16.9	10.0	12.8	7.9	2.8
2010	17.8	10.5	13.6	7.3	4.0

Note: The measure reflects the 2008 Federal Physical Activity Guidelines for Americans to perform 1) at least 150 minutes a week of moderate-intensity or 75 minutes a week of vigorous-intensity aerobic physical activity, and 2) moderate- to high-intensity muscle-strengthening activities for major muscle groups at least two days a week. The measure shows the percentage who met both guidelines.

Reference population: These data refer to the resident noninstitutionalized population.

Source: Federal Interagency Forum on Age-Related Statistics (compiled from CDC, National Center for Health Statistics, National Health Interview Survey).

When assessing an older patient for a disease management plan, the CDSMP model is useful; it has been effective with both physical and mental health conditions. An integrative approach that incorporates evidence-based non-pharmacologic complementary modalities has been found to improve health outcomes. In our high-tech age, with new drugs coming out every few months, it is tempting to rely on medication as the first and primary defense against chronic disease. Even the most effective medications have some side effects, especially after long-term use. It is wise to keep in mind the old medical dictum, "To do no harm." It might take a little longer to train a patient to learn MBSR or a Benson relaxation technique than it does to pop a pill, but in the end, it is worth the effort. It saves money and reduces potential harm to the patient.

CONCLUSION

Disease is a function of interaction among three entities—host, agent, and environment. Self-management of chronic diseases deals primarily with the host and the environment. For example, to manage the host (mind-body), a patient with T2DM follows a healthy low-fat, low-sodium, non-AGE diet, exercises moderately, avoids tobacco and alcohol, and monitors blood sugar and insulin therapy, all under physician supervision. To manage the environment, a person suffering from asthma or COPD avoid triggers such as pet dander or industrial pollutants that might provoke an exacerbation. Self-management of chronic diseases is a growing concern for both patients and healthcare providers. The CDSMP model reminds us that "one size does not fit all." A detailed needs assessment of each group and topic is recommended to help the supervising physician tailor the CDSMP for each patient. The problem-solving model of CDSMP is useful in identifying the underlying issue that is bothering the patient. After identifying the issue, the provider can help the patient to make decisions about daily activities, such as how much exercise is enough for a given session, or whether a pain in the lumbar spine is a severe enough to call the doctor. The patient and doctor form a partnership, or management team. The doctor provides the patient with knowledge about his or her conditions and steers the patient toward resources to support self-management.

To persevere at self-management, patients need to believe in themselves and their ability to take care of the multi-faceted job of management, including following dietary and exercise recommendations, avoiding tobacco, and practicing some form of relaxation, meditation, or stress-reduction technique to deal with the emotional toll of living with a chronic disease. This self-efficacy should be coupled with a positive psychology outlook that sees things from an optimistic point of view.

There are many medical and complementary therapy websites that offer patients free information on their specific conditions. *Caveat emptor* (buyer beware) of infomercials that are selling supplements, not health promotion. Major medical centers and research studies recommend sticking to safe, evidence-based complementary modalities. Before using any complementary modality, patients should ask their supervising doctor about it to make sure that it is safe and appropriate. Alternative treatments may be harmful, interacting with medical treatments.

The last century saw enormous medical advances, with the life expectancy increasing 60%, the development of antibiotics, organ transplants, and artificial limbs. Who knows what the next century will bring? We may see paralyzed patients walk, artificial skin on burn victims, and a life expectancy of 120 years. Health-related quality of life should to continue to improve in the U.S. thanks to the information revolution on the Internet and social media, advances in medical technology and electronic record-keeping, and proactive patient self-management of health conditions.

REFERENCES

Agarwal, M., Dalal, A., Agarwal, D., & Agarwal, R. (1995). Positive life orientation and recovery from myocardial infarction. *Social Science & Medicine*, *40*(1), 125–130. doi:10.1016/0277-9536(94)E0058-Z PMID:7899916

Allen, K., Golden, L. H., Izzo, J. L. Jr, Ching, M. I., Forrest, A., Niles, C. R., ... Barlow, J. C. (2001). Normalization of hypertensive responses during ambulatory surgical stress by perioperative music. *Psychosomatic Medicine*, *63*(3), 487–492. doi:10.1097/00006842-200105000-00019 PMID:11382277

American Diabetes Association. (2015). Making healthy food choices. Retrieved from: http://www.diabetes.org/food-and-fitness/food/what-can-i-eat/making-healthy-food-choices/?loc=ff-slabnav

American Heart Association. (2015). Prevention and treatment of high blood pressure. Retrieved from: www.heart.org/HEARTORG/Conditions/HighBloodPressure/PreventionTreatmentofHighBloodPressure

American Music Therapy Association (AMTA). (2015). About Music Therapy & AMTA. Silver Spring, MD: AMTA. Retrieved from http://www.musictherapy.org/about/musictherapy/

Americans with Disabilities Act (ADA). (1990). Washington, D.C.: U.S. Department of Justice.

Ángeles Ruiz, M.; Sanjuan, P.; Pérez-García, A.M.; Rueda, B.& (2011). Relations between life satisfaction, adjustment to illness, and emotional distress in a sample of men with ischemic cardiopathy. *Spanish Journal of Psychology*, 14(1), 356.

Anh, S., Basu, R., Smith, M. L., Jiang, L., Lorig, K., Whitelaw, N., & Ory, M. G. (2013). The impact of chronic disease self-management programs: Healthcare savings through a community-based intervention. *BMC Public Health*, *13*(1), 1141. doi:10.1186/1471-2458-13-1141 PMID:24314032

Appel, L.J., Moore, T.J., Obarzanek, E., Vollmer, W.M., Svetkey, L.P., Sacks, F.M., Bray, G.A., Vogt, T.M., Cutler, J.A., & Windhauser, M.M., Lin-P-H, & Karanja, N. (1997). A clinical trial of the effects of dietary patterns on blood pressure. *N ENlg. Journal of Medicine*, *336*, 1117–1124.

Bandura, A. (1977). Self-efficacy: Toward a unifying theory of behavioral change. *Psychological Review*, *84*(2), 191–215. doi:10.1037/0033-295X.84.2.191 PMID:847061

Bandura, A. (1982). Self-efficacy mechanism in human agency. *The American Psychologist, 37*(2), 122–147. doi:10.1037/0003-066X.37.2.122

Bandura, A. (1989). Human agency in social cognitive theory. *The American Psychologist, 44*(9), 1175–1184. doi:10.1037/0003-066X.44.9.1175 PMID:2782727

Bandura, A. (1991). Social-cognitive theory of self-regulation. *Organizational Behavior and Human Decision Processes, 50*(2), 179–211. doi:10.1016/0749-5978(91)90022-L

Bao, T. (2014). Integrative oncology: 65+ workshop. Treating symptoms & improving well- being. Memorial Sloan Kettering Cancer Center. Retrieved from: https://www.mskcc.org/cancer-care/treatments/symptom-management/integrative- medicine.

Barasch, M. I. (1994). The amazing power of visualization. *Natural Health, 24*(4), 64.

Benson, H., & Klipper, M. (1975/2001). *The relaxation response*. New York: HarperCollins.

Benson, H., & Proctor, W. (2010). *Relaxation revolution: Enhancing your personal health through the science and genetics of mind body healing*. New York: Scribner.

Benson, H., Rosner, B. A., Marzetta, B. R., & Klemchuk, H. M. (1974). Decreased blood pressure in pharmacologically treated hypertensive patients who regularly elicited the relaxation response. *Lancet, 303*(7852), 289–291. doi:10.1016/S0140-6736(74)92596-3 PMID:4130474

Blumenthal, J. A., Babyak, M. A., Hinderliter, A., Watkins, L. L., Craighead, L., Lin, P.-H., ... Sherwood, A. (2010). Effects of the DASH diet alone and in combination with exercise and weight loss on blood pressure and cardiovascular biomarkers in men and women with high blood pressure: The ENCORE study. *Archives of Internal Medicine, 170*(2), 126–135. doi:10.1001/archinternmed.2009.470 PMID:20101007

Bongo therapy. (2011). *Einstein: The Magazine for Alumni and Friends of Albert Einstein College of Medicine*. Summer/fall, 9. Retrieved from https://www.einstein.yu.edu/docs/publications/einstein-magazine/einstein-magazine-summer-fall-2011.pdf

Brown, K. W., & Ryan, R. M. (2003). The benefits of being present: Mindfulness and its role in psychological well-being. *Journal of Personality and Social Psychology, 84*(4), 822–848. doi:10.1037/0022-3514.84.4.822 PMID:12703651

Brownson, R. C., Chang, J. C., Davis, J. R., & Smith, C. A. (1991). Physical activity on the job and cancer in Missouri. *American Journal of Public Health, 81*(5), 639–642. doi:10.2105/AJPH.81.5.639 PMID:2014869

Buffart, L. M., van Uffelen, J. G., Riphagen, B. J., & Brown, W. J. (2012). Physical and psychosocial benefits of yoga in cancer patients and survivors, a systematic review and meta-analysis of randomized controlled trials. *BMC Cancer*, *12*(1), 559. doi:10.1186/1471-2407-12-559 PMID:23181734

Calenda, E. (2006). Massage therapy for cancer pain. *Current Pain and Headache Reports*, *10*(4), 270–274. doi:10.100711916-006-0031-1 PMID:16834941

Camacho, T. C., Roberts, R. E., Lazarus, N. B., Kaplan, G. A., & Cohen, R. D. (1991). Physical activity and depression: Evidence from the Alameda County Study. *American Journal of Epidemiology*, *134*, 220–231. PMID:1862805

Carney, C. P., & Jones, L. E. (2006). Medical comorbidity in women and men with bipolar disorders: A population-based controlled study. *Psychosomatic Medicine*, *68*(5), 684–691. doi:10.1097/01.psy.0000237316.09601.88 PMID:17012521

Carney, C. P., Jones, L. E., & Woolson, R. F. (2006). Medical comorbidity in women and men with schizophrenia: A population-based controlled study. *Journal of General Internal Medicine*, *21*(11), 1133–1137. doi:10.1111/j.1525-1497.2006.00563.x PMID:17026726

Carver, C., Pozo, C., Harris, S., Noriega, V., Scheier, M., Robinson, D., ... Clark, K. (1993). How coping mediates the effect of optimism on distress: A study of women with early stage breast cancer. *Journal of Personality and Social Psychology*, *65*(2), 375–390. doi:10.1037/0022-3514.65.2.375 PMID:8366426

Cassileth, B. R. (2011). Green Tea (Camellia sinensis). *Oncology (Williston Park)*, *14*, 1432–1433. PMID:22329195

Cassileth, B. R., & Vickers, A. J. (2004). Massage therapy for symptom control: Outcome study at a major cancer center. *Journal of Pain and Symptom Management*, *28*(3), 244–249.

Centers for Disease Control and Prevention. (2000). *Measuring healthy days: Population assessment of health-related quality of life*. Atlanta, GA: Centers for Disease Control and Prevention.

Centers for Disease Control and Prevention. (2013). Death and Mortality. NCHS FastStats Web Site. Retrieved from: http://www.cdc.gov/nchs/fastats/deaths.htm

Centers for Disease Control and Prevention, National Center for Health Statistics. (2015). Underlying Cause of Death 1999-2013.

Chapman, B. P., Hampson, S., & Clarkin, J. (2014). Personality-informed interventions for healthy aging: Conclusions from a National Institute on Aging work group. *Developmental Psychology, 50*(5), 1426–1441. doi:10.1037/a0034135 PMID:23978300

Chen, L.-C., Wang, T.-F., Shih, Y.-N., & Wu, L.-J. (2013). Fifteen-minute music intervention reduces pre-radiotherapy anxiety in oncology patients. *European Journal of Oncology Nursing, 17*(4), 436–441. doi:10.1016/j.ejon.2012.11.002 PMID:23218591

Constantino, M. I., Molyneaux, L., Limacher-Gisler, F., Al-Saeed, A., Luo, C., Wu, T., ... Wong, J. (2013). Long-term complications and mortality in young-onset diabetes: Type 2 diabetes is more hazardous and lethal than type 1 diabetes. *Diabetes Care, 36*(12), 3863–3869. doi:10.2337/dc12-2455 PMID:23846814

Cooperative Program Centers for Disease Control and Prevention. (2016). *Self-management education. CDC- recommended programs. Chronic Disease Self-Management Program (CDSMP)*. Atlanta, GA: Centers for Disease Control and Prevention.

Corbin, J., & Strauss, A. (1988). *Unending work and care: Managing chronic illness at home*. San Francisco: Jossey-Bass.

Cramer, H., Lange, S., Klose, P., Paul, A., & Dobos, G. (2012a). Yoga for breast cancer patients and survivors: A systematic review and meta-analysis. *BMC Cancer, 12*(1), 412. doi:10.1186/1471-2407-12-412 PMID:22988934

Cramer, H., Lauche, R., Haller, H., & Dobos, G. (2013a). A Systematic review and meta- analysis of yoga for low back pain. *The Clinical Journal of Pain, 29*(5), 450–460. doi:10.1097/AJP.0b013e31825e1492 PMID:23246998

Cramer, H., Lauche, R., Klose, P., Langhorst, J., & Dobos, G. (2013b). Yoga for schizophrenia: A systematic review and meta-analysis. *BMC Psychiatry, 13*(1), 32. doi:10.1186/1471-244X-13-32 PMID:23327116

Cramer, H., Lauche, R., Paul, A., & Dobos, G. (2012b). Mindfulness-based stress reduction for breast cancer-a systematic review and meta-analysis. *Current Oncology (Toronto, Ont.), 19*(5), e343–e352. doi:10.3747/co.19.1016 PMID:23144582

Creer, T., Renne, C., & Christian, W. (1976). Behavioral contributions to rehabilitation and childhood asthma. *Rehabilitation Literature, 37*, 226–232, 247. PMID:959645

Deng, G., & Cassileth, B. R. (2014). *Integrative oncology: An overview. American Society of Clinical Oncology Education Book* (pp. 233–242). New York: Integrative Medicine Service, Memorial Sloan Kettering Cancer Center.

Dickinson, H. O., Mason, J. M., Nicolson, D. J., Campbell, F., Beyer, F. R., Cook, J. V., ... Ford, G. A. (2006). Lifestyle interventions to reduced raised blood pressure: A systematic review of randomized control trials. *Journal of Hypertension*, *24*(2), 215–233. doi:10.1097/01.hjh.0000199800.72563.26 PMID:16508562

DiMeglio, L. (2013). *Help yourself form healthy habits*. Alexndria, VA: American Diabetes Association. Retrieved from http://www.diabetesforecast.org/2013/jul/help-yourself-form-healthy-habits.html

Druss, B. G., Zhao, L., von Esenwein, S. A., Bona, J. R., Fricks, L., Jenkins-Tucker, S., ... Lorig, K. (2010). The health and recovery peer (HARP) program: A peer-led intervention to improve medical self-management for persons with serious mental illness. *Schizophrenia Research*, *118*(1-2), 264–270. doi:10.1016/j.schres.2010.01.026 PMID:20185272

Dunbar, J. (2015). Qigong Therapy. Magic Tortoise Taichiquan School. Retrieved from: http://www.magictortoise.com/qigong_therapy.htm

Elmer, P. J., Obarzanek, E., Vollmer, W. M., Simons-Morton, D., Stevens, V. J., Young, D. R., ... Svetkey, L. P. (2006). Effects of Comprehensive lifestyle modification on diet, weight, physical fitness, and blood pressure control: 18-month results of a randomized trial. *Annals of Internal Medicine*, *144*(7), 485–495. doi:10.7326/0003-4819-144-7-200604040-00007 PMID:16585662

Esch, T., Fricchione, G. L., & Stefano, G. B. (2003). The therapeutic use of the relaxation response in stress-related diseases. *Medical Science Monitor*, *9*, RA23–RA34. PMID:12601303

Everett, B., Salamonson, Y., & Davidson, P.M. (2009). Bandura's exercise self-efficacy scale: Validation in an Austrian cardiac rehabilitation setting. *Int. J. Nurs. Stud.*, *46*(6), 824-829.

Ezzo, J., Vickers, A., & Richardson, M. A. (2005). Acupuncture-point stimulation for chemotherapy-induced nausea and vomiting. *Journal of Clinical Oncology*, *23*(28), 7188–7198. doi:10.1200/JCO.2005.06.028 PMID:16192603

FAO/WHO. (1998). Carbohydrates in human nutrition. *FAO Food and Nutrition Paper*, 1998, 66.

Federal Interagency Forum on Aging-Related Statistics. (2012). *Older Americans 2012: Key indicators of well-being*. Washington, D.C.: U.S. Government Printing Office.

Foster, C., Hillsdon, M., Thorogood, M., Kaur, A., & Wedatilake, T. (2005). Interventions for promoting physical activity. *Cochrane Database of Systematic Reviews*, (1): CD003180. PMID:15674903

Fox, K. R. (1999). The influence of physical activity on mental well-being. *Public Health Nutrition*, *2*(3a3A), 411–418. doi:10.1017/S1368980099000567 PMID:10610081

Fulton-Kehoe, D., Hamman, R. F., Baxter, J., & Marshall, J. (2001). A case-control study of physical activity and non-insulin dependent diabetes mellitus (NIDDM). The San Luis Valley Diabetes Study. *Annals of Epidemiology*, *11*(5), 320–327. doi:10.1016/S1047-2797(01)00218-6 PMID:11399446

Galvin, J. A., Benson, H., Deckro, G. R., Fricchione, G. L., & Dusek, J. A. (2006). The relaxation response: Reducing stress and improving cognition in healthy aging adults. *Complementary Therapies in Clinical Practice*, *12*(3), 186–191. doi:10.1016/j.ctcp.2006.02.004 PMID:16835029

Gerteis, J., Izrael, D., Deitz, D., LeRoy, L., Ricciardi, R., Miller, T., & Basu, J. (2014). *Multiple chronic condition chartbook: 2010 medical expenditure panel survey data*. Rockville, MD: Agency for Healthcare Research and Quality.

Giovannucci, E., Ascherio, A., Rimm, E. B., Colditz, G. A., Stampfer, M. J., & Willett, W. C. (1995). Physical activity, obesity, and risk for colon cancer and adenoma in men. *Annals of Internal Medicine*, *122*(5), 327–334. doi:10.7326/0003-4819-122-5-199503010-00002 PMID:7847643

Good, M., Anderson, G. C., Stanton-Hicks, M., Grass, J. A., & Makii, M. (2002). Relaxation and music reduce pain after gynecologic surgery. *Pain Management Nursing*, *3*(2), 61–70. doi:10.1053/jpmn.2002.123846 PMID:12050837

Gorelick, P. B., Sacco, R. L., Smith, D. B., Alberts, M., Mustone-Alexander, L., Rader, D., ... Rhew, D. C. (1999). Prevention of a first stroke: A review of guidelines and a multidisciplinary consensus statement from the National Stroke Association. *Journal of the American Medical Association*, *281*(12), 1112–1120. doi:10.1001/jama.281.12.1112 PMID:10188663

Hart, K. E., Turner, S. H., & Cardozo, S. R. (1987). Ongoing research. Stress, personality, coping and well-being: A four-wave longitudinal process study. *Personality and Individual Differences*, *8*(4), 591–593. doi:10.1016/0191-8869(87)90226-1

Healthy People 2020. (n. d.). Physical activity. Washington, D.C.: U.S. Department of Health & Human Services.

Hu, F. B., Manson, J. E., Stampfer, M. J., Colditz, G., Liu, S., Solomon, C. G., & Willett, W. C. (2001). Diet, lifestyle, and the risk of type 2 diabetes mellitus in women. *The New England Journal of Medicine*, *345*(11), 790–797. doi:10.1056/NEJMoa010492 PMID:11556298

Hu, F. B., Stampfer, M. J., Colditz, G. A., Ascherio, A., Rexrode, K. M., Willett, W. C., & Manson, J. E. (2000). Physical activity and risk of stroke in women. *Journal of the American Medical Association*, *283*(22), 2961–2967. doi:10.1001/jama.283.22.2961 PMID:10865274

Jaglal, S. B., Kreiger, N., & Darlington, G. (1993). Past and recent physical activity and risk of hip fracture. *American Journal of Epidemiology*, *138*, 107–118. PMID:8342529

Kallio, P., Kolehmainen, M., Laaksonen, D. E., Kekäläinen, J., Salopuro, T., Sivenius, K., ... Uusitupa, M. (2007). Dietary carbohydrate modification induces alterations in gene expression in abdominal subcutaneous adipose tissue in persons with the metabolic syndrome: The FUNGENUT Study. *The American Journal of Clinical Nutrition*, *85*, 1417–1427. PMID:17490981

Karadag, F., Ozcan, H., Eskin, M., Karul, A. B., Ceylan, E., Tufek, Y., & Cildag, O. (2008). Psychological distress in chronic obstructive pulmonary disease patients. *Stress and Health*, *24*(2), 115–122. doi:10.1002mi.1178

Kelley, G. A., & Kelley, K. S. (2015). Meditative movement therapies and health-related quality- of-life in adults: A systematic review of meta-analyses. *PLoS ONE*, *10*(6), e129181. doi:10.1371/journal.pone.0129181 PMID:26053053

Kiecolt-Glaser, J. K., Christian, L., Preston, H., Houts, C. R., Malarkey, W. B., Emery, C. F., & Glaser, R. (2010). Stress, inflammation, and yoga practice. *Psychosomatic Medicine*, *72*(2), 113–121. doi:10.1097/PSY.0b013e3181cb9377 PMID:20064902

Kohrt, W. M., Snead, D. B., Slatopolsky, E., & Birge, S. J. Jr. (1995). Additive effects of weight- bearing exercise and estrogen on bone mineral density in older women. *Journal of Bone and Mineral Research*, *10*(9), 1303–1311. doi:10.1002/jbmr.5650100906 PMID:7502701

Laaksonen, D. E., Toppinen, L. K., Juntunen, K. S., Autio, K., Liukkonen, K. H., Poutanen, K. S., ... Mykkänen, H. M. (2005). Dietary carbohydrate modification enhances insulin secretion in persons with the metabolic syndrome. *The American Journal of Clinical Nutrition*, *82*, 1218–1227. PMID:16332654

Ledesma, D., & Kumano, H. (2009). Mindfulness-based stress reduction and cancer: A meta- analysis. *Psychooncology, 18,* 571-579. Leeds, A.R. (1979). The dietary management of diabetes in adults. *The Proceedings of the Nutrition Society*, *98*, 365–371.

Lenker, S. L., Lorig, K., & Gallagher, G. (1984). Reasons for the lack of association between changes in health behavior and improved health status: An exploratory study. *Patient Education and Counseling*, *6*(2), 69–72. doi:10.1016/0738-3991(84)90036-3 PMID:10268098

Lin, K. Y., Hu, Y. T., Chang, K. J., Lin, H. F., & Tsauo, J. Y. (2011). Effects of yoga on psychological health, quality of life, and physical health of patients with cancer: A meta- analysis. *Evidence-Based Complementary and Alternative Medicine*. PMID:21437197

Lopez, A. D., Shibuya, K., & Rao, C. (2006). Chronic obstructive pulmonary disease: Current burden and future projections. *The European Respiratory Journal*, *27*(2), 397–412. doi:10.1183/09031936.06.00025805 PMID:16452599

Lorig, K. R., Chastain, R. L., Ung, E., Shoor, E., & Holtman, H. R. (1989). Development and evaluation of a scale to measure perceived self-efficacy in people with arthritis. *Arthritis and Rheumatism*, *32*(1), 37–44. doi:10.1002/anr.1780320107 PMID:2912463

Lorig, K. R., & Holman, R. H. (2003). Self-management education: History, definition, outcomes, and mechanisms. *Annals of Behavioral Medicine*, *26*(1), 1–7. doi:10.1207/S15324796ABM2601_01 PMID:12867348

Lorig, K. R., Sobel, D. S., Stewart, A. L., Brown, B. W. Jr, Ritter, P. L., González, V. M., ... Holman, H. R. (1999). Evidence suggesting that a chronic disease self-management program can improve health status while reducing utilization and costs: A randomized trial. *Medical Care*, *37*(1), 5–14. doi:10.1097/00005650-199901000-00003 PMID:10413387

Lorig, K. R., Stewart, A. L., Gonzalez, V. M., Laurent, D. D., & Lynch, J. (1996). *Outcome Measures for Health Education and Other Health Care Interventions*. Thousand Oaks, CA: Sage Publications.

Magidson, J. F., Roberts, B. W., Collado-Rodriguez, A., & Lejuez, C. W. (2014). Theory driven intervention for changing personality: Expectancy value theory, behavioral activation, and conscientiousness. *Developmental Psychology*, *50*(5), 1442–1450. doi:10.1037/a0030583 PMID:23106844

Mathieu, R.A., Powell-Wiley, T.M., Ayers, C., McGuire, D.K., Khera, A., & Das, S.R., & Lakoski, S. G. (2012). Physical activity participation, health perceptions, and cardiovascular disease mortality in a multiethnic population: The Dallas Heart Study. *American Heart Journal*, *163*(6), 1037–1040. doi:10.1016/j.ahj.2012.03.005 PMID:22709758

McDermott, M. S., & While, A. E. (2013). Maximizing the healthcare environment: A systematic review exploring the potential of computer technology to promote self-management of chronic illness in healthcare settings. *Patient Education and Counseling*, *92*(1), 13–22. doi:10.1016/j.pec.2013.02.014 PMID:23566427

Melchior, M. A., Seff, L. R., Albatineh, A. N., McCoy, H. V., Page, T. F., & Palmer, R. C. (2014). Intermediate outcomes of chronic disease self-management program offered by members of the Healthy Aging Regional Collaborative in South Florida. *Research on Aging*, *36*(4), 431–449. doi:10.1177/0164027513500054 PMID:25651315

Memorial Sloan Kettering Cancer Center (MSKCC) Bendheim Integrative Medicine Center. (2015). Nutritional and dietary-supplement counseling. Retrieved from: https://www.mskcc.org/locations/bendheim-integrative-medicine

Memorial Sloan Kettering Cancer Center (MSKCC) Integrative Medicine. (2015). About herbs, botanicals, and other products. Retrieved from https://www.mskcc.org/cancer-care/treatments/symptom-management/integrative-medicine/expertise

Mentgen, J. (2002). Healing touch. *The Nursing Clinics of North America*, *36*(1), 143–157.

Meyer, H.E., Tverdal, A., & Falch, J.A. (1993). Risk factors for hip fracture in middle-aged Norwegian women and men. *American Journal of Epidemiology*, *137*, 1203–1211.

Michel, A., Bosch, C., & Rexroth, M. (2014). Mindfulness as a cognitive-emotional segmentation strategy: An intervention promoting work-life balance. *Journal of Occupational and Organizational Psychology*, *87*(4), 733–754. doi:10.1111/joop.12072

Miner, W. (2007). Training massage therapists to work in oncology. *Journal of the Society for Integrative Oncology*, *5*(4), 163–166. doi:10.2310/7200.2007.015 PMID:19087760

Mirmiran, P., Bahadoran, Z., & Azizi, F. (2014). Functional foods-based diet as a novel dietary approach for management of type 2 diabetes and its complications: A review. *World J. Diabetes*, *5*(3), 267–281. doi:10.4239/wjd.v5.i3.267 PMID:24936248

Moadel, A. (2010). *Einstein on Cancer: Dr. Alyson Moadel. Psychosocial oncology: Coping with cancer*. Bronx, NY: Albert Einstein College of Medicine. Retrieved from http://www.einstein.yu.edu/video/?VID=259#top

Moadel, A. B., Shah, C., & Sisco, R. (2009). Description of the Yoga-based Cancer Rehabilitation Program of the Montefiore-Einstein Cancer Center. Retrieved from: https://www.einstein.yu.edu/docs/faculty/profiles/479-alyson-moadel/integral-hatha-yoga-protocol-description-MECC-rehab-ca-pgm.pdf

Mroczek, D. (2014). Personality plasticity, healthy aging, and interventions. *Developmental Psychology*, *50*(5), 1470–1474. doi:10.1037/a0036028 PMID:24773109

Murray, C. J. L., & Lopez, A. D. (1997). Alternative projections of mortality and disability by cause 1990-2020; Global Burden of Disease Study. *Lancet*, *349*(9064), 1498–1504. doi:10.1016/S0140-6736(96)07492-2 PMID:9167458

National Heart, Lung, and Blood Institute. (2015). Description of the DASH eating plan. National Institutes of Health. U.S. Department of Health & Human Services. Retrieved from http://www.nhlbi.nih.gov/health/health-topics/topics/dash/

National Institute on Drug Abuse (NIDA). (2015). *DrugFacts: Prescription and over-the-counter medications*. Washington, D.C.: National Institute of Health.

Neithercott, T. (2014). *A Mediterranean food plan can protect health. Diabetes Forecast: The Healthy Living Magazine*. Alexandria, VA: American Diabetes Association. Retrieved from http://www.diabetesforecast.org/2014/08-aug/a-mediterranean-food-plan-can.html?loc=ymal

Ogden, C. L., Carroll, M. D., Kit, B. K., & Flegal, K. M. (2014). Prevalence of Childhood and Adult Obesity in the United States, 2011-2012. *Journal of the American Medical Association*, *311*(8), 806–814. doi:10.1001/jama.2014.732 PMID:24570244

Ory, M. G., Anh, S. N., Jiang, L., Lorig, K., Ritter, P., Laurent, D. D., ... Smith, M. L. (2013). National Study of Chronic Disease Self-Management: Six-Month Outcome Findings. *Journal of Aging and Health*, *25*(7), 1258–1274. doi:10.1177/0898264313502531 PMID:24029414

Pan, L., Yan, J., Guo, Y., & Yan, J. (2013). Effects of Tai Chi training on exercise capacity an quality of life in patients with chronic heart failure: A meta-analysis. *European Journal of Heart Failure*, *15*(3), 316–323. PMID:23099355

Panda, A., Arjona, A., Sapey, E., Bai, F., Fikrig, E., Montgomery, R. R., ... Shaw, A. C. (2009). Human innate immunosenescence: Causes and consequences for immunity in old age. *Trends in Immunology, 30*(7), 325–333. doi:10.1016/j.it.2009.05.004 PMID:19541535

Parks, J., & Svedsen, D. (2006). *Morbidity and mortality in people with serious mental illness*. Alexandria, VA: National Association of State Mental Health Program Directors.

Pauwels, R. A., Buist, A. S., Calverley, P. M. A., Jenkins, C. R., & Hurd, S. S. (2001). Global strategy for the diagnosis, management, and prevention of chronic obstructive pulmonary disease: National Heart Lung and Blood Institute and World Health Organization Global Initiative for Chronic Obstructive Lung Disease (GOLD): executive summary. *Respiratory Care, 46*(8), 798–825. PMID:11463370

Peters, R. K., Benson, H., & Peters, J. M. (1977). Daily relaxation response breaks in a working population: 2. Blood pressure. *American Journal of Public Health, 67*(10), 954–959. doi:10.2105/AJPH.67.10.954 PMID:333958

Pfohl, M., & Schatz, H. (2001). Strategies for the prevention of type 2 diabetes. *Experimental and Clinical Endocrinology & Diabetes, 109*(Suppl. 2), S240–S249. doi:10.1055-2001-18585 PMID:11460574

Piet, J., Wurtzen, H., & Zachariae, R. (2012). The effect of mindfulness-based therapy on symptoms of anxiety and depression in adult cancer patients and survivors: A systematic review and meta-analysis. *Journal of Consulting and Clinical Psychology, 80*(6), 1007–1020. doi:10.1037/a0028329 PMID:22563637

Pimouguet, C., LeGoff, M., Thiebaut, R., Dartigues, J.F., & Helmer, C. (2011). Effectiveness of disease-management programs for improving diabetes care: A meta-analysis. *Canadian Medical Association Journal, 183(2)*, E115.

Prasad, K., Sharma, V., Lackore, K., Sarah, M., Jenkins, S. M., Prasad, A., & Sood, A. (2010). Use of complementary therapies in cardiovascular disease. *The American Journal of Cardiology, 111*(3), 339–345. doi:10.1016/j.amjcard.2012.10.010 PMID:23186602

Racine, E., Troyer, J. L., Warren-Findlow, J., & McCauley, W. J. (2011). The effect of medical nutrition therapy on changes in dietary knowledge and DASH diet adherence in older adults with cardiovascular disease. *The Journal of Nutrition, Health & Aging, 15*(10), 868–876. doi:10.100712603-011-0102-9 PMID:22159775

Reig-Ferrer, A., Ferrer-Cascales, R., Santos-Ruiz, A., Campos-Ferrer, A., Prieto-Seva, A., Velasco-Ruiz, I., ... Albaladejo-Blazquez, N. (2014). A relaxation techniques enhances psychological well-being and immune parameters in elderly people from a nursing home: A randomized controlled study. *BMC Complementary and Alternative Medicine*, *14*(1), 311. doi:10.1186/1472-6882-14-311 PMID:25151398

Rosén, L. A., Silva, L. O., Andersson, U. K., Holm, C., Ostman, E. M., & Björck, I. M. (2009). Endosperm and whole grain rye breads are characterized by low post-prandial insulin response and a beneficial blood glucose profile. *Nutrition Journal*, *8*(1), 42. doi:10.1186/1475-2891-8-42 PMID:19781071

Salamon, E., Bernstein, S. R., Kim, S. A., Kim, M., & Stefano, G. B. (2003). The effects of auditory perception and musical preference on anxiety in naïve human subjects. *Medical Science Monitor*, *9*, R396–CR399. PMID:12960929

Santaguida, P. L., Balion, C., Hunt, D., Morrison, K., Gerstein, H., Raina, P., ... Yazdi, H. (2005). Diagnosis, prognosis, and treatment of impaired glucose tolerance and impaired fasting glucose. *Evidence Report/Technology Assessment (Summary)*, 128, 1–11. PMID:16194123

Scheier, M., Matthews, J., Owens, J., Magovern, G., Lefebvre, R., Abbott, R., & Carver, C. (1989). Dispositional optimism and recovery from coronary artery bypass surgery: The beneficial effects on physical and psychological well-being. *Journal of Personality and Social Psychology*, *57*(6), 1024–1040. doi:10.1037/0022-3514.57.6.1024 PMID:2614656

Seligman, M. E. P. (2011). *Flourish: A visionary new understanding of happiness and well- being*. New York: Simon and Schuster.

Seligman, M. E. P. (2015). Authentic happiness. University of Pennsylvania Positive Psychology Center. Retrieved from https://www.authentichappiness.sas.upenn.edu/content/about-us

Seligman, M. E. P., & Csikszentmihalyi, M. (2000). Positive psychology: An introduction. *The American Psychologist*, *55*(1), 5–14. doi:10.1037/0003-066X.55.1.5 PMID:11392865

Sesso, H. D., Paffenbarger, R. S. Jr, & Lee, I. M. (2000). Physical activity and coronary heart disease in men: The Harvard Alumni Health Study. *Circulation*, *102*(9), 975–980. doi:10.1161/01.CIR.102.9.975 PMID:10961960

Shakespeare, W. (1602/1623). Twelfth Night, Act 1, scene 1, 1-3. First Folio. British Library.

Shen, R. L., Cai, F. L., Dong, J. L., & Hu, X. Z. (2011). Hypoglycemic effects and biochemical mechanisms of oat products on streptozotocin-induced diabetic mice. *Journal of Agricultural and Food Chemistry*, *59*(16), 8895–8900. doi:10.1021/jf200678q PMID:21749041

Shennan, C., Payne, S., & Fenlon, D. (2011). What is the evidence for the use of mindfulness- based interventions in cancer care? A review. *Psycho-Oncology*, *20*(7), 681–697. doi:10.1002/pon.1819 PMID:20690112

Shneerson, C., Taskila, T., Gale, N., Greenfield, S., & Chen, Y. F. (2013). The effect of complementary and alternative medicine on the quality of life of cancer survivors: A systematic review and meta-analyses. *Complementary Therapies in Medicine*, *21*(4), 417–429. doi:10.1016/j.ctim.2013.05.003 PMID:23876573

Sokal, J., Dickerson, F. B., Kreyenbuhl, J., Brown, C. H., Goldberg, R. W., & Dixon, L. B. (2004). Comorbidity of medical illnesses among adults with serious mental illness who are receiving community psychiatric services. *The Journal of Nervous and Mental Disease*, *192*(6), 421–427. doi:10.1097/01.nmd.0000130135.78017.96 PMID:15167405

Spurlock, M. (Writer & Dir.). (2004). *Supersize Me.*

Stanczyk, M. M. (2011). Music therapy in supportive cancer care. *Reports of Practical Oncology and Radiotherapy*, *16*(5), 170–172. doi:10.1016/j.rpor.2011.04.005 PMID:24376975

Stanton, A., Revenson, T., & Tennen, H. (2007). Health psychology: Psychological adjustment to chronic disease. *Annual Review of Psychology*, *58*(1), 565–592. doi:10.1146/annurev.psych.58.110405.085615 PMID:16930096

U.S. Census Bureau. (2010). Facts for features: Older Americans month. May 2010. Retrieved from http://www.census.gov/newsroom/releases/pdf/cb10-ff06.pdf

Venn, B. J., & Mann, J. I. (2004). Review: Cereal grains, legumes, and diabetes. *European Journal of Clinical Nutrition*, *58*(11), 1443–1451. doi:10.1038j.ejcn.1601995 PMID:15162131

Verwey, R., van der Weegen, S., Spreeuwenberg, M., Tange, H., van der Weijden, T., & de Witte, L. (2014a). A monitoring and feedback tool embedded in a counseling protocol to increase physical activity of patients with COPD or type 2 diabetes in primary care: Study protocol of a three-arm cluster randomized controlled trial. *BMC Family Practice*, *15*(1), 93. doi:10.1186/1471-2296-15-93 PMID:24885096

Verwey, R., van der Weegen, S., Tange, H., Spreeuwenberg, M., van der Weijden, T., & de Witte, L. (2014b). A pilot study of a tool to stimulate physical activity in patients with COPD or type 2 diabetes in primary care. *Journal of Telemedicine and Telecare*, *20*(1), 29–34. doi:10.1177/1357633X13519057 PMID:24414397

Vickers, A. J., Cronin, A. M., Maschino, A. C., Lewith, G., MacPherson, H., Foster, N. E., ... Linde, K. (2012). Acupuncture for chronic pain: Individual patient data meta-analysis. *Archives of Internal Medicine*, *172*(19), 1444–1453. doi:10.1001/archinternmed.2012.3654 PMID:22965186

Vickers, A. J., & Linde, K. (2014). Acupuncture for chronic pain. *Journal of the American Medical Association*, *311*(9), 955–956. doi:10.1001/jama.2013.285478 PMID:24595780

Volpato, E., Banfi, P., Rogers, S. M., & Pagnini, F. (2015). Relaxation techniques for people with chronic obstructive pulmonary disease: A systematic review and a meta-analysis. *Evidence-Based Complementary and Alternative Medicine*, *2015*, 1–22. doi:10.1155/2015/628365 PMID:26339268

Wang, F., Man, J. K., Lee, E. K., Wu, T., Benson, H., & Fricchione, G. L. (2013). The effects of qigong on anxiety, depression, and psychological well-being: A systematic review and meta-analysis. *Evidence-Based Complementary and Alternative Medicine*. PMID:23401706

Wannamethee, S. G., & Shaper, A. G. (1999). Physical activity and the prevention of stroke. *Journal of Cardiovascular Risk*, *6*(4), 213–216. doi:10.1177/204748739900600404 PMID:10501271

Wannamethee, S. G., & Shaper, A. G. (2001). Physical activity in the prevention of cardiovascular disease: An epidemiological perspective. *Sports Medicine (Auckland, N.Z.)*, *31*(2), 101–114. doi:10.2165/00007256-200131020-00003 PMID:11227978

Ward, B. W., Schiller, J. S., & Goodman, R. A. (2014). Multiple chronic conditions among US adults: A 2012 update. *Preventing Chronic Disease*, 2014, 11. PMID:24742395

Wardell, D. W., & Weymouth, K. F. (2004). Review of studies of Healing Touch. *Journal of Nursing Scholarship*, *36*(2), 147–154. doi:10.1111/j.1547-5069.2004.04012.x PMID:15227762

Weisenberger, J. (2014). *Foods high in AGEs. Diabetes Forecast: The Healthy Living Magazine*. Alexandria, VA: American Diabetes Association. Retrieved from http://www.diabetesforecast.org/2014/11-nov/foods-high-in-ages.html?loc=ymal

Weyerer, S. (1992). Physical inactivity and depression in the community. Evidence from the Upper Bavarian Field Study. *International Journal of Sports Medicine*, *13*(06), 492–496. doi:10.1055-2007-1021304 PMID:1428382

Yang, Y. C., Lu, F.-H., Wu, J.-S., Wu, C.-H., & Chang, C.-J. (2004). The protective effect of habitual tea consumption on hypertension. *Archives of Internal Medicine*, *164*(14), 1534–1540. doi:10.1001/archinte.164.14.1534 PMID:15277285

Zainal, N. Z., Booth, S., & Huppert, F. A. (2013). The efficacy of mindfulness-based stress reduction on mental health of breast cancer patients: A meta-analysis. *Psycho-Oncology*, *22*(7), 1457–1465. doi:10.1002/pon.3171 PMID:22961994

Zeng, Y., Luo, T., Xie, H., Huang, M., & Cheng, A. S. (2014). Health benefits of qigong or tai chi for cancer patients: A systematic review and meta-analyses. *Complementary Therapies in Medicine*, *22*(1), 173–186. doi:10.1016/j.ctim.2013.11.010 PMID:24559833

Zhang, J., Yang, K. H., Tian, J. H., & Wang, C. M. (2012). Effects of yoga on psychologic function and quality of life in women with breast cancer: A meta-analysis of randomized controlled trials. *Journal of Alternative and Complementary Medicine*, *18*(11), 994–1002. doi:10.1089/acm.2011.0514 PMID:22909345

Zimmerman, L., Pozehl, B., Duncan, K., & Schmitz, R. (1989). Effects of music in patients who had chronic cancer pain. *Western Journal of Nursing Research*, *11*(3), 298–309. doi:10.1177/019394598901100304 PMID:2750142

KEY TERMS AND DEFINITIONS

Alternative Medicine: If a non-mainstream healing or therapeutic practice is used in place of conventional medicine, it's considered "alternative."

Complementary Medicine: When a non-mainstream healing or therapeutic practice is used together with conventional medicine, it's considered "complementary."

DASH Diet: Dietary Approach to Stop Hypertension (DASH) diet. The Dash diet reduces intake of saturated fat, total fat, sodium, and cholesterol, increases intake of fruits and vegetables, and increases consumption of potassium, calcium, magnesium, fiber, and protein.

Integrative Medicine: Healing-oriented medicine that takes account of the whole person (body, mind, and spirit), including all aspects of lifestyle. It emphasizes the therapeutic relationship and makes use of all appropriate therapies, both conventional and complementary.

Positive Psychology: The scientific study of the strengths that enable individuals and communities to thrive, a branch of psychology whose aim is authentic happiness and flourishing.

Self-Efficacy: A person's belief that he or she can successfully execute a particular behavior to achieve a certain outcome.

This research was previously published in Healthcare Community Synergism between Patients, Practitioners, and Researchers edited by Valerie C. Bryan and Jennifer Lynne Bird, pages 176-212, copyright year 2017 by Medical Information Science Reference (an imprint of IGI Global).

Chapter 11
Research-Based Applied Psychophysiology:
Yoga for Occupational Stress and Health

Ned Hartfiel
Bangor University, UK

Rhiannon Tudor Edwards
Bangor University, UK

ABSTRACT

Recent research indicates that yoga can be effective for reducing both musculoskeletal conditions and stress. In the workplace, musculoskeletal conditions and stress are the two most common reasons for sickness absence. The World Health Organisation has identified the workplace as a priority area for promoting good health. As a result, yoga is increasingly being offered in workplace settings to improve the physical health and mental wellbeing of employees. In September 2014, a comprehensive search of relevant electronic databases was performed to determine the effectiveness of yoga in workplace settings. Eight randomised trials met the inclusion criteria. The results showed that the effectiveness of yoga in the workplace was strong for musculoskeletal conditions, moderate for perceived stress, limited for sleep quality and conflicting for heart rate variability. Overall, this evidence is promising, yet limited due to a lack of high quality studies of yoga in workplace settings.

DOI: 10.4018/978-1-7998-1680-5.ch011

BACKGROUND: HEALTH CHALLENGES IN THE WORKPLACE

The health of the workforce is vital to the economy. Sickness absence from work is costly to employees, employers and the wider society. In many industrialized countries, the two most common reasons for sickness absence include musculoskeletal disorders (such as back and neck pain) and stress-related illness (such as anxiety and depression) (Office of National Statistics, 2014; Black & Frost, 2011).

The World Health Organization identifies the workplace is a priority area for promoting health and addressingthe challenges of musculoskeletal disorders and stress (WHO, 1997). The average person spends more than a third of their waking hours at work and up to 40 years of their life in the workplace (Jones & Barham, 2009).

Employers are thus well-placed to support workers not only by promoting health (e.g., physical activity and healthy eating), but also by helping employees integrate lifestyle changes into their daily life. Research indicates that workplace physical activity interventions can reduce absenteeism by up to 30%, and therefore deliver value for money to employers (Mackett & Brown, 2011). By investing in workplace health, employers can play a fundamental role in preventing illness, promoting good health and improving productivity.

YOGA FOR MANAGING MUSCULOSKELETAL CONDITIONS, BACK PAIN, AND STRESS

Recent research suggests that yoga is one form of physical activity that can reduce musculoskeletal disorders and stress. Developed in India nearly 3,000 years ago, yoga is considered a means for promoting physical, mental and spiritual wellbeing (Cramer, et al., 2013a). Yoga often includes four main components: physical movement, breathing exercises, relaxation methods and meditation/mindfulness techniques (Collins, 1998; Woodyard, 2011; Ward, Treharne, & Stebbings, 2011; NIH, 2013; Cramer, Krucoff, & Dobos, 2013a).

In recent years, yoga has gained popularity as a therapeutic practice for improving mental and physical health. In 2012, approximately 20 million people in the United States practiced yoga with the specific intention to improve their overall health (Yoga Journal, 2012). Today, yoga is practiced in the United States by more than 36 million people (Yoga Journal and Yoga Alliance, 2016). Yoga is now commonplace in western countries and taught in community centers, health clubs, schools, hospitals and workplaces (Cramer et al., 2013a).

Yoga for Musculoskeletal Conditions

Two recent systematic reviews of 'yoga for musculoskeletal conditions' found yoga to be a safe, acceptable and feasible intervention, superior to usual care in reducing pain and improving functional outcomes (McCaffrey & Park, 2012; Ward, Stebbings, Cherkin, & Baxter, 2013). McCaffrey and Park (2012) reviewed the evidence from 31 randomized and non-randomized studies. They found yoga to be 'moderately feasible' and likely to reduce both pain and the use of medication for pain.

Ward et al. (2013) found 17 randomized controlled trials covering yoga for low back pain, osteoarthritis, osteoporosis, rheumatoid arthritis and fibromyalgia. The authors concluded that the yoga produced clinically meaningful reductions in pain and improvements in functional outcomes across a range of musculoskeletal conditions (Ward et al., 2013).

Yoga for Back Pain

Three additional systematic reviews on 'yoga for back pain' found strong evidence of yoga's effectiveness for relieving short-term back pain and moderate evidence of yoga's effectiveness for reducing long-term back pain (Posadski & Ernst, 2011; Holzman & Beggs, 2013; Cramer, Lauche, Haller, & Dobos, 2013). Posadksi and Ernst (2011) reviewed seven randomized controlled trials and concluded that yoga generated significantly greater reductions in low back pain compared with usual care, education or conventional therapeutic exercise.

Holzman and Beggs (2013) found eight randomized controlled trials of yoga for assessing back pain and functional disability. In their meta-analysis, the authors reported that at post-treatment, yoga had a medium to large effect in reducing both pain (Cohen's d=0.623) and functional disability (Cohen's d=0.645). Although follow-up effect sizes were smaller, they were still significant for both pain (d=0.486) and functional disability (d=0.397).

More recently, Cramer et al. (2013b) found 10 randomized trials on yoga for patients with back pain. Eight of the ten studies were rated low risk of bias and most showed significant reductions in pain when compared with usual care or education groups.

Yoga for Stress Management

Chong et al. (2011) identified eight randomized controlled trials and clinical controlled trials that assessed the effect of yoga on healthy adults. The results showed an overall positive effect of yoga in reducing stress levels or stress symptoms, although most of the studies had methodological limitations due to a short intervention duration and limited follow-up data.

EFFECTIVENESS OF YOGA IN THE WORKPLACE

Although there are no published systematic reviews of randomized controlled trials of yoga in workplace settings, a comprehensive search of relevant electronic databases was performed in September 2014 (systematic review in press). Eight randomized trials met the inclusion criteria.

The results indicated that yoga's effectiveness in the workplace was strong for musculoskeletal conditions, moderate for perceived stress, limited for sleep quality and conflicting for heart rate variability. Overall, the evidence was promising, yet limited due to a lack of high quality studies of yoga in workplace settings.

The findings from these eight yoga studies were grouped into four main categories: musculoskeletal conditions, perceived stress, sleep quality and heart rate variability.

Musculoskeletal Conditions

Five randomized controlled trials assessed the effectiveness of yoga for alleviating musculoskeletal conditions at work. Garfinkel et al. (1998) reported significant pain reduction among 22 yoga participants with carpal tunnel syndrome. Garfinkel et al. (1998) found that yoga was effective for improving grip strength. Telles et al. (2009) and Joshi and Bellad (2009) reported that yoga was effective for reducing musculoskeletal discomfort among computer users in India.

In the UK, Hartfiel et al. (2012) found that yoga helped to alleviate back pain among government employees. In India and Australia, Cheema et al. (2013) and Telles et al. (2009) reported that yoga significantly improved hip flexibility. These results were promising and provided strong evidence for the effectiveness of yoga for improving musculoskeletal conditions in the workplace (Table 1).

Stress Reduction

Three randomized trials evaluated yoga for reducing perceived stress. Granath et al. (2006), Wolever et al. (2012) and Hartfiel et al. (2012) all reported significant reductions in perceived stress from practicing yoga in the workplace. Both Wolever and Hartfiel used the more common 10-item Perceived Stress Scale, while Granath used the 14-item version (Cohen, 1983) (REF not in the list).

Different types of yoga were used in these studies and the length of the programs varied. Granath et al. (2006) used a ten-week program of *Kundalini yoga* in Sweden, Wolever a twelve-week *Viniyoga* intervention in the United States and Hartfiel et al. (2012) used an eight-week Dru Yoga program in the UK. Although these results were consistently favorable toward yoga, they indicated only moderate evidence for reducing perceived stress at work. This was due to the lack of high quality studies (Table 1).

Sleep Quality

Two randomized controlled studies measured the effect of yoga on sleep quality. In the Wolever et al. (2012) study of 90 *Viniyoga* participants, significant improvements in sleep quality were reported. In the Garfinkel et al. (1998) study of 22 *Iyengar yoga* participants, reductions in sleep disturbance were noted in participant diaries. However, because the reduction in sleep disturbance was not statistically significant in the Garfinkel study, there appears to be only limited evidence on the effectiveness of yoga for improving sleep quality among employees (Table 1).

Heart Rate Variability

Two randomized trials measured the effects of yoga on heart rate variability. In the United States, Wolever et al. (2012) found a significant improvement in heart rate variability. In Australia, Cheema et al. (2013) reported no significant improvement for the yoga group compared to the control group. Thus, conflicting evidence is reported for the effectiveness of yoga in improving heart rate variability (Table 1).

COST-EFFECTIVENESS OF YOGA

Although research indicates that yoga can be effective for managing musculoskeletal conditions and perceived stress in the workplace, few studies have explored the cost-effectiveness of yoga. Two recent studies, however, suggest that yoga can be cost-effective, for patient populations with chronic or non-specific low back pain (Chuang et al., 2012; Aboagye, Karlsson, Hagberg, & Jensen, 2015).

The Chuang and Aboagye studies found that a series of 12 yoga classes had a favorable impact on sickness absence days for patients with both chronic low back pain (Chuang et al., 2012) and non-specific low back pain (Aboagye et al., 2015).

Chuang reported that yoga participants missed an average of 3.8 days off work compared to 12.3 in a usual care group over a one-year period. In addition, patients who were offered yoga treatment for their back pain gained 0.037 quality-adjusted life years (QALYs) more than those patients offered usual care.

Similarly, Aboagye reported that patients offered yoga treatment missed an average of 12.4 days of work over a one year period compared to 29.6 days missed by patients offered usual care. Aboagye found that patients offered yoga for their back pain gained 0.036 QALYs more than those patients offered usual care.

Table 1. Comparing studies (Source: Cheema, 2013)

	Initial (n=)	Age (Years)	Yoga Style	Control Group(s)	Time Period	Frequency	Home Practice	Rate of Completion	Adverse Events	Quality Rating	Risk of Bias	Outcome Measures	Mean Difference (SD)	Result
	37	mean=38	*Hatha*	Wait-list	10 weeks	3 x per week 50 min class	No	34 of 37 92%	No	High	Low	Heart rate variability	0.20 (±0.26)	p= 0.48
												Sit and reach	4.1 (±1.04)	p< 0.001
Garfinkel, 1998	51	24 to 77	*Iyengar*	Wrist Splint	8 weeks	2 x per week 90 min class	No	42 of 51 82%	Not reported	High	Low	Grip strength Sleep quality	19.2 (± 2.12) Not reported	p= 0.009 p= 0.26
Granath, 2006	37	working age	*Kundalini*	CBT	10 weeks	1 x per week # of minutes unreported	No	33 of 37 89%	Not reported	Medium	Medium	Perceived stress	-0.39 (± 0.24)	p< 0.01
Hartfiel, 2011	48	mean=39	Dru	Wait-list	6 weeks	1 x per week 60 min class	Yes	40 of 48 83%	Not reported	Medium	Medium	Self-confidence in dealing with stress	1.04 (± 0.32)	p= 0.001
Hartfiel, 2012	74	mean=45	Dru	Wait-list	8 weeks	1 x per week 50 min class	Yes	59 of 74 80%	Not reported	Medium	Medium	Back pain Perceived stress	1.17 (±0.35) -2.40 (±0.66)	p< 0.01 p< 0.01
Joshi, 2009	60	mean=33	*Iyengar*	Counselling	12 weeks	3 x per week 60 min class	No	58 of 60 97%	Not reported	Low	High	Symptom Severity Functional Status	-0.17 (±0.11) -0.06 (±0.08)	p= 0.002 p= 0.06
Telles, 2009	291	21 to 49	Not specified	Wait-list	8 weeks	5 x per week 60 min class	No	118 of 291 41%	Not reported	Medium	Medium	Musculoskeletal Discomfort Grip strength Sit and reach	-10.07 (±0.54) 0.65 (±0.54) 10.4 (±0.53)	p< 0.001 p< 0.05 p< 0.001
Wolever, 2012	239	mean=42	*Viniyoga*	Mindfulness Usual care	12 weeks	1 x per week 60 min class	Yes	205 of 239 86%	Not reported	Medium	Medium	Perceived stress Sleep Quality Heart rate variability	-4.01 (±0.14) -1.11 (±0.11) 0.50 (±0.04)	p< 0.001 p< 0.05 p< 0.001

Cost-Effectiveness and Return on Investment of Yoga in the Workplace

In the United Kingdom, a recent randomized controlled trial (in press) involving 151 National Health Service employees investigated the cost-effectiveness and return on investment of an eight-week yoga program in the workplace. Cost and effect data was collected at baseline, eight weeks and six months. Outcome measures included back pain, health-related quality of life and sickness absence related to musculoskeletal conditions.

During this six month study, yoga participants missed only 2 days due to musculoskeletal conditions, while the usual care group missed 43 days. In addition, yoga participants gained 0.032 QALYs more than those participants offered usual care. These results indicated that when compared with usual care, yoga was cost-saving for the employer with benefit-cost ratios ranging between 1.62 and 3.71, depending on whether the extra costs associated with sickness absence and/or employee co-payments for the yoga sessions were included in the analysis.

The results from this study (in press) along with the findings from Chuang et al. (2012) and Aboagye et al. (2015) showed that yoga could substantially improve health-related quality of life and provide significant cost savings from sickness absence days averted.

CONCLUSION

Yoga can be an effective workplace intervention, especially for managing musculoskeletal disorders and stress.In addition, cost-effectiveness studies suggest that yoga can save employers sickness absence days due to musculoskeletal disorders and back pain.

Although the evidence for yoga is promising, it is limited due to a lack of high quality studies both for effectiveness and cost-effectiveness. To strengthen the evidence base, more high-quality randomized controlled trials of yoga interventions in different workplace settings are required.

REFERENCES

Aboagye, E., Karlsson, M. L., Hagberg, J., & Jensen, I. (2015). Cost-effectiveness of early interventions for non-specific low back pain: A randomized controlled study investigating medical yoga, exercise therapy and self-care advice. *Journal of Rehabilitation Medicine*, *47*(2), 167–173. doi:10.2340/16501977-1910 PMID:25403347

Black, C. D., & Frost, D. (2011). *Health at work- an independent review of sickness absence*. London: The Stationery Office.

Cheema, B. S., Houridis, A., Busch, L., Raschke-Cheema, V., Melville, G. W., Marshall, P. W., ... Colagiuri, B. (2013). Effect of an office worksite-based yoga program on heart rate variability: Outcomes of a randomized controlled trial. *BMC Complementary and Alternative Medicine*, *13*(1), 82. doi:10.1186/1472-6882-13-82 PMID:23574691

Chong, C. S., Tsunaka, M., & Chan, E. P. (2011). Effects of yoga on stress management in healthy adults: A systematic review. *Alternative Therapies in Health and Medicine*, *17*(1), 32–38. PMID:21614942

Chuang, L. H., Soares, M. O., Tilbrook, H., Cox, H., Hewitt, C. E., Aplin, J., ... Torgerson, D. J. (2012). A pragmatic multicentered randomized controlled trial of yoga for chronic low back pain: Economic evaluation. *Spine*, *37*(18), 1593–1601. doi:10.1097/BRS.0b013e3182545937 PMID:22433499

Collins, C. (1998). Yoga: Intuition Preventive Medicine Treatment. *Journal of Obstetric, Gynecologic, and Neonatal Nursing*, *27*(5), 563–568. doi:10.1111/j.1552-6909.1998.tb02623.x PMID:9773368

Cramer, H., Krucoff, C., & Dobos, G. (2013). Adverse events associated with yoga: A systematic review of published case reports and case series. *PLoS ONE*, *8*(10), e75515. doi:10.1371/journal.pone.0075515 PMID:24146758

Cramer, H., Lauche, R., Haller, H., & Dobos, G. (2013). A systematic review and meta-analysis of yoga for low back pain. *The Clinical Journal of Pain*, *29*(5), 450–460. doi:10.1097/AJP.0b013e31825e1492 PMID:23246998

Garfinkel, M. S., Singhal, A., Katz, W. A., Allan, D. A., Reshetar, R., & Schumacher, H. R. Jr. (1998). Yoga-based intervention for carpal tunnel syndrome: A randomized trial. *Journal of the American Medical Association*, *280*(18), 1601–1603. doi:10.1001/jama.280.18.1601 PMID:9820263

Granath, J., Ingvarsson, S., von Thiele, U., & Lundberg, U. (2006). Stress management: A randomized study of cognitive behavioural therapy and yoga. *Cognitive Behaviour Therapy*, *35*(1), 3–10. doi:10.1080/16506070500401292 PMID:16500773

Hartfiel, N., Burton, C., Rycroft-Malone, J., Clarke, G., Havenhand, J., Khalsa, S. B., & Edwards, R. T. (2012). Yoga for reducing perceived stress and back pain at work. *Occupational Medicine*, *62*(8), 606–612. doi:10.1093/occmed/kqs168 PMID:23012344

Hartfiel, N., Havenhand, J., Khalsa, S. B., Clarke, G., & Krayer, A. (2011). The effectiveness of yoga for the improvement of well-being and resilience to stress in the workplace. *Scandinavian Journal of Work, Environment & Health*, *37*(1), 70–76. doi:10.5271jweh.2916 PMID:20369218

Holtzman, S., & Beggs, R. T. (2013). Yoga for chronic low back pain: A meta-analysis of randomized controlled trials. *Pain Research & Management*, *18*(5), 267–272. doi:10.1155/2013/105919 PMID:23894731

Joshi, V., & Bellad, A. (2011). Effect of yogic exercises on symptoms of musculoskeletal disorders of upper limbs among computer users: A randomised controlled trial. *Indian Journal of Medical Sciences*, *65*(10), 424–428. doi:10.4103/0019-5359.109256 PMID:23511042

Mackett, R. L., & Brown, B. (2011). Transport, Physical Activity and Health: Present knowledge and the way ahead.

McCaffrey, R., & Park, J. (2012). The benefits of yoga for musculoskeletal disorders: A systematic review of the literature. *J Yoga Phys Ther*, *2*(122), 2.

National Institute for Health. (2013). *Yoga for health*. U.S. Department of Health and Human Sciences: National Institute of Health, National Center for Complimentary and Alternative Medicine.

Office for National Statistics. (2014). *Full report: Sickness absence in the labour market*. London: Office for National Statistics.

Posadski, P. & Ernst, E. (2011). Yoga for low back pain: a systematic review of randomized clinical trials. *Clinical Rheumatology*, *30*, 1257–1262.

Sherman, K. J., Cherkin, D. C., Wellman, R. D., Cook, A. J., Hawkes, R. J., Delaney, K., & Deyo, R. A. (2011). A randomized trial comparing yoga, stretching, and a self-care book for chronic low back pain. *Archives of Internal Medicine*, *171*(22), 2019–2026. doi:10.1001/archinternmed.2011.524 PMID:22025101

Telles, S., Dash, M., & Naveen, K. V. (2009). Effect of yoga on musculoskeletal discomfort and motor functions in professional computer users. *Work (Reading, Mass.)*, *33*(3), 297–306. PMID:19759428

Tilbrook, H. E., Cox, H., Hewitt, C. E., Kangombe, A. R., Chuang, L. H., Jayakody, S., ... Torgerson, D. J. (2011). Yoga for Chronic Low Back Pain: A Randomized Trial. *Annals of Internal Medicine*, *155*(9), 569–578. doi:10.7326/0003-4819-155-9-201111010-00003 PMID:22041945

Vaughan-Jones, H., & Barham, L. (2009). *Health work: challenges and opportunities to 2030*. London: Bupa.

Ward, L., Stebbings, S., Cherkin, D., & Baxter, G. D. (2013). Yoga for Functional Ability, Pain and Psychosocial Outcomes in Musculoskeletal Conditions: A Systematic Review and Meta-Analysis. *Musculoskeletal Care*, *11*(4), 203–217. doi:10.1002/msc.1042 PMID:23300142

Ward, L., Treharne, G. J., & Stebbings, S. (2011). The suitability of yoga as a potential therapeutic intervention for rheumatoid arthritis: A focus group approach. *Musculoskeletal Care*, *9*(4), 211–221. doi:10.1002/msc.217 PMID:21800407

Wolever, R. Q., Bobinet, K. J., McCabe, K., Mackenzie, E. R., Fekete, E., Kusnick, C. A., & Baime, M. (2012). Effective and viable mind-body stress reduction in the workplace: A randomized controlled trial. *Journal of Occupational Health Psychology*, *17*(2), 246–258. doi:10.1037/a0027278 PMID:22352291

Woodyard, C. (2011). Exploring the therapeutic effects of yoga and its ability to increase quality of life. *International Journal of Yoga*, *4*(2), 49–54. doi:10.4103/0973-6131.85485 PMID:22022122

World Health Organization (WHO). (1997). WHO's global healthy works approach. Division of Health Promotion, Education & Communication and Office of Occupational Health, Geneva.

Yoga Journal and Yoga Alliance. (2016). *Yoga in America Study*. Retrieved from www.yogajournal.com/yogainamericastudy.

Yoga Journal. (2012). *Yoga in America Market Study*. Retrieved from http://www.yoga journal.com/article/press-releases/yoga-journal-releases-2012-yoga-in-america-market-study

KEY TERMS AND DEFINITIONS

Cost-Effectiveness of Yoga: Cost-effectiveness is the degree to which something is effective or productive in relation to its cost.

Dru Yoga: Dru yoga is a style of yoga that works with postures, breath work, relaxation and meditation. Its series or sequences are called Energy Block Release.

Health Related Quality of Life: Health-Related Quality of Life (HRQoL) is a multi-dimensional concept that includes domains related to physical, mental, emotional, and social functioning.

Heart Rate Variability: Heart rate variability (HRV) is the physiological phenomenon of variation in the time interval between heartbeats. It is measured by the variation in the beat-to-beat interval.

Musculoskeletal Disorders: Musculoskeletal Disorders or MSDs are injuries and disorders that affect the human body's movement or musculoskeletal system (i.e. muscles, tendons, ligaments, nerves, discs, blood vessels, etc.). Common MSDs include: Carpal Tunnel Syndrome, Tendonitis, and Muscle / Tendon strain.

Non-Specific Low Back Pain: Non-specific low back pain is usually categorized in 3 subtypes: acute, sub-acute and chronic low back pain. This subdivision is based on the duration of the back pain.

Occupational Stress: Occupational stress is a major hazard for many workers. Increased workloads downsizing, overtime, hostile work environments, and shiftwork are just a few of the many causes of stressful working conditions.

Perceived Stress: Perceived psychological stress has been defined as the extent to which persons perceive (appraise) that their demands exceed their ability to cope.

Quality Adjusted Life Years: The quality-adjusted life year or quality-adjusted life-year (QALY) is a generic measure of disease burden, including both the quality and the quantity of life lived. It is used in economic evaluation to assess the value for money of medical interventions. One QALY equates to one year in perfect health.

Quality of Sleep: The Sleep Cycle's Sleep Quality is affected by two factors: (i) Sleep quantity and (ii) Frequency of movement. In short, the more you sleep and the less you move, the higher Sleep Quality you will get.

This research was previously published in Research-Based Perspectives on the Psychophysiology of Yoga edited by Shirley Telles and Nilkamal Singh, pages 175-183, copyright year 2018 by Medical Information Science Reference (an imprint of IGI Global).

Chapter 12
Whole-Body Cryotherapy as a Tool to Improving of Infrared Thermography Diagnostics

Armand Cholewka
University of Silesia, Poland

Karolina Sieroń-Stołtny
Medical University of Silesia, Poland

Agata Stanek
Medical University of Silesia, Poland

Joanna Kajewska
University of Silesia, Poland

ABSTRACT

The use of low temperature on the whole human body switched on beneficial physiological reactions. Whole-body cryotherapy is used as a part of rehabilitation. There were reported studies of thermal imaging performed due to whole body cooling in case of patients suffering from different diseases that showed a significant enhancement of the skin temperature gradient observed after cryotherapy. That explains that such therapeutic technique like whole-body cryotherapy can be used as a part of infrared thermography diagnostic procedure.

INTRODUCTION

Skin Temperature as the Physical Parameter

Body temperature is used as an indicator of diseases processes. It is usually measured by contact thermometers which must be stick to the skin or put inside the body orifices i.e. mouth, ear or rectum. It is very important factor describing our health state. But what about the skin temperature? Does it give us some important information about our health state too? Nowadays, we can say that it is very important to measure not

DOI: 10.4018/978-1-7998-1680-5.ch012

only internal organism temperature, but also, in many cases, body surface temperature which might be sensitive indicator of metabolism changes beneath the skin what might be related to health state. This was proved by Hipocrates. However, his experiments were performed with poor precision and had only qualitative character. Can we measure it very precisely? Can we use such parameter like body surface temperature to evaluate or even diagnose some diseases? Maybe it is possible to use thermal maps of the body to differentiate diseases?

However, first we should take into consideration that body surface temperature can give us very important information about tissue's health state – especially soft tissues just beneath the skin. Hippocrates was the first one who proved and showed how important skin temperature is. He did it using wet soil which was put on patient's skin in vicinity of abdomen. Wet soil while drying changing its color and Hippocrates was able to see in a sense the temperature gradient. Now it is obvious that skin temperature gradient is also a very important physical parameter that can be used in medical diagnosis. There is no doubt that the skin temperature and its variation can also be a symptom of disease in living organism. It is very important that the skin temperature change can be easily detected by infrared imaging. Temperature gradient is a very good diseases indicator because local blood flow and metabolism changes cause temperature change of the skin Therefore, infrared thermography imaging which is completely non-invasive diagnostic technique can be widely and easily used in medical diagnosis (Ring, Jung, Kalicki, Zuber, Rustecka, & Vardasca, 2013; Cholewka & Drzazga, 2006).

Maybe it will be possible to combine body cooling with thermal imaging and use it as a diagnostics method. However, before we present the achieves and possibilities of use the infrared thermography as a tool of diagnosis in whole body cryotherapy, we should first explain a little what the whole – body cryotherapy is and how it is used in medicine.

Whole Body Cooling in Sport and Medicine

In last few decades, very popular modern forms of wellness in sport has become using the whole body cooling as a part not only the rehabilitation but also as a part of normal training program as well as in recovering after injuries. Properly dosed and applied treatments renewing athletes, give a chance to reduce the negative effects of overloads and prepare the sportsman for the next train. The aim of wellness in sportsmen is to speed up the healing process and rise the efficiency level of the body (Vardasca, Ring, Plassmann, & Jones, 2012). Cryotherapy may cause circulatory and metabolic better exercise tolerance and delay the accumulation of tiredness while working muscle. In addition, the subjective feelings of the athletes after using a series of sessions in the cryochamber show a faster regeneration after training, and higher motivation to re-repetition training (Ring & Ammer, 2012). Cryotherapy has been also considered as an excellent treatment method in many fields of sports. Many clinical studies have reported that the use of cryotherapy has a beneficial effect on pain reduction and recovery of various injuries. Additionally, results of various studies are coherent on the effects on pain and neuromuscular processes (Ring, Jung, Kalicki, Zuber, Rustecka, & Vardasca, 2013). Whole-body cryotherapy, as well as the local one, are methods used for the treatment of acute soft tissue injuries. As part of the therapy can be used various methods such as ice towels, ice packs, ice massage, refrigerant gases, gel packs and inflatable splints. The chosen method of cooling the tissue directly influences the obtained therapeutic effect (Ring & Ammer, 2012).

It is known the biochemical and physiological processes in the human body are highly sensitive due to temperature change. The internal temperature of the body is constant and is kept at 37 °C with primary typical daily changes approximately 0.7 °C. But the surface temperature of the body changes in a wide range because of changes in ambient temperature.With all energy generated by the tissues mentioned, only 15-25% is converted into kinetic energy. The rest of the energy is converted into heat and distributed by the blood supply to the whole body (Ganong, 2009; Traczyk, 2007; Ronikier, 2008; Ammer, 2008). There are three main ways to heat loss: convection, conduction and infrared radiation. Instead, an important mechanism of the body's cooling process is evaporating water from the mouth and the mucous membranes of the respiratory system. The exchange of water or water vapor is an endothermic process which resulted in the body is cooled during sweating. Evaporation of one gram of water is approximately 0.6 kcal heat removal (Podbielska & Skrzek, 2014).

The average temperature of human body surface *Tsurf* is calculated based on the empirical formula (1) (Pilawski, 1983):

$$T_{surf} = 0.32 \cdot T_{tibia} + 0.18 \cdot T_{chest} + 0.14 \cdot T_{arms} + 0.07 \cdot T_{foot} + 0.07 \cdot T_{head} + 0.05 \cdot T_{hands} + 0.17 \cdot T_{back} \quad (1)$$

where: T_{tibia} is legs surface temperature; T_{chest}, chest surface temperature; T_{arms}, arms surface temperature; T_{foot}, foot surface temperature; T_{head}, head surface temperature; T_{hands}, hands surface temperature; T_{back}, back surface temperature.

Food delivered to the body is transformed by the process of digestion, which is directly related to metabolism (Ammer (2008)). The amount of heat losses ΔQ is associated with changes energy ΔE_M and the work done by the muscles ΔW, in relation to the first law of thermodynamics to biological processes, this dependence can written as (Equation 2):

$$\Delta Q = \Delta E_M + \Delta W \quad (2)$$

The moment when the body is in repose, work is not performing ($\Delta W = 0$) there is a possibility to change the Equation 2 into the Equation 3. Then the heat flux φ transferred to the environment can be calculated from Equation 3, which is called the Basal Metabolism Rate BMR0 and is presented below (Hulbert & Else, 2004; Ammer, 2008; Cholewka, Kasprzyk, Stanek, Sieroń-Stołtny, & Drzazga, 2015; Cholewka, Kasprzyk, Stanek, Sieroń-Stołtny, & Drzazga, 2015):

$$\phi = \frac{\Delta E}{\Delta t} \Leftrightarrow BMR_0 = mM^{\frac{3}{4}} \tag{3}$$

where: M – body weight; m – the factor for mammals with the value 3.4 W*kg$^{-3/4}$.

It should be also noted that many different diseases which symptoms are manifested as an increase or decrease of internal temperature as well as the skin temperature can be found (Ring, Jung, Kalicki, Zuber, Rustecka, & Vardasca, 2013; Cholewka, Drzazga, Sieroń, & Stanek, 2010). On the other hand, there are many different physical factors used in the medicine, mostly in physical medicine that can influence skin temperature of human body. This is the reason why in this chapter authors focused on some experiences of the influence of very low temperature (below -100 °C) used in the whole body cryotherapy on human organism as not only part of rehabilitation, but as a part of medical procedure used in thermovision diagnostic. It was found that the use of very low temperature before thermal imaging, can influence on thermal map by increasing the diagnostic value. When we say about cold treatment we should explain that whole body cryotherapy is a medical specialty that is widely used in medicine. However, the main goal of whole body cryotherapy is using the lower temperature in short periods of time to stimulate different organism reactions by triggering the defense mechanisms against the cold. In this kind of treatment, whole body of patient is influenced by temperature lower than -100°C for a period of 2-3 minutes in a special room, called cryogenic chamber, in order to cause some physiological and biochemical reactions in the organism. The treatment takes usually 10-20 sessions of cryotherapy – day by day (excluded weekends). Use of extremely low temperature in such way leads to shortening the process of treatment of some diseases (Podbielska & Skrzek, 2012; Sieroń & Cieślar, 2003; Sieroń, Cieślar, & Stanek, 2010; Sieroń, Stanek, Cieślar, & Pasek, 2007). Applying of cryogenic temperature on the whole human body evokes in human body beneficial physiological reactions such as: analgesic, neuro-muscular, antiodematous and anti-inflammatory effects as well as circulatory, hormonal and immunological reactions. Moreover, whole - body cryotherapy procedures have also a beneficial influence on human psyche through relaxation action and decrease level of anxiety, as well as excretion and increase of different hormones what undoubtedly is also very important in treatment. Whole – body cryotherapy is used as a part of rehabilitation programme with kinesiotherapy (physical exercises) what leads to shortening of the recovery time and makes the rehabilitation most efficient. This therapy is applied in different motion organs diseases: degeneration and inflammatory states of joints (monoarthritis and oligoarthritis) and periarthritis, rheumatism, low back pain diseases and inflammatory, degeneration states of spinal vertebrae joints, fibromialgia and osteoporosis. It was also reported positive influence of whole – body cryotherapy on mental health what is connected with increase of concentration of some hormones and destroying the free radicals. Cold treatment may be beneficial also in tiredness and dream disturbance. Moreover, the cryotherapy has wide application in spine and nervous system diseases, like sciatica and spondyloarthrosis, as well as sclerosis multiplex. It should be underline that all of mentioned diseases are treated by used whole – body cryotherapy correlated with kinesitherapy procedures. Such procedures allow intensification of the training and extension of its duration by several times. Therefore, procedures of whole body cryotherapy and kinesiotherapy are altogether main components of so - called cryorehabilitation. Such influence is very useful in treatment of many different diseases what was reported in literature through last decades (Bauer, Hurnik, Zdziarski, Mielczarek, Skrzek, Podbielska, & Zagrobelny, 1997; Biały, Zimmer, Skrzek, & Zagrobelny, 1998).

It was also reported that whole - body cryotherapy causes only a slight change in blood morphology parameters within the range of reference values, different in patients with ankylosing spondylitis and healthy volunteers. In patients with ankylosing spondylitis after the end of a cycle of whole - body cryotherapy a significant decrease in hematocrit value and mean capacity of single blood corpuscle (MCV), as well as an increase in mean concentration of haemoglobin in blood corpuscle (MCHC) were observed. In patients with ankylosing spondylitis it seems to be a safe method leading to improvement of rheologic properties of blood. On the other hand, in healthy volunteers a significant increase in erythrocytes, hemoglobin concentration, hematocrit value and mean capacity of single blood corpuscle, decrease in mean concentration of haemoglobin in blood corpuscle as well as an increase in platelets count and proportion of monocytes in differential cell count (Stanek, Sieron, Cieslar, Matyszkiewicz, & Rozmus-Kuczia, 2005).

The whole - body cryotherapy procedures are performed in special rooms called cryochambers. There are two main types of cryochambers: closed one (two-step, so called Wroclawska cryochamber) and cryochamber with cold retention (in some papers called chamber with lingering cold). Cryochamber may be cooled by liquid nitrogen fumes and liquid synthetic air. Synthetic air is easier in exploitation and its use reduces costs of cryochamber construction up to 40%. First type of cryogenic chambers consists of two parts: a pre-chamber with temperature up to - 60°C and a proper chamber, where main therapy takes place and temperature inside ranges from

-110°C to -160°C. Pre-chamber is the place where patient adapt to extremely low temperature. Adaptation time in pre-chamber is up to 30s, then patients enter to a main chamber, where whole - body cryotherapy procedures are performed and patient is influenced at least by -100°C. Temperature and time of whole body cryotherapy procedure depends on patient's health and sometimes individual reaction to the cold. Usually the main therapy in the proper chamber lasts 3 minutes. Cryochamber operation is completely automatic and may be operated by only one person. However, there are physician as well as technician or rehabilitant always inside the chamber during the patients treatment. Moreover, cryochambers are usually covered with wood and have swing doors that a subject may easily open at any time to interrupt a procedure when a temporary indisposition occurs. In some versions of cryochambers treatment may be carried out for 4-6 subjects simultaneously. It is observed for bigger ones like two-stepped cryochambers (Stanek, Cieslar, & Sieron, 2007; Sieroń, Stanek, Cieślar, & Pasek, 2007; Stanek, Cholewka, Cieslar, Rosmus-Kuczia, Drzazga, & Sieron, 2011; Stanek, Cieslar, Strzelczyk et al., 2010). In the case of cryochamber with lingering cold, its principle of operation on the physical phenomenon of lingering cold in the basin. Therefore, the cryogenic chamber is placed underground. In this case, to get very low temperature, the liquid air with modified composition (21% to 30% oxygen) is usually used which is pumped from the tank outside the chamber by the pipes into the sprayer nozzles inside the cryogenic chamber.

There is another type of cryochamber called cryosauna which is designates for only one patient. Despite the basis of functioning being similar to the other cryochambers, there is one big difference – in this case it is possible to change the height of the platform on which patient stay, what gives possibility to take a cryotherapy by patients suffering from claustrophobia.

It was proved that that the application of 10 - days of whole – body cryotherapy sessions leads to health improvement. It was also reported that the good health state increases with the number of sessions. That is why patients sometimes take another cycle of cold treatment. Patient's health state improves relatively quickly what is manifested by the reduction of the level of pain, improvement of health condition and the feeling of well-being what was reported in literature (Cholewka & Drzazga, 2005; Cholewka & Drzazga, 2006). The very important thing is that every kind of the cryochamber gives similar positive results in patients' health. The first and most important thing is that it leads to reduction of pain level what is the result of increased excretion of β-endorphins, the switching off the feeling receptors non-active due to cold and their connection with pro-prioreceptors and slower conduction in feeling fibres (Sieroń, Cieślar & Stanek, 2010; Stanek, Sieron, Cieslar, Matyszkiewicz, & Rozmus-Kuczia, 2005; Stanek, Cieslar, & Sieron, 2007). Another aspect of cold treatment, is the improvement of physical fitness what is important in sport's medicine.

It was also reported that whole – body cooling has similar positive influence on increase of the pain level for all studied patients - regardless of their age. The situation was quite different in the case of influence of whole – body cryotherapy on patients' shape. In this case, the effects are better seen for younger patients than for older ones. The cryotherapy effects for older patients were also beneficial however there were some patients that did not reported any physical shape improvement. However, body cryotherapy is beneficial and after each session patients felt better and relaxed. Thus patients took willingly the next cryotherapy sessions and there were patients that took even several times cryotherapy sessions during few years. Some studies showed that patients indicate similar reception of the whole – body cryotherapy, regardless of cryogenic chamber type what seems to be obvious when we keep strictly to the protocol and physical parameters conditions like time of treatment and magnitude of the temperature inside the chamber.

It should also be noted that there are differences in cold influence on different parts of human body. It is caused mostly by set-up and physiology of their organs as well as their geometry. That is why during whole - body cryotherapy procedures a temperature of organs in chest, abdominal cavity, skull inside and blood is steady. One only observes the changes of body surface temperature. The biggest heat losses is observed on parts of the body, which are relatively big in relation to theirs volume (mainly fingers, toes, limbs). Heat loss in fingers and toes is nearly ten times higher than in trunk what also has a meaning in diagnostic value of thermal imaging (Sieroń, Cieślar, & Stanek, 2010; Stanek, Sieron, Cieslar, Matyszkiewicz, & Rozmus-Kuczia, 2005; Stanek, Cieslar, & Sieron, 2007; Stanek, Cieślar, Mrowiec, & Sieroń, 2006; Biały, Zimmer, Skrzek, & Zagrobelny, 1998).

Every patient before whole - body cryotherapy procedures always have to be examined and qualified to procedure by a physician. For each patient qualified to whole body cryotherapy, procedure therapeutic parameters and individual program of kinesiotherapy are determined (Sieroń, Cieślar, & Stanek, 2010; Stanek, Sieron, Cieslar, Matyszkiewicz, & Rozmus-Kuczia, 2005; Stanek, Cieslar, & Sieron, 2007; Stanek, Cieślar, Mrowiec, & Sieroń, 2006; Biały, Zimmer, Skrzek, & Zagrobelny, 1998).

In a cryochamber some parts of the body that are most sensitive to extremely low temperature and mostly exposed to cryogenic temperature have to be particularly protected against injury. Hands are protected by gloves, shanks and feet - by woolen knee length socks and feet additionally by wooden clogs. Then auricles are protected by a cap or headband and mouths - by gauze - lined surgical masks. During the procedure, woman wear swimming costumes and men shorts. The main idea of whole body cooling is to expose as big as possible, body surface to cold. The above-described outfit allows for contact of bigger body area with low temperature what leads to overcooling as more as possible receptors of the body.

Before the subjects are instructed how to behave in cryochamber during whole - body cryotherapy procedure. Patient should pay special attention to the way of breathing in the chamber during the procedure. Inhaling should be two times shorter than exhaling due to decompression of cooled air in lungs. It is also forbidden to touch other subjects or rub own skin. Each time before whole - body cryotherapy procedure, patients should dry thoroughly their skin with a towel in order to remove sweat, as sweat drops turn into crystals they cause frostbite. Immediately after leaving a cryochamber, patients underwent kinesiotherapy procedures, usually lasting 30-60 minutes what is dependent on the health state of the patient and predicted by physician (Sieroń, Cieślar, & Stanek, 2010; Stanek, Sieron, Cieslar, Matyszkiewicz, & Rozmus-Kuczia, 2005; Stanek, Cieslar, & Sieron, 2007; Stanek, Cieślar, Mrowiec, & Sieroń, 2006; Biały, Zimmer, Skrzek, & Zagrobelny, 1998).

Cryotherapy treatment has rapidly developing during last 30 years. Nowadays it is being widely used in many applications, mostly in medicine i.e.: degeneration and inflammatory states of joints (monoarthritis and oligoarthritis) and periarthritis, rheumatism, low back pain diseases, inflammatory, in degeneration states of spinal vertebrae joints and fibromyalgia as well as in osteoporosis preventive treatment. It has also application in nervous system diseases like sclerosis multiplex and sciatica, discopathy and many other spine lesions that are connected with perturbations of nervous system. The very common spine diseases treated by whole- body cryotherapy are ankylosing spondylitis, sciatica and spondyloarthrosis.. Whole - body cryotherapy is also applied in sports' medicine in the treatment of both, acute and chronic injuries of soft tissue in sportsmen as well as, adjunctive method in biological regeneration (biostimulating effect, endurance and strength training, acceleration of post-endurance restitution, and prophylaxis of locomotor system overloading (Sieroń, Cieślar, & Stanek, 2010; Stanek, Sieron, Cieslar, Matyszkiewicz, & Rozmus-Kuczia, 2005; Stanek, Cieslar, & Sieron, 2007; Stanek, Cieślar, Mrowiec, & Sieroń, 2006; Gregorowiczv & Zagrobelny, 1998).

Nowadays more and more often healthy subjects start to use whole - body cryotherapy to keep good health and well-being, prevention of stresses and their consequences, revitalize and harden the body as well as a method of anti - aging (Gage & Baust, 2002).

In turn, absolute contraindications for applying whole - body cryotherapy procedures include: intolerance of cold, cold utricaria, cryoglobulinemia, cryofibrynogemia, Raynaud's symptom, hypothyroidism, severe anemia, acute diseases of respiratory tract, neoplastic disease, purulent-gangrenous skin lesions, vegetative neuropathies, local blood flow disturbances, cachexia, hypothermia, claustrophobia (Sieroń, Cieślar, & Stanek, 2010; Stanek, Sieron, Cieslar, Matyszkiewicz, & Rozmus-Kuczia, 2005; Stanek, Cieslar, & Sieron, 2007).

Assessment of Whole Body Cryotherapy by Infrared Thermography

Influence of cold on the human body leads primarily to reduce the temperature of the skin and tissues subsurface. Different parts of the body are cooling in different ways (Sieroń & Cieślar, 2003; Sieroń, Cieślar, & Stanek, 2010; Sieroń & Cieślar, 2007; Sieroń & Cieślar, 2003; Zagrobelny, 2003). Human as a warm-blooded organism - characterized by homeostasis, strives to maintain a constant temperature inside the body. Therefore, in the analysis of the thermal response to the cooling of the body must distinguish internal and surface layers' temperature. The internal temperature is necessary for the correct functioning of the body and the temperature of the surface layer depends on the ambient temperature (Cholewka, Stanek, Sieroń, & Drzazga, 2011; Sieroń & Cieślar, 2003; Sieroń, Cieślar, & Stanek, 2010; Sieroń & Cieślar, 2007; Sieroń & Cieślar, 2003; Zagrobelny, 2003; Cholewka, Drzazga, Borgieł, & Kurpas, 2005).

With some approximation, it can be assumed that the heat map observed on the surface of the body presents a thermodynamic state of the body. This state is caused by the influence of external conditions on the internal environment of the body - the metabolically active tissue producing internal heat in a living organism. This fact is illustrated on thermal images of patients treated by whole body cryotherapy (Figures 1-3). One can see that thermal images performed immediately after body cooling are different and show some detailes not seen before one what was discussed in literature (Cholewka, Stanek, Sieroń, & Drzazga, 2011; Cholewka & Drzazga, 2005; Cholewka, Drzazga, & Sieroń, 2006; Cholewka, Drzazga, Kajewski, Bogucki, & Wiśniowska, 2004; Cholewka, Drzazga, Kajewski, Bogucki, & Wiśniowska, 2004; Cholewka, Drzazga, Sieroń, Stanek, Knefel, Kawecki, & Nowak, 2010; Cholewka, Drzazga, Borgieł, & Kurpas, 2005; Cholewka, Drzazga, Kajewski, Sieroń, & Wiśniowska, 2004).

Analysis of thermal images and temperature parameters collected in the tables draws (Figure 1) attention to decrease in the surface temperature of the body as a result of cryotherapy and changing the temperature gradient by cooling the body. On thermograms can be seen a slight thermal asymmetry of the body related to the anatomical asymmetry. Also, by comparing the average temperature obtained for the extremities from thermal parameters of thorax it is easy to see greater decreases of the temperature of these parts of the body where the surface to volume ratio is relatively large. It is easy to notice that the higher temperature with skin areas directly with blood vessels and blood flow, which will have a temperature close to 37°C (e.g. subclavian veins, around the mediastinum). The average temperature is lower in areas where blood flow and metabolic processes are less intensive e.g. knees. Analysis of the thermal images of the chest taken before, and immediately after cooling of the body showed

Figure 1. Representative thermal images of the chest and tables of temperatures from areas of interest received for a healthy man made before and after cryotherapy

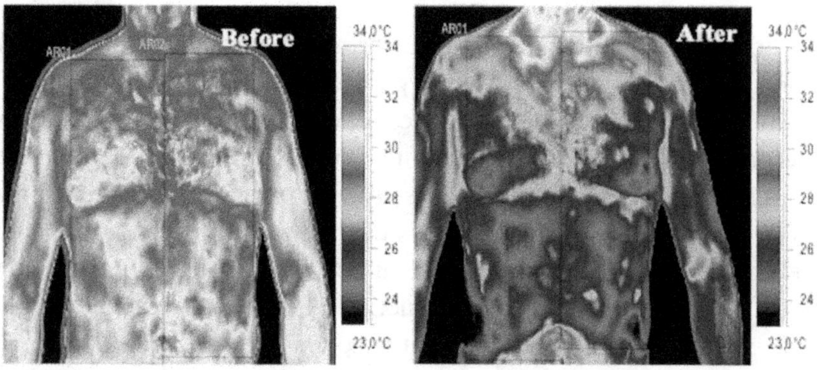

Area	Temperature °C Before cryotherapy	Temperature °C After cryotherapy
AR01 : T_{mean}	31,2	26,4
AR02 : T_{mean}	31,4	26,6
AR01: T_{max}	33,9	31,9
AR01: T_{min}	28,9	22,7
AR02: T_{max}	33,5	22,8
AR02: T_{min}	29,0	32,0

that the greatest cooling was observed on large batches of muscles: musculus pectoralis major and minor and the musculus rectus abdominis as opposed to the area of the breastbone where the pulmonary trunk and large blood vessels (Cholewka, Stanek, Sieroń, & Drzazga, 2011; Cholewka, Drzazga, Sieroń, & Stanek, 2010; Cholewka, Drzazga, & Sieroń, 2006; Cholewka, Drzazga, Sieroń, Stanek, Knefel, Kawecki, & Nowak, 2010; Cholewka, Drzazga, Sieroń, & Wiśniowska, 2004; Cholewka, Drzazga, Kajewski, Sieroń, & Wiśniowska, 2004). The study showed that the internal temperature of the body due to cryotherapy decreases slightly ($\Delta T_{org} = 0.8$ °C) which proves that a short stay in a cryochamber may not cause any negative effects (Cholewka, Drzazga, Michalik, & Sieroń, 2006; Cholewka & Drzazga, 2006; Ring, 1999). The use of thermal imaging allowed the calculation of the average temperature from the selected areas of the body surface to estimate the average temperature of the total body surface area (T_{body}) before and after cryotherapy based on empirical Equation 1. It was the subject of the researches presented in literature (Cholewka, Stanek, Sieroń, & Drzazga, 2011; Cholewka, Drzazga, Kajewski, Bogucki & Wiśniowska, 2004). According to the empirical formula (1) the main role in the mean temperature of the total body have the back, legs, chest and arms.

Table 1. The average skin surface temperature before (Ta ± SD) and after (Tb ± SD) cryotherapy for research group

Temperature (°C)	**Temperature ± SD (°C)** *Before Cryotherapy*	**Temperature ± SD (°C)** *After Cryotherapy*	$\Delta T = T^{before} - T^{after}$ (°C)
T_{head}	30.0 ± 0.9	27.7 ± 0.9	2.3
T_{chest}	31.9 ± 1.0	27.0 ± 1.8	4.9
T_{back}	31.6 ± 1.1	27.5 ± 1.8	4.1
T_{arms}	30.1 ± 1.3	24.5 ± 2.6	5.6
T_{shin}	28.0 ± 1.8	19.3 ± 3.9	8.7
T_{hands}	24.2 ± 2.7	20.7 ± 2.8	3.5
T_{feet}	23.4 ± 2.8	18.2 ± 2.2	5.2
T_{body}	29.2 ± 0.9	23.4 ± 2.0	5.8
$T_{internal\ body}$ ($T_{int.}$)	35.6 ± 0.6	34.8 ± 0.6	0.8

Source: Cholewka, Drzazga, Kajewski, Bogucki, & Wiśniowska, 2004; Cholewka, Stanek, Sieroń, & Drzazga, 2011

The calculations of average temperatures of regions of interest are summarized in Table 1.

The temperature parameters summarized in Table 1 show that, as a result of cryotherapy, surface of the body is cooling what is obvious but the average temperature of the whole body surface calculated from the equation (1) decreased almost 6°C. Different body parts got cooled at different rates. The occurrence of high standard deviation (SD) providing for differences between individuals in terms of the body's response to cryotherapy.

Analyzing the changes of the average of whole body surface temperature due to cryotherapy, an interesting effect associated with varying degrees of cooling the body depending on obesity factor (Body mass index) was observed and discussed in literature (Cholewka, Stanek, Sieroń & Drzazga, 2011; Cholewka, 2005). It was obtained that the average temperature decrease (ΔT) of whole surface of the body is correlated with the BMI (Cholewka, Stanek, Sieroń, & Drzazga, 2011; Cholewka, 2005).

The obtained positive correlation indicates that the body's response to low temperature depends on the physical characteristics (weight and height) of the patient. Obtained result may suggest that parameters such as exposure time and the absolute value of the temperature in the cryogenic chamber should be selected according with the BMI. It can have a potential impact on the therapeutic effect carried out cryotherapy.

Thermal imaging performed immediately after cooling the body in a cryogenic chamber have reflected some anatomical details that were not visible on the thermograms taken before cryotherapy at standard conditions. It is easier to observe some of the muscles on the thermograms of the chest and back. For example, on the back thermograms (Figure 2 and Table 2) it can be seen the entire range of dorsal region of upper back with the lumbar area allows to see trapezius muscle and monotonic changes in temperature along the spine. In this case, it can be seen areas with significantly lower (cold spot) or higher temperature (hot spot) on the line of the spine, which can be linked to the vertebrae, or whole sections of the spine and surrounding area. The effect of increasing the accuracy of the thermal images is associated with a nearly double increase in the temperature gradient ($\Delta T = Tmax - Tmin$) between the maximum and minimum temperatures obtained from selected areas (Cholewka, Stanek, Sieroń, & Drzazga, 2011; Cholewka, Drzazga, Sieroń, & Stanek, 2010; Cholewka, Drzazga, & Sieroń, 2006; Cholewka, Drzazga, Sieroń, Stanek, Knefel, Kawecki, & Nowak, 2010; Cholewka, 2005; Cholewka, Drzazga, Sieroń, & Wiśniowska, 2004). This is caused by the intensification of metabolic processes of various tissues or whole muscle groups. Therefore, the low temperature impact differentiates a thermal map of the body showing details not visible or less visible in the classical thermography (Cholewka, Stanek, Sieroń, & Drzazga, 2011; Cholewka, Drzazga, Sieroń, & Stanek, 2010; Cholewka, Drzazga, & Sieroń, 2006; Cholewka, Drzazga, Sieroń, Stanek, Knefel, Kawecki, & Nowak, 2010; Cholewka, 2005; Cholewka, Drzazga, Sieroń, & Wiśniowska, 2004).

Thermography as a technique for imaging the surface of the body presents a temperature gradient on the patients skin. Heat map of the skin is connected with changes in blood supply and metabolism changes in soft tissues. Imaging is more accurate if these changes are related to the tissues located closer to the surface of the skin (Cholewka, Stanek, Sieroń, & Drzazga, 2011; Cholewka, Drzazga, Sieroń, & Stanek, 2010; Cholewka, 2005; Nowakowski et al., 2001; Żuber & Jung, 1997).

Figure 2. Representative thermograms of the back

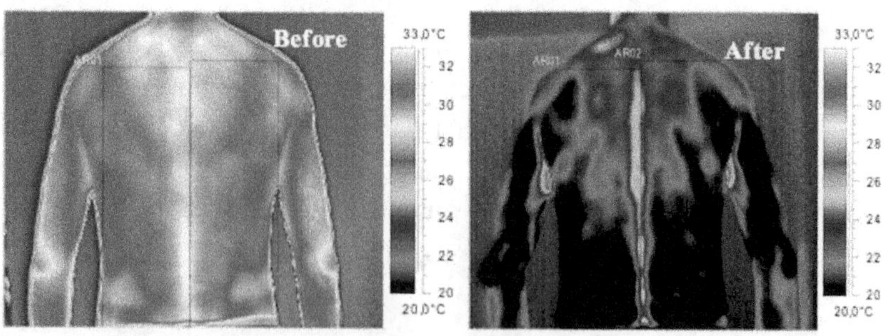

Table 2. Temperatures of regions of interest received for healthy patients taken before and after cryotherapy

Area	Temperature °C Before Cryotherapy	Temperature °C After Cryotherapy
AR01: T_{mean}	31.5	21.0
AR02: T_{mean}	31.1	20.9
AR01: T_{max}	33.7	25.9
AR01: T_{min}	27.7	14.3
AR02: T_{max}	33.1	25.6
AR02: T_{min}	28.1	15.1

Figure 3. The thermograms lower extremity with marked areas the lower leg and tables temperatures of the areas of interest for the health of the patient taken before and after cryotherapy
Source: Cholewka & Drzazga, 2005; Cholewka, Drzazga, Sieroń, Stanek, Knefel, Kawecki, & Nowak, 2010

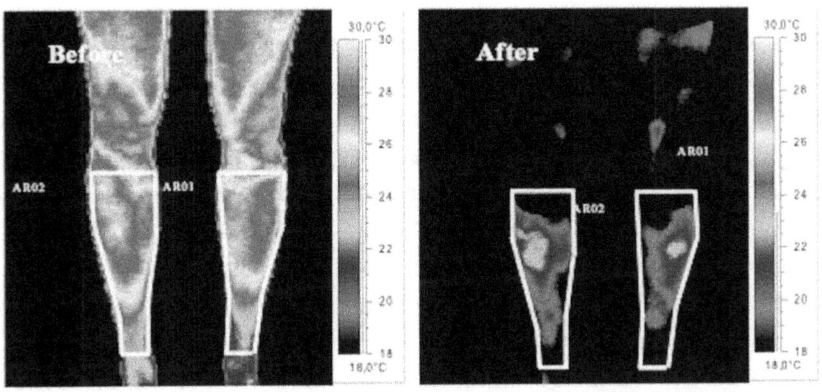

Area	Temperature (°C) Before cryotherapy	Temperature (°C) After cryotherapy
AR01 : T_{mean}	26.2	19.1
AR02 : T_{mean}	27.0	18.5
AR01: T_{max}	28.9	23.6
AR01: T_{min}	19.8	12.6
AR02: T_{max}	30.1	23.1
AR02: T_{min}	21.3	12.6

Figure 4. A scatterplot parameters presented dependence of temperature decrease as a function of body mass index

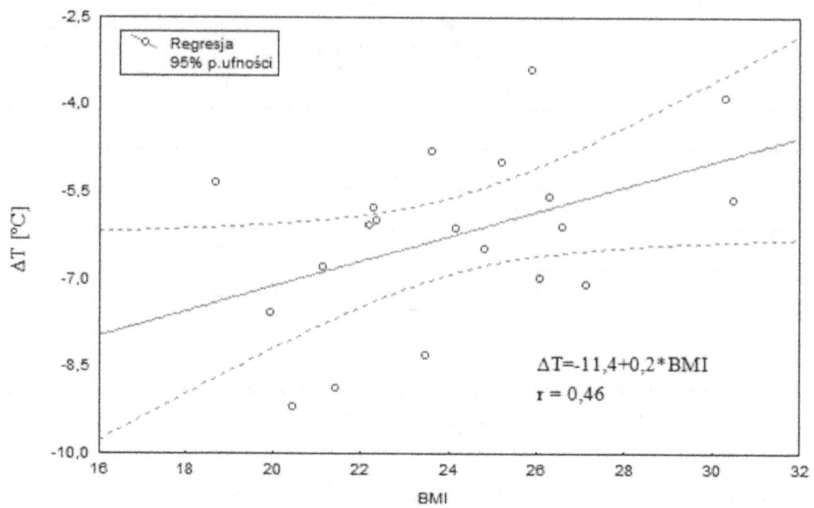

This allows to use in the evaluation of various diseases. Thermal imaging performed before and after cryotherapy is a one of application in various disease entities. An example might be palm thermograms of a patient with a chronic bacterial infection left hand performed before and after cryotherapy (Figure 5) (Cholewka, Stanek, Sieroń, & Drzazga, 2011; Cholewka, Drzazga, Sieroń, & Stanek, 2010; Cholewka, 2005; Nowakowski et al., 2001; Żuber & Jung, 1997; Ring, 2001; Ammer, 2004).

The evaluation of thermal images after performing cryotherapy allows to see a strong asymmetry in the temperature of both hands. Analysis of the temperature data presented in the tables shows that, prior to cryotherapy, the difference in average temperatures between selected areas was only 0.2°C. While the difference after cryotherapy increases more than 10 times to the value 2.7°C. Healthy hand has cooled as a result of staying in a cryogenic chamber while the hand with a bacterial infection did not show significant cooled. This confirms inflammation of patient hand (Cholewka, 2005; Cholewka, Drzazga, Kajewski, Sieroń, & Wiśniowska, 2004; Cholewka, Drzazga, Sieroń, Stanek, Knefel, Kawecki, & Nowak, 2010; Cholewka & Drzazga, 2005).

Another very interesting example of application of thermography and cryotherapy is related to venous insufficiency and has been discussed in literature (Cholewka, 2005; Cholewka, Drzazga, Kajewski, Sieroń, & Wiśniowska, 2004; Cholewka, Drzazga, Sieroń, Stanek, Knefel, Kawecki, & Nowak, 2010; Cholewka & Drzazga, 2005). The case refers to a patient complaining about the pain in the left thigh. The patient was diagnosed as saphenous vein insufficiency of the left thigh. In this case,

Figure 5. The thermograms of hands (left with chronic bacterial infection) performed before and after cryotherapy

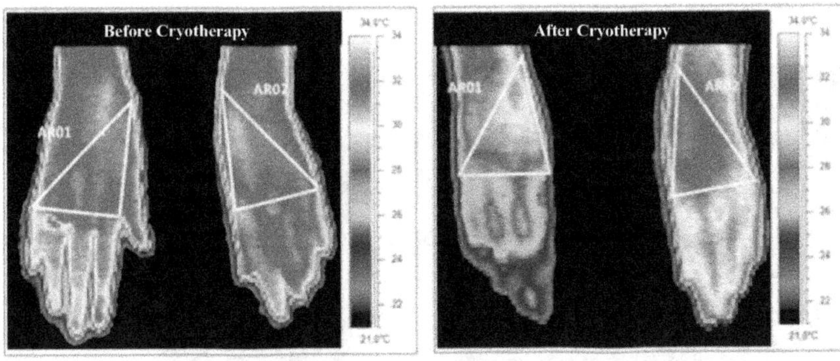

Parameter	$\Delta T = T_{mean}^{AR01} - T_{mean}^{AR02}$
ΔT_{befor}	0.2
ΔT_{after}	2.7

classic thermography performed before cooling the body revealed an elongated area characterized by higher temperature near the medial left thigh. Such a thermal asymmetry in relation to the other limb may indicate the existing inflammatory state of soft tissue or other lesion associated with venous stasis of blood in the area of the limb. Owever the thermogram taken after the cooling of the body is much more detailed and shows three additional areas of high temperature - indicated in Figure 6 by arrows. They are probably the areas of location of bad working venous valves in the saphenous vein of the left thigh (bad blood flow) which results in a local increase in the surface temperature of the body. In the examined patients it was diagnosed inflammation of the saphenous vein in the course of its valves insufficiency. Saphenous vein in the thigh has 2 to 5 valves, which may lead to malfunction of the deformation and extension of the vessel as a result of stagnation in the blood.

This example shows that thermal imaging diagnostics in combination with cooling the body can bring helpful information, for example, to a vascular surgeon. This is a quick and completely safe method that can be used in the screening of venous diseases.

This research used thermal imaging for the diagnosis of various diseases in combination with cooling body and the assessment of the effects of cryotherapy. Performed studies showed that the application of a short-term (up to 3 minutes) pulse cold affecting the entire human body significantly increases the temperature range of the analyzed areas. This leads to a better differentiation of the surface temperature of the skin and thus increase the contrast of temperature demonstrating the details of which the classic thermography is not able to see accurately.

Figure 6. The thermograms of the lower limbs of the patient diagnosed with insufficiency saphenous vein left thigh performed after whole – body cryotherapy
Source: Cholewka & Drzazga, 2005; Cholewka, Drzazga, Sieroń, Stanek, Knefel, Kawecki, & Nowak, 2010

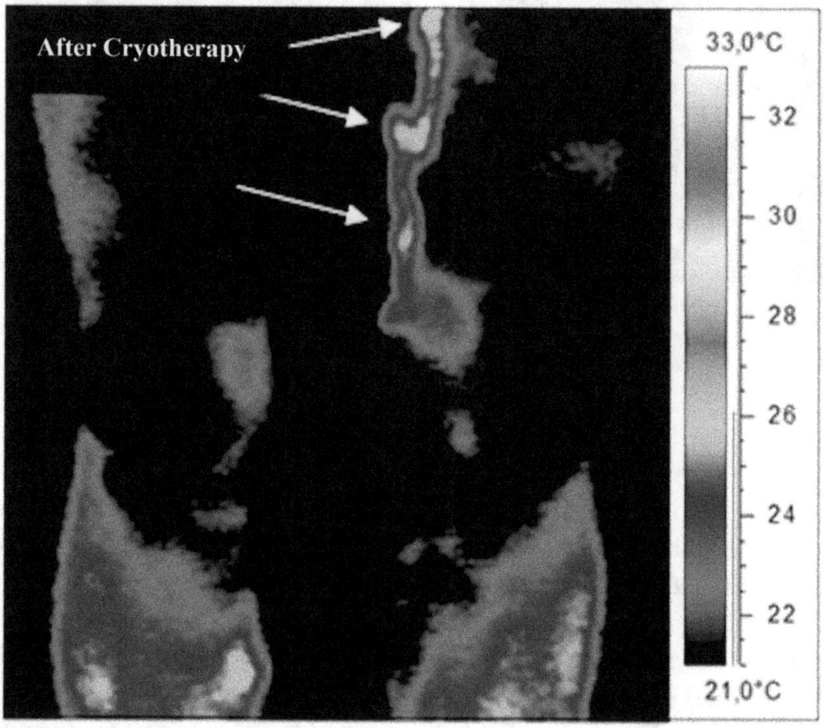

WHOLE BODY COOLING AS A TOOL TO IMPROVING OF THERMOVISION DIAGNOSTICS

Most of the diseases that are treated by whole – body cryotherapy – especially locomotory diseases are connected with metabolism changes so they can be seen in thermal imaging. Moreover, it was proved that decrease of body surface temperature differentiates thermal map of the body what reveals the details. When we consider metabolism increase or decrease of some tissues especially in the very superficial layers of the body it is possible to see then very clearly on thermograms performed just after body cooling. One can find that there have been many papers about cold treatment and application of whole body cryotherapy (Podbielska & Skrzek, 2012; Jiménez-Balderas & Mintz, 1993). However, there are not so many papers concerning data of using the thermal imaging due to cold impact on human body to determine diagnostics value of thermovision (Cholewka, 2005; Cholewka, Ciszek, & Drzazga, 2012). That is why this chapter concerns the use of body cooling as a tool to improving of thermovision diagnostics.

It was found that the use of thermal imaging after whole-body cryotherapy for patients with different diseases indicate the marked changes of thermal map of the body surface. The increase of difference between maximum and minimum (ΔT), called temperature contrast, derived from chosen Region of Interest obtained after cold impact point out significant increase of thermal imaging diagnostics value what was reported in literature mostly for patients with spine diseases (Cholewka, Stanek, Sieroń, & Drzazga, 2011; Cholewka, Drzazga, Sieroń, & Stanek, 2010).

The effect of increase the diagnostic value of thermal imaging can be easily shows on thermograms performed before and after body cooling. This fact is presented in Figure 7. Representative thermograms of patients suffering from spine diseases (low back pain) performed before and after whole - body cryotherapy session in the same temperature scale are presented in Figures 7 and 8. The bigger differentiation of thermal maps is easy seen on thermograms performed after whole – body cryotherapy (images on the right side) in comparison to thermograms performed before one.

Figure 7. Representative thermograms of patient's backs suffering from back pain performed before (left column) and after (right column) 3 minutes of body cooling with temperature inside the cryochamber set as -120°C. There are no lines marked along spinal for Patient No. 1 opposite for Patients No. 2 for whom in the range of Th1/Th2 – L5/S1 was marked line. Moreover thermograms are performed in two common scales of pseudocolors – rain and medical, for Patient No. 1 and 2, respectively

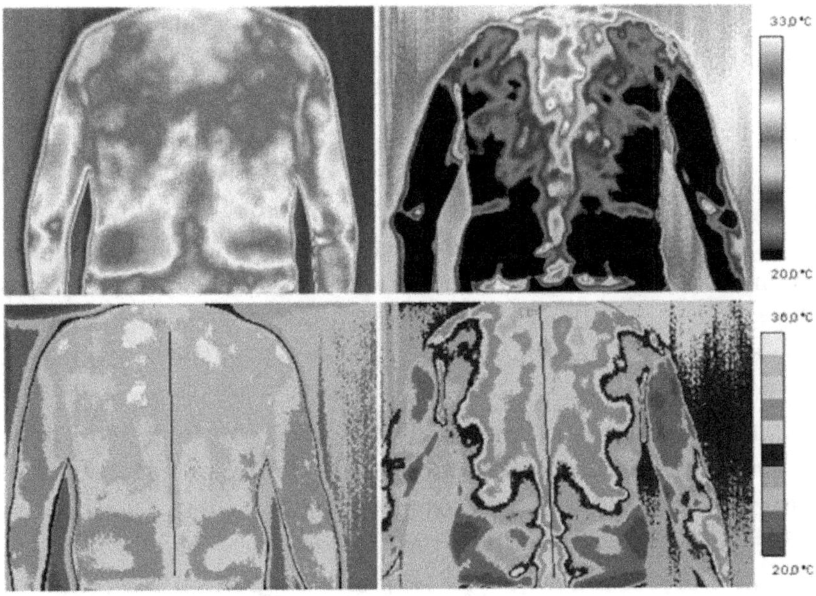

It is clearly seen in Figure 7 that the body surface thermal maps obtained after extremely low temperature impact on whole human body reveal significant temperature differentiation on it. It was reported in literature that there are details not seen in classic thermography which become more visible on the thermograms performed only after body cooling. It led to increase the diagnostics value of thermal imaging what was reported in some papers (Cholewka, Stanek, Sieroń, & Drzazga, 2011; Cholewka, Drzazga, Sieroń, & Stanek, 2010). On the other hand, it follows from comparison of temperature variation along spine that there are no temperature anomalies along spinal column for healthy (both before and after cold impact) unlike patient with spine diseases (Cholewka, Stanek, Sieroń, & Drzazga, 2011; Cholewka, Drzazga, Sieroń, & Stanek, 2010). This is other interesting fact that gives opportunity to differentiation between healthy and patients – in this case patients with spine diseases. It is also important that thermograms performed after whole body cryotherapy, while taking into consideration all tissues observed on the whole back, reveal the decrease of whole body surface temperature. There are hot spots observed in thermograms suggest inflammatory states connected with strict vertebrates. It seems that important advantages of thermal diagnostics connected with body cooling gives possibilities to see some temperature gradient changes in different part of the body i.e. occurred on the both side of spinal cord what may suggest the inflammatory states of soft tissues characterized sciatica. That fact was also reported in literature (Cholewka, Stanek, Sieroń, & Drzazga, 2011; Cholewka, Drzazga, Sieroń, & Stanek, 2010). It was also reported that of temperature variations depends on severity as well as the kind of illness. Moreover, the temperature plots performed on thermograms obtained after cold impact give additional and important information. The temperature plots obtained i.e. along spinal cord indicate very clearly the inflammatory states connected with concrete vertebrates (Cholewka, Stanek, Sieroń, & Drzazga, 2011; Cholewka, Drzazga, Sieroń, & Stanek, 2010). What seems to be interesting diagnostic fact for physician or rehabilitation.

We can influence on skin thermal map by using cold impact on human body but the question was - can we see significant differences in thermal images performed after body cooling for different spine diseases and differentiate them just using thermograms? That was the aim of the different work where authors focused on possibilities of differentiation between thermal maps of patients suffering from ankylosing spodylitis, sciatica and spondyloarthrosis (Cholewka, Drzazga, Sieroń, & Stanek, 2010).

In those studies chosen spine region (Th1/Th2–L5/S1) was taken into consideration for all groups of patients and healthy. Representative thermograms of the back for healthy man (H), patient suffering from ankylosing spodylitis (AS), suffering from sciatica (Sc) and spondyloarthrosis (Sp) performed after whole body cryotherapy in the same time of rehabilitation cycle (in presented results it was after 5th day of treatment) are presented in Figure 8. We should focus on thermograms performed after body cooling. These thermograms are more clear and reveal some hot spots not seen in thermograms performed in classic thermography what undoubtedly increase a diagnostic value of thermal imaging. Such effect was presented and commented widely in literature. But the more important thing which seemed to conclude from thermograms analysis that obtained thermal maps seem to be specific for studied back diseases. It could be seen that obtained thermograms suggest standard maps for chosen spine diseases (Cholewka, Stanek, Sieroń, & Drzazga, 2011; Cholewka, Drzazga, Sieroń & Stanek, 2010). That is why it was interesting to compare the thermograms of the back of patient suffering from ankylosing spodylitis (Figure 8 AS) with representative thermograms of patients suffering from sciatica (Figure 8 Sc) and spondyloarthrosis (Figure 8 Sp) all performed after cold impact.

Thermal studies are a useful diagnostic tool in many fields of medicine, including arthritis, venous insufficiency spine diseases or even in cancer diagnosis. The idea of thermal diagnosis in different diseases relies on bigger differentiation of the thermal body map due to differences in metabolism intensity in soft tissues in the region of interest. Usually the biggest metabolism is observed in the areas where the inflammatory state or intensity blood supply occurred. When these processes are amplified by some physical factor, like cold influenced on the body, it leads to a wider range of thermal maps and allows to see more details.

For example, the thermograms obtained for patients with ankylosing spondylitis points out the areas of higher temperature are observed almost along the whole spinal column. This is a chronic inflammatory arthritis connected with almost all vertebrates in spinal column (Jiménez-Balderas & Mintz, 1993; Brooks, Bogduk, & Bellamy, 2003). Arthritis is a common condition that apart from pain, causes inflammation of the joints and tissue around them. Therefore, the area characterized by higher temperature is connected with whole spine and has elongated shape. On the other hand, sciatica is the disease where all symptoms including pain may be caused by compression and irritation of one of five nerve roots that give rise to the sciatic nerve, or the sciatic nerve itself. The pain is felt usually in lower back, one leg or even foot. It is generally caused by the compression of lumbar nerves L4 or L5 or sacral nerves S1, S2 or S3 and far less commonly by compression of the sciatic nerve itself. Pain is not the only symptom of sciatica. There could be seen also inflammatory states of soft tissues in the vicinity of loins. It usually occurs on the both sides of the spine what seems to be typical symptom of this disease. Thermal imaging of patients back with sciatica showed temperature anomalies mainly in the lower lumbar region. The increase of skin temperature occurred not only along the spine in lumbar region but also in the areas over the tissues adjacent to the spine on both sides in the lower lumbar region (Cholewka, Drzazga, Wiśniowska, & Sieroń, 2002; Cholewka, Drzazga, Kajewski, Sieroń, & Wiśniowska, 2004; Cholewka,

Drzazga, & Sieroń, 2006; Cholewka, Drzazga, Sieroń, & Stanek, 2010). This fact is presented in Figure 8 *Sc* where the hot spots are clearly seen in the lower lumbar region on the both sides of the spine. Such thermal maps seem to correspond with medical report. However, in the case of spondyloarthrosis, the inflammatory state also occurs mainly in the lumbar region of spine and in the cervical. From medical point of view, this is a progressive destruction of the facet joint sand and is characterized by loss of articular cartilage and production of osteophytes. This disease can lead to narrowing of the neural foramina in the lumbar regions and a stenosing of spinal canal causing inflammatory state and back pain (Jiménez-Balderas & Mintz, 1993; Brooks, Bogduk & Bellamy, 2003). Probably that is why the situation is similar to that observed in the thermograms of patients suffering from sciatica but in the case of spondyloarthrosis the inflammatory state as well as the area characterized by higher temperature of the spine (Figure 8, *Sp*) is usually observed in wider/longer area than in sciatica but is also connected with lower lumbar region. However, the tissues adjacent to the spine are less affected than in sciatica what can be also clearly seen in Figure 8 *Sp* in comparison to the Figure 8 *Sc*.

Thermal images of other diseases i.e. crura ulceration can also give bigger differentiation due to processes that are localized in very superficial tissue or even on the skin surface. However, thermal map evaluation may be difficult to describe when we consider oncology changes like breast cancer due to different depth of localized the cancerous tissue what influences on heat transfer to the body surface, so the temperature map observed in thermovision. The similar situation may be seen in the case of blood supply system evaluation. That is why the easiest to see in thermal imaging are superficial veins.

It was reported in literature that temperature plots derived from the thermograms show changes of skin temperature more clearly than plots derived from thermograms performed before body cooling in normal conditions – from classic thermograms. It was wide discussed in previous papers (Cholewka, 2012; Cholewka, Drzazga, Kajewski, Sieroń, & Wiśniowska, 2004; Cholewka, Drzazga, Sieroń, & Stanek, 2010). Such phenomenon confirms the increase of thermal imaging diagnostic value. The anomalies of temperature (increase and decrease) in different ranges of vertebrates seen, in the cases of patients with spondyloarthrosis and ankylosing spondylitis, or seen in the soft tissues on both sides of spine in vicinity of loins, in the case of patient with sciatica, can be treated as connected with different pathology states. Thermogram of patient with sciatica (Sc) reveals increase of temperature only in the lower lumbar region. So the temperature plots performed for patient with spondyloarthrosis also point out the marked inflammatory states in the corresponding range. For example, in patient thermogram presented in Figure 8 Sc, the inflammatory state will be seen from L2/L3 to L5/S1, the degeneration state in the vicinity of Th11/Th12 and the weak inflammatory state from Th6/Th7 to Th9/

Figure 8. Thermograms of patients' backs of healthy man (H) and patient suffering from ankylosing spodylitis (AS), sciatica (Sc) and spondyloarthrosis (Sp) performed after whole body cryotherapy at the same period of rehabilitation cycle

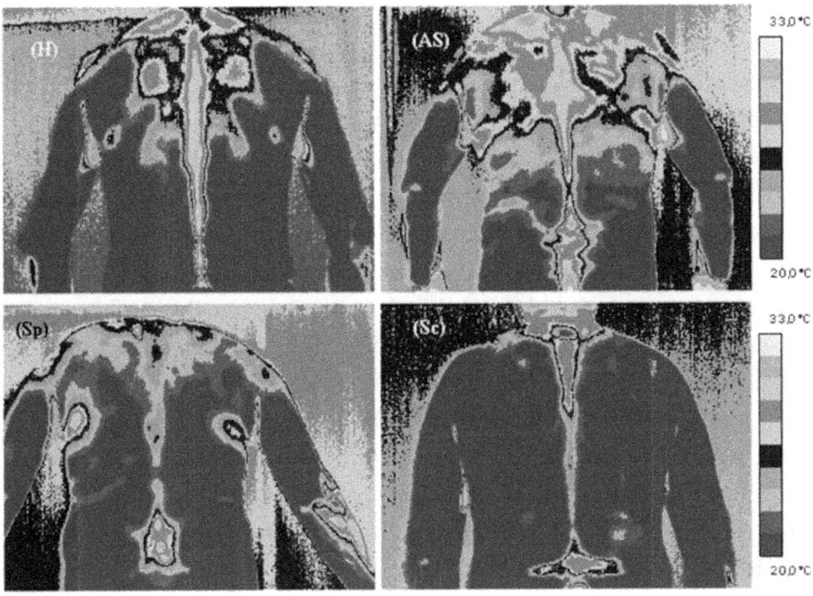

Th10. Moreover, the temperature plots along the lines performed perpendicular to spinal column will be corresponding with specific of the disease as well as health state of patient showing increase of temperature on both sides of spine. It was also presented on thermogram of patient with sciatica. Increased temperature on both sides of spine confirms the inflammatory state of tissues adjacent to the spine, what is a characteristic symptom for this kind of disease. Thermogram after body cooling in the case of patient with ankylosing spondylitis revealed increased temperature on almost all spinal column, however the levels Th5/Th6 – Th8/Th9 and Th11/Th12 – L2/L3 seem to indicate bigger inflammatory states thanother spine regions. It was also showed and discussed in previous papers that such increased temperature in adjacent tissues in the vicinity of loins can be seen not only for patients with sciatica but also in the case of spondyloarthrosis

(Cholewka, Drzazga, Sieroń, & Stanek, 2010). However, the inflammatory state in spondyloarthrosis seems to have a bigger range than in the case of sciatica. In presented thermograms the range of increased temperature is observed from Th12/L1 to L5/S1 what is clearly seen in thermogram of patient with spondyloarthrosis (Figure 8 Sp).

Moreover it follows from the results of the thermal imaging in spine diseases that using only such parameters like mean temperature as well as maximum or minimum temperature seem to be not adequate to analyze and differentiation the diseases. This is because diseases are dependent on magnitude of temperature inside the cryochamber, level of decrease of the body surface temperature, number of cryotherapy sessions taken by patient, the health state of patients and also individual sensitivity of patient to body cooling (Cholewka, Drzazga, Sieroń, & Stanek, 2010).

For the better inside into the problem, the contrast temperature has been defined as $\Delta T = Tmax - Tmin$ (difference between maximum and minimum temperature from chosen Region of Interest). Moreover the relative contrast ratio defined as temperature contrast and mean temperature derived from chosen Region of Interest ratio $(\Delta T)/(Tmean)$ was introduced. Results showed that the difference between maximum and minimum temperature obtained from chosen lines along the spine is about 3°C for healthy while for patients with back diseases is markedly larger and even crossed 4.5°C and it was statistically significant. The differences become more visible when we consider the relative contrast ratio $\Delta T/Tmean$. For the group of healthy people its value was 0.12 ± 0.03 while it increases up till 0.19 ± 0.06 for the patients with back pain. Such increase of this parameter was also statistically significant for all groups of patients. It seems that the temperature contrast and relative contrast ratio should be more proper in thermal characteristics of back pain diseases due to theirs independency of conditions of body cooling (Cholewka, Drzazga, Sieroń, & Stanek, 2010).

Thermal imaging as a completely noninvasive and safe for patients diagnostic technique can be used not only to diagnosis, but also to evaluate the effects of therapy. In this case thermal imaging was the tool to lead the study on back's temperature changes along the spinal column in the case of patients with spine diseases treated by whole body cryotherapy and kinesiotherapy.

The region of increased temperature in the lower lumbar region connected with inflammatory state is observed during the whole therapy cycle when it is considered patients suffering from Spondyloarthrosis. The other important thing is that when we take into consideration the temperature plots as a function of number of rehabilitation cycles (2, 5 and 10) obtained results suggest that a wide peak connected with the inflammatory state observed after 2nd day of whole body cryotherapy becomes more clear and better visible and reveals not one big area but two smaller peaks what may be connected with the shrink inflammatory states or points out that bigger decrease of body surface temperature lead to better differentiation of thermal maps. However, it is noteworthy that temperature plots did not show the significant differences in size of area characterized with higher temperature with number of cryotherapy sessions although people reported decrease of pain and increase of fitness (Cholewka, Drzazga, Sieroń, & Stanek, 2010; Cholewka & Drzazga, 2005; Cholewka & Drzazga, 2006).

Avail oneself of possibility of thermal imaging it was checked the correlation between the whole body skin temperature decrease caused by whole body cryotherapy and body mass index (BMI), what was presented and discussed in literature (Cholewka, Drzazga, Sieroń, & Stanek, 2010; Cholewka & Drzazga, 2005; Cholewka & Drzazga, 2006). Obtained results showed medium positive correlation between BMI and the decrease of mean body temperature due to cold impact in cryogenic chamber. The results gave clear information that the response of organisms on whole body cryotherapy depends on the physical conditions of the organism (i.e. mass and height). Moreover, the magnitude of body temperature response on cooling is also dependent on the state of health as well as the individual features of the patient. By analyzing such results, it comes one important question - do such parameters like the magnitude of the low temperature used in the cryogenic chamber or time of stay in cryogenic chamber should be selected with regards to body mass index. It may have a potential meaning on the range of body cooling as well as the therapy effects. It seems that due to wider application of thermovision in medicine it could be possible to match the time of lasting and the magnitude of temperature inside the cryochamber according to body mass index of patient as well as health state (Cholewka, Drzazga, Sieroń, & Stanek, 2010; Cholewka & Drzazga, 2005; Cholewka & Drzazga, 2006).

CONCLUSION

The results of discussed works and presented representative analysis showed clearly that the thermal imaging performed after whole-body cryotherapy has a potential diagnostics value in case of back diseases i.e. spondyloarthrosis, ankylosing spondylitis and sciatica. Moreover, it seems that thermovision is not only the qualitative technique but also can give some quantitative data. Temperature plots performed along, as well as, perpendicular to spine and temperature parameters such as temperature contrast and relative contrast ratio are objective and useful in differentiating between some spine diseases. Additionally, thermal imaging studies in combination with cryotherapy show improved diagnostic possibilities of many diseases. The combination of these two methods is perfect for sportsmen - improves the athlete performance and allows him to faster recovery.

REFERENCES

Ammer. (2004). Temperature effects of thermotherapy determined by infrared measurements. *Physica Medica, 20*(S1), 64-66.

Ammer. (2008). The Glamorgan Protocol for recording and evaluation of thermal images of the human body. *Thermology International*.

Banfi, L., Lombardi, G., Colombini, A., & Melegati, G. (2010). Whole-body cryotherapy in athletes. *Sports Medicine (Auckland, N.Z.)*, *40*(6), 509–517. doi:10.2165/11531940-000000000-00000 PMID:20524715

Bauer, Hurnik, & Zdziarski, Mielczarek, & Podbielska. (1997). Thermovision and its applications in medicine. *Acta Bio-Optica et Informatica Medica*, *3*(2-4), 121–131.

Bauer, Hurnik, Zdziarski, Mielczarek, & Skrzek, Podbielska, & Zagrobelny. (1997). Thermovison evaluation of cryotherapy effects. *Acta Bio-Optica et Informatica Medica*, *3*(2-4), 133–140.

Bauer & Skrzek. (1997). Physiological basis of cryotherapy. *Acta Bio-Optica et Informatica Medica*, *3*(2-4), 115–120.

Bauer & Skrzek. (1999). Fizjologiczne podstawy krioterapii. *Medycyna sportowa, 94*, 3-7. (in Polish)

Biały, Zimmer, Skrzek, & Zagrobelny. (1998). Cryogenic Chamber – Possibilities Of Use In Rehabilitation. *Baln. Pol*, *40*(3-4), 44–47.

Biały, Zimer, & Zagrobelny. (1999) Acta Bio-Optica et Informatica Medica. *Inżynieria Biomedyczna Wpływ ogólnoustrojowej krioterapii na parametry krwi obwodowej zawodników kadry narodowej lekkoatletów, 5*(1-2), 7-10. (in Polish)

Birkner, Sieroń, Beck, Jagodziński, & Romuk, Skrzep-Poloczek, & Stanek. (2003). Application of cryogenic temperatures in medicine. *Wiadomosci Lekarskie (Warsaw, Poland)*, *56*(1-2), 53–56. PMID:12901269

Brengelmann. (1989). Body temperature regulation In H. D. Patron, A. F. Fuchs, B. Hill, A. M. Scher, & R. Steiner (Eds.), *Textbook of Physiology*. Academic Press.

Brooks, Bogduk, & Bellamy. (2003). *Evidence based – Management of acute muscosceletal pain.* Australian Academic Press.

Cholewka, Ciszek, & Drzazga. (2012). Cryogenic chamber used in physical medicine and their comparison. *W: Zastosowanie niskich temperatur w medycynie, redakcja: Anna Skrzek i Halina Podbielska 2012*. Oficyna Wydawnicza Politechniki Wrocławskiej, Wrocław.

Cholewka, Drzazga, Wiśniowska, & Sieroń. (2002). The temperature changes of the skin surface during whole body cryotherapy. *IFMBE Proceedings of 2nd EMBEC, 2*, 1330-31.

Cholewka, Drzazga, Sieroń, & Wiśniowska. (2004). Temperature effect of whole body cryotherapy determined by thermography. *Thermology International*, 57-63.

Cholewka, Drzazga, Borgieł, & Kurpas. (2005). Cold penetration of the fourth layer tissue model in the whole body cryotherapy conditions. *IFMBE Proceedings of 3rd EMBEC*.

Cholewka, Drzazga, Michalik, & Sieroń. (2006). Whole Body Cryotherapy and Magnetotherapy Influence on Some Cardiac Parameters. *Pol J of Environ Stud, 15*(4A), 19-21.

Cholewka, Drzazga, Sieroń, & Stanek. (2010). Thermovision diagnostics in chosen spine diseases treated by whole body cryotherapy. *Journal of Thermal Analysis and Calorymetry*.

Cholewka, D., Drzazga, Z., & Sieroń, A. (2006). Monitoring of whole body cryotherapy effects by thermal imaging – preliminary report. *Physica Medica, 22*(2), 57–62. doi:10.1016/S1120-1797(06)80054-2 PMID:17643893

Cholewka, D., Drzazga, Z., Sieroń, A., & Stanek, A. (2010). Thermovision diagnostics in chosen spine diseases treated by whole body cryotherapy. *Journal of Thermal Analysis and Calorimetry, 102*(1), 113–119. doi:10.100710973-010-0873-y

Cholewka, Drzazga, & Kajewski, Bogucki, & Wiśniowska. (2004). The thermal imaging of skin body surface due to whole body cryotherapy – preliminary report. *Physica Medica, 20*(Suppl. I), 70–72.

Cholewka, Drzazga, Kajewski, Sieroń, & Wiśniowska. (2004). Thermographic assessment of cryotherapy effects. *VI Konferencja Krajowa TTP2004 Ustroń-Jaszowiec, Proceedings*, (pp. 143 – 148).

Cholewka, Drzazga, Knefel, Kawecki, & Nowak. (2010). Thermal Imaging In Hyperbaric Oxygen Therapy (HBO). *Inżynieria Biomedyczna*.

Cholewka, Drzazga, Sieroń, Stanek, Knefel, Kawecki, & Nowak. (2010). Some Applications Of Thermal Imaging In Medicine. *Monographs of Polish Journal of Environmental Studies*.

Cholewka, Knefel, Stanek, Kawecki, & Nowak, Sieroń, & Drzazga. (2011). Thermal imaging and TC oximetry measurements of hyperbaric oxygen therapy (HBO) effects on trophic ulceration of the crura. *Journal of Thermal Analysis and Calorimetry*. doi:10.100710973-011-1934-6

Cholewka, Kasprzyk, & Stanek, Sieroń-Stołtny, & Drzazga. (2015). May thermal imaging be useful in cyclist endurance tests? *Journal of Thermal Analysis and Calorimetry*. doi:10.100710973-015-4662-5

Cholewka, Stanek, Sieroń, & Drzazga. (2011). Thermography study of skin response due to whole-body cryotherapy. *Skin Research and Technology*. PMID:21507075

Cholewka, Sieroń, & Drzazga. (2014). Application thermal imaging in diseases of the blood vessels. W: Biomedyczne zastosowania termowizji, pod redakcją H. Podbielska i A. Skrzek, Biomedyczne zastosowania termowizji. Oficyna Wydawnicza Politechniki Wrocławskiej.

Cholewka, Stanek, Kasprzyk, Urbańczyk, Jagodziński, Sieroń, & Drzazga. (2013). The application of thermography in research efficiency athletes, pilot studies. *PAK, 9*, 871-874.

Cholewka, S., & Klimas, S. (2014). Thermal imaging application in chronic venous disease: Pilot study. *Journal of Thermal Analysis and Calorimetry, 115*(2), 1609–1618. doi:10.100710973-013-3356-0

Cholewka, Stanek, Kwiatek, Sieroń, & Drzazga. (2011). The use of thermography in the diagnosis of selected changes to skin cancer - preliminary study. *Application of thermovision to diagnosis of chosen skin cancer changes – preliminary studies*. PAK.

Cholewka, S., & Kwiatek, S. (2013). Does the temperature gradient correlate with the photodynamic diagnosis parameter numerical colour value (NCV)? *Photodiagnosis and Photodynamic Therapy, 10*(1), 33–38. doi:10.1016/j.pdpdt.2012.07.001 PMID:23465370

Cholewka & Drzazga. (2005a). Diagnostic value of thermal imaging due to whole body cryotherapy. *IFMBE Proceedings of 3rd EMBEC*.

Cholewka & Drzazga. (2005b). Krioterapia ogólnoustrojowa w kriokomorze dwustopniowej oraz kriokomorze z zaleganiem zimna. *Acta Bio-Optica et Informatica Medica*, 57-63. (in Polish)

Cholewka & Drzazga. (2006). Comparison Of Some Parameters Of Two-Stepped Cryogenic Chamber And Chamber With Lingering Cold. *Biomedical Engineering Acta Indygo, 11*, 103–110.

Cholewka. (2005). *The impact of low temperatures on the body - in vivo and in vitro studies*. Rozprawa doktorska Uniwersyetet Śląski w Katowicach, Katowice.

Cholewka. (2012). Meaning of thermal diagnostic analysis of the whole body cryotherapy. *W: Zastosowanie niskich temperatur w medycynie*. Redakcja: Anna Skrzek i Halina Podbielska.

Chwalbińska-Moneta. (2003). Wpływ kriostymulacji ogólnoustrojowej na niektóre reakcje wysiłkowe u sportowców. *Sport Wyczynowy, 5/6*, 50-54. (in Polish)

Ganong. (2009).FizjologiaPZWL.

Gage & Baust. (2002). Cryosurgery – a review of recent advances and current issues. *Cryo Letters*, *23*(2), 30–32. PMID:12050774

Goodman, Murphy, Siltanen, Kelley, & Rucker. (1986). Normal temperature asymmetry of the back and extremities by computer-assisted infrared imaging. *Thermology, 1*, 195-202.

Góralczyk, Mikuła, & Jagodzińska. (2002). Osteoarthritis. Choroba zwyrodnieniowa stawów. *Medycyna Rodzinna*, *10*, 2.

Gregorowicz & Dalidowski. (1998). Cryotherapy In Sclerosis Multiplex (Sm) Treatment Acta Bio-Opt. *Inform. Med.*, *4*(4), 173 – 174.

Gregorowicz. (1992). *The influence of whole body cryotherapy on chosen haemodynamic and lungs ventilation markers in rheumatoid diseases.* Praca Doktorska AM.

Gregorowiczv & Zagrobelny. (1998). Whole body cryotherapy, indications and contraindications, treatment and its physiological and clinical effects. Acta Bio-Optica et Informatica Media, 4, 120-131.

Hoffman & Bischo. (2002). The cryobiology of cryosurgical injury. *Urology, 60*(2), 40-49.

Hrycaj & Łącki. (2002). Od zwyrodnienia do zapalenia – współczesne poglądy na patogenezę choroby zwyrodnieniowej stawów. *Nowa Medycyna*, (2), 115.

Hulbert & Else. (2004). Basal Metabolic Rate: History, Composition, Regulation and Usefulness. *Physiol Biochem Zool., 77*(6), 869-76.

Jagodziński, Kubacka, & Wiśniowska, Puszer, & Stanek. (2001). Whole Body Cryotherapy Part 1 Priv. [In Polish]. *Cab*, *4*(92), 10–11.

Jagodziński, S., & Gmyrek, C. (2007). Evaluation of whole - body cryotherapy on the circulatory system in patients with ankylosing spondylitis by analysis of duration and QT interval dispertion. *Fizjoterapia Polska*, *7*(3), 362–369.

Jazienicka, Pietrzak, & Toruniowi. (1991). New indications for cryotherapy. *Przeglad Dermatologiczny, 78*(3), 190–194.

Jiménez-Balderas & Mintz. (1993). Ankylosing Spondylitis: Clinical Course In Women And Men. *J Rheumatol, 20*(12), 2069–72.

Johnston, S., Schoenfeld, P., Mysore, J. V., & Dubois, A. (1999, July). Endoscopic spray cryotherapy: a new technique for mucosal ablation in the esophagus. *Gastrointestinal Endoscopy, 50*(1), 86–92. doi:10.1016/S0016-5107(99)70352-4 PMID:10385730

Jonderko. (1990). Current state of knowledge about the application of cryotherapy for treatment of musculoskeletal diseases. *Chir Narzadow Ruchu Ortop Pol, 55*, 31-5.

Kasprzyk, Wójcik, Cholewka, Sieroń-Stołtny, Piętka, Drzazga, & Stanek. (2015). *The applications of thermal imaging in energy cost rating during Aerobic Circuit Training*. QIRT.

Kerschan-Schindl, Uher, Zauner-Dungl, & Fialka-Moser. (1998). V Cold And Cryotherapy. A Review Of The Literature On General Principles And Practical Applications Acta Med. *Austriaca, 25*(3), 73 – 8.

Knight. (1995). *Cryotherapy in sport injury management*. Human Kinetics.

Korzonek-Szlacheta, Wielkoszynski, & Stanek. (2007). Influence of whole - body cryotherapy on the levels of some hormones in professional footballers. *Endokrynologia Polska, 58*(1), 27–32. PMID:17354202

Kozielski & Ziora. (1997). Bronchoscopic cryotherapy. *Pneumonologia i Alergologia Polska, 65*(5-6), 411–416. PMID:9340073

Księżpolska-Pietrzak. (1998). Krioterapia W Osteoporozie: Polski Merkuriusz Lekarski, D. [In Polish]. *Polski Tygodnik Lekarski, 28*, 222–224.

Księżpolska-Pietrzak, Cygler, Lesiak, & Noniewicz. (1993). The Influence Of Low Temperature Treatment On Reumatoid Arm. *Reumatologia, 31*(2), 179–183.

Leppaluto, W. (2008). Effect of long-term whole-body cold exposures on plasma concentrations of ACTH, beta-endorphin, cortisol, catecholamines and cytokines in healthy females. *Scandinavian Journal of Clinical and Labolatory Investstigation, 68*(2), 145–153. doi:10.1080/00365510701516350

Maraso, B., Gai, G., & Massaglia, O. (1998). Radiofrequency resection of bronchial tumours in combination with cryotherapy: Evaluation of a new technique. *Thorax, 53*(2), 106–109. doi:10.1136/thx.53.2.106 PMID:9624294

Meeusen & Lievens. (1986). The use of cryotherapy in sports injuries. *Sports Med., 3*(6), 398-414.

Metzger, Zwingmann, Protz, & Jackel. (2000). Die Bedeutung Der Ganzkorperkaltetherapie Im Rahmen Der Rehabilitation Bei Patienten Mit Rheumatishen. *Erkrank. Rehabil., 39*, 93–100. doi:10.1055-2000-14442

Misztela, Kuliński, & Rybak. (1995). Ocena Krioterapii Miejscowej W Reumatoidalnym Zapaleniu Stawów Baln. [In Polish]. *Pol, 37*(3-4), 38–41.

Mraz, Skrzek, & Gruszka, Chamela-Bilińska, Drak-Wojakiewicz, & Dutkiewicz. (2001). The influence of physiotherapy and whole body cryotherapy on standing position balance of patients with sclerosis multiplex. *Physiotherapy, 9*(1), 26–29.

Nowakowski. (2001). *Postępy termografii – aplikacje medyczne*. Gdańsk: Academic Press.

O'Keefe, M., OReilly, J., & Lanigan, B. (1998). Longer term visual outcome of eyes with retinopathy of prematurity treated with cryotherapy or diode laser. *The British Journal of Ophthalmology, 82*(11), 1246–1248. doi:10.1136/bjo.82.11.1246 PMID:9924326

Pasricha, Hill, Wadwa, Gislason, & Okolo. (1999). Endoscopic cryotherapy: experimental results and first clinical use. *Gastrointest. Endosc., 49*(5), 627-631.

Pilawski. (1983). *Podstawy biofizyki*. PZWL. (in Polish)

Podbielska & Skrzek. (Eds.). (2012). The application of low temperatures in biomedicine. Oficyna Wydawnicza Politechniki Wrocławskiej, Wrocław.

Podbielska & Skrzek. (2014). *Biomedical application of thermography, Biomedyczne zastosowania termowizji, praca zbiorowa*. Wrocław: Oficyna Wydawnicza Politechniki Wrocławskiej.

Raczkowski & Zagrobelny. (1990). *Technical and physiological aspects of whole body cooling*. Materials of IV Science and Training Conference of Polish Cryomedical Society.

Ring, Jung, Kalicki, Zuber, Rustecka, & Vardasca. (2013). New Standards For Fever Screening With Thermal Imaging Systems. *Journal of Mechanics in Medicine and Biology, 13*(2).

Ring & Ammer. (2000). The technique of infrared imaging in medicine. *Thermol. Intern., 10*(1), 7-14.

Ring & Ammer. (2012a). Infrared thermal imaging in medicine. *Physiological Measurement, 33*(3), R33-46.

Ring & Ammer. (2012b). Thermal imaging in rheumatology - An overview. *Thermology International, 22*(2), 68-69.

Ring. (1999). Thermal Symmetry of Human Skin Temperature. *Thermology International, 9*(2), 53-55.

Ring. (2001). Provocation tests in thermal imaging. *Abs. Thermology Int., 11*, 2.

Ronikier. (2008). *Physiology of exercise in sports, physiotherapy and recreation.* Centralny Ośrodek Sportu, Warszawa.

Rybak, Kuliński, Misztela, & Podgórski. (1995). Zastosowanie Krioterapii W Leczeniu Następstw Blizn Kanału Kręgowego Baln. [In Polish]. *Pol, 37*(3-4), 29–30.

Rymaszewska, Biały, Zagrobelny, & Kiejna. (2000). The Influence Of Whole Body Cryotherapy On Mental Health. *Psychiatria Polska, 34*(4), 649 – 653.

Rymaszewska, R., Ramsey, D., & Chładzińska-Kiejna, S. (2008). Whole - body cryotherapy as adjunct treatment of depressive syndrome and anxiety disorders. *Archivum Immunologiae et Therapiae Experimentalis, 56*(1), 63–68. doi:10.100700005-008-0006-5 PMID:18250970

Schroder & Anderson. (1995). *Kryo- und Thermotherapie. Grundlangen und praktische Anwendung*. New York: Gustaw Hischer Verlag.

Sieroń, Cieślar, & Stanek. (2010). *Cryotherapy. Theoretical bases, biological effects, clinical applications*. α-Medica Press Bielsko Biała.

Sieroń, Pastuszka, Marniok, Wiśniowska, & Jagodziński, Ślusarczyk, … Stanek. (2004). Influence of low temperature on lymph formation and lymph flow velocity in mice. *Thermol. Int., 14*, 127–130.

Sieroń, Stanek, Cieślar, & Pasek. (2007). Cryorehabilitation - the role cryotherapy in modern rehabilitation. *Fizjoterapia, 15*(2), 3–8.

Sieroń, Stanek, & Cieślar. (Eds.). (2014). *Wellness, Spa, Anti-aging*. PZWL.

Sieroń & Cieślar. (2003a). *The Application Of Cold In Medicine - Cryosurgery And Cryotherapy*. A-Medica Press Bielsko-Biala Poland. (in Polish)

Sieroń & Cieślar. (2003b). The theoretical basis for cooling treatment. The application of cold medicine - cryosurgery and cryotherapy. α-Medica Press.

Sieroń & Cieślar. (2007). Cryotherapy – cold treatment. α-Medica Press.

Silverman, Tuncali, Adams, von Sonnenberg, Zou, Kacher, ... Jolesz. (2000). MR imaging-guided percutaneous cryotherapy of liver tumors: Initial experience. *Radiology, 217*, 657-664.

Stanek, Cieslar, & Matyszkiewicz. (2005). Subjective estimation of therapeutic efficacy of whole - body cryotherapy in patients with ankylosing spondylitis. *Balneolologia Polska*, *47*(1-2), 24–32.

Stanek, Cieślar, & Matyszkiewicz. (2006). Changes in antioxidant status in patients with ankylosing spondylitis during cryotherapy. *European Journal of Clinical Investigation*, *36*(Suppl.1), 20.

Stanek, Cieslar, & Rosmus-Kucza. (2006). Influence of whole - body cryotherapy on blood morphology parameters in patients with ankylosing spondylitis and in healthy volunteers. *Acta Bio-Optica et Informatica Medica*, *12*(3), 207-210.

Stanek, Cieślar, Mrowiec, & Sieroń. (2006). Cryotherapy in clinical practice. *Rehabilitacja w Praktyce*, *1*, 27–31.

Stanek, Cieslar, & Sieron. (2007). Therapeutic application of cryotherapy in clinical practice. *Balneologia Polska*, *49*(1), 37–45.

Stanek, Cieślar, & Sieroń. (2008). Application of cryotherapy in sport medcine. *Rehabilitacja w Praktyce*, *2*, 34–35.

Stanek, Cieslar, & Strzelczyk. (2010). Influence of cryogenic temperatures on inflammatory markers in patients with ankylosing spondylitis and healthy volunteers. *Polish Journal of Environmental Studies*, *19*(1), 167–175.

Stanek, Cholewka, & Cieslar, Rosmus-Kuczia, Drzazga, & Sieron. (2011). The assessment of the analgesic action of whole - body cryotherapy in patients with ankylosing spondylitis. *Fizjoterapia Polska*, *11*(1), 49–55.

Stanek, Sieron, & Cieslar, Matyszkiewicz, & Rozmus-Kuczia. (2005). Influence of whole-body cryotherapy on parameters of spine mobility in patients with ankylosing spondylitis. *Ortopedia, Traumatologia, Rehabilitacja*, *5*(7), 549–554. PMID:17611448

Stanek, Wielkoszynski, & Cholewka. (2011). Influence of whole - body cryotherapy on some chosen non - enzymatic parameters of antioxidant status in patients with ankylosing spondylitis. *Acta Balneolgica*, *53*(4), 264–269.

Styczyński, Gasik, Krzemińska-Dąbrowska, & Pyskło. (2001). Ocena Przydatności Krioterapii U Chorych Na Bóle Krzyża Związane Z Dyskopatią I Zmianami Zwyrodnieniowymi Kręgosłupa Baln. *Pol.*, *43*(1-2), 50 – 55. (in Polish)

Swenson, S., Swärd, L., & Karlsson, J. (1996). Cryotherapy in sports medicine. *Scandinavian Journal of Medicine & Science in Sports*, *6*(4), 193–200. doi:10.1111/j.1600-0838.1996.tb00090.x PMID:8896090

Traczyk. (2007). *Fizjologia człowieka w zarysie*. PZWL.

Vardasca, Ring, Plassmann, & Jones. (2012). Thermal symmetry of the upper and lower extermities in healthy subjects. *Thermology International, 22*(2), 53-60.

Wiącek, Rzymska-Klicha, Kaszuba, & Drobnik. (1999). The use of cryosurgical techniques in dermatology – own experiences. *Nowa. Klin.*, *6*(12), 1178–1184.

Wozniak, M.-K., Drewa, D., & Wozniak, O. (2001). Activity of chosen lisosome's enzymes in plasma of canoeists after whole - body cryotherapy. *Med Sport, 17*, 322–327.

Yamauchi, Nogami, & Miura. (1981). Various applications of extreme cryotherapy and strenuous exercise program - focusing on chronic rheumatoid arthritis. *Physiother Rehab*, *5*, 35–39.

Zagrobelny, Halawa, Jegierski, & Wawrowska. (1993). The influence of whole body cooling in cryogenic chamber on chosen haemodynamic markers and hormone concentration in serum of healthy people. *Physician Polish Weekly, 48*(14-15), 303-305.

Zagrobelny & Zimmer. (1999). The application of of cryogenic temperatures in medicine and physical sports therapy. *Med. Sport.*, *15*(94), 8–13.

Zagrobelny. (Ed.). (2003a). *Whole-body and local cryotherapy*. Urban & Partner.

Zagrobelny. (Ed.). (2003b). *Local and wholebody cryotherapy*. Urban & Partner.

Żuber & Jung. (1997). *Thermographic methods in medical diagnostics*. Warszawa: Academic Press.

This research was previously published in Innovative Research in Thermal Imaging for Biology and Medicine edited by Ricardo Vardasca and Joaquim Gabriel Mendes, pages 93-118, copyright year 2017 by Medical Information Science Reference (an imprint of IGI Global).

Section 5
Virtual Reality and Video Games

Chapter 13
Uses of Virtual Reality (VR) for Chronic Pain

Bradley Chi
Zucker School of Medicine at Hofstra/Northwell, USA

Brian Chau
Loma Linda University Health, USA

Phillip Ta
Loma Linda University Health, USA

ABSTRACT

Chronic pain affects many people worldwide with significant individual impact and societal cost. One such area involves the psychiatric co-morbidities associated with chronic pain. Despite its prevalence, the underlying mechanism of chronic pain is not fully understood although evidence suggests the importance of biologic, psychologic, and social factors in the perception of pain. Virtual reality has the potential to be a powerful therapeutic option for chronic pain. This may be due to its impact on attention, emotion, and potentially central nervous system plasticity. Virtual reality therapy has been used successfully for a variety of chronic pain conditions showing its potential. It has also been safely used in pediatric populations. However, the major current limitation is quality of evidence; therefore, future studies should aim to address this issue.

DOI: 10.4018/978-1-7998-1680-5.ch013

INTRODUCTION

Chronic pain is highly prevalent worldwide but our current understanding of the condition, its influences, and its consequences are not fully understood. Despite this, clinicians and scientists have recognized multiple factors influencing chronic pain including biological, psychological, and social factors (Katz, Rosenbloom, & Fashler, 2015). As understanding of this complex subject has improved, alternative therapeutic methods have been developed to target the various factors believed to play a role in the chronic pain experience. This chapter presents the relationship between chronic pain and mental health, outlines the mechanisms underlying chronic pain and virtual reality (VR) therapy, and then reviews the expanding role of VR in the treatment of chronic pain.

BACKGROUND

While acute pain has an intuitive role in human adaptation, the role of chronic pain is ill-defined and maladaptive. Initially, biologically-driven theories of chronic pain, such as the gate-control theory, were used to explain chronic pain (Ehde, Dillworth, & Turner, 2014; Melzack & Wall, 1965). Shortly thereafter, researchers began to realize the complexity and multi-faceted issues involved with chronic pain. Observations of the psychologic and social effects of chronic pain became apparent. This led psychologists to apply behavioral and cognitive therapy to these patients (Ehde et al., 2014; Fordyce & Company, 1977). With the success of these therapies, recognition of chronic pain has evolved to encompass the variety of areas it can impact patients' lives. One way to capture this complexity is describing chronic pain as a perceptual phenomenon, therefore encompassing the biologic, psychologic, and social influences and impacts (Songer, 2005).

Before the next section discusses the biologic component, the following will touch on the equally important psychologic and social aspects. Chronic pain is highly correlated with negative emotions such as depression, anxiety, anger, isolation, and demoralization (Gatchel, Peng, Peters, Fuchs, & Turk, 2007). This can lead to the psychologic impacts described later but can also impact the relationship between patient and healthcare system. These negative emotions impact motivation for treatment and compliance with therapies (Gatchel et al., 2007). Furthermore, patients suffering from chronic pain often deal with repeated failures of treatment, which can lead to frustration and irritation with the healthcare system (Gatchel et al., 2007). This emotional distress is compounded by rejection from the medical system as healthcare providers may label these patients as "complainers" or "symptom magnifiers" (Gatchel et al., 2007). Therefore, the psychosocial components of chronic pain described below should be viewed holistically, keeping mindful of their interconnected relationships.

Evidence that chronic pain is highly comorbid with mental health conditions is strong. In particular, comorbidity with mood disorders and anxiety disorders are prevalent. Large surveys recording 12-month prevalence of comorbid chronic pain and mood disorders are as high as 17.5%, with major depression being the most common comorbid condition (Demyttenaere et al., 2007; Von Korff et al., 2005). In a survey of Canadian patients with chronic pain, over 80% had symptoms of depression, as measured by the Beck Depression Inventory, of which over half were moderate to extremely severe levels (Choinière et al., 2010). Additionally, over one third expressed suicidal ideation. Similarly, these surveys found significant correlations between chronic pain and almost all anxiety disorders. The highest odds ratios were for generalized anxiety disorder (OR 2.6-2.7) and post-traumatic stress disorder (OR 2.6) (Demyttenaere et al., 2007; Von Korff et al., 2005). Patients with chronic pain are also at increased risk of suicidal ideation and death (Hassett, Aquino, & Ilgen, 2014). While some of this is attributed to the psychiatric comorbidities, current evidence supports chronic pain as an independent risk factor for suicide(Ilgen et al., 2013). In addition to these comorbidities, patients suffering from chronic pain are associated with other challenges, including financial, functional, occupational, and psychosocial. A large survey of people suffering from chronic pain, two-thirds had sleep disruption, half had difficulty walking and with household chores, and one-third had a dependent lifestyle (Breivik, Collett, Ventafridda, Cohen, & Gallacher, 2006). Other significant findings included difficulty with sexual relations (40%) and feeling inadequate as a spouse or partner (20%) (Breivik et al., 2006). All of which shows the wide-ranging impact chronic pain has on people's lives.

Further evidence of the link between chronic pain and comorbid psychiatric disorders is the efficacy found with psychological-based approaches such as cognitive behavioral therapy (CBT), meditation, operant conditioning, and insight-cased approaches (Turk, Swanson, & Tunks, 2008). Of these, the most robust evidence is for CBT which was been shown in multiple studies to result in small to moderate improvements in pain intensity, pain disability, mood, and catastrophizing (Ehde et al., 2014). A 2012 Cochrane review of studies comparing CBT to treatment as usual or wait-list control conditions for patients with chronic pain found mild improvements in the four outcomes mentioned above, but at 6 months follow up, only improvement in mood persisted. When comparing CBT to active control, the review found mild improvement of pain disability and catastrophizing persisting to 6 months follow up, but no improvement in pain intensity or mood (Williams, Eccleston, & Morley, 2012). Multiple other randomized control trials (RCT) focused on specific pain conditions such as migraine headache, orofacial pain, fibromyalgia, and arthritis.

In totality, the studies support the conclusion that CBT is effective as treatment for chronic pain with the treatment effect being mild to moderate improvement in pain and mood (Ehde et al., 2014). Again, these findings support a strong link between chronic pain and mental health.

MAIN FOCUS OF THE CHAPTER

Theories of Pain

In its evolutionary role, pain is in an important adaptive defense mechanism that allows humans to protect themselves from potential dangers (Melzack & Wall, 1965). Despite this, maladaptive pain is now a common problem significantly impacting millions of people worldwide. A basic understanding of how the body perceives pain is important to discuss the potential mechanisms explaining the role of VR in pain reduction. While the current understanding of pain is complex and incomplete, the following section aims to outline our current understanding of the mechanisms governing pain. Pain can be viewed as a sensation and/or a perception. The sensation of pain refers to the biologic process of sensing pain (Turk & Okifuji, 2002). This differs from perception of pain, which refers to the brains processing and interpretation of pain sensation (Turk & Okifuji, 2002).

Initially, the sensation of pain requires stimuli activating peripheral pain receptors. When activated, these receptors transmit signals through the peripheral nervous system (PNS) back to the central nervous system (CNS), specifically the spinal cord. Within the spinal cord, these signals are transmitted along pain-specific neural tracts up to the brain stem and cortex where the pain is interpreted and enters our consciousness. Two main types of fibers carry the pain signal from receptor to CNS: a-delta and c fibers. This is an important distinction as the fibers carry different types of pain (Gold, Belmont, & Thomas, 2007). A-delta fibers allow rapid conduction along the nerve and therefore are ideal for carrying signals of acute pain, while c-fibers have limited conduction velocity making them useful for chronic pain (Gold et al., 2007). In addition to the ascending pain pathway described, there is also a descending pain modulatory pathway. This cortical pathway is part of a complex pain modulatory system in which multiple factors both peripherally and centrally affect an individual's perception of pain. All of this is important because of the synergistic relationship between understanding the pain pathway and development of therapeutic options. For example, attempts to understand the analgesic effect of opioid medications led to the discovery of mu opioid receptors at various levels of the nervous system (Akil, Mayer, & Liebeskind, 1976). Conversely, understanding of c-fibers allowed development of targeted medications such as NSAIDs and capsaicin cream, both of which reduce c-fiber activation (Gold et al., 2007; Heppelmann, Messlinger, Neiss, & Schmidt, 1990). Finally, the understanding of the pain pathway may help us explain potential mechanisms underlying the analgesic effects of VR therapy.

While the difference between pain sensation and perception is recognized, the mechanism controlling pain perception is not fully understood. This is significant because pain perception impacts people, not pain sensation. Throughout history, multiple theories have been proposed to explain the human pain perception system. These include the specificity theory, first described by Von Frey in 1895, which postulated that the perception of pain was simply a result of summation of sensory pain stimuli (Moayedi & Davis, 2013). The major flaw in this theory is the observation that identical stimuli can produce varying reactions ranging from painful to non-painful. For example, American soldiers returning from war expressed that they did not feel pain despite having severe wounds from battle (Melzack & Wall, 1965). Their lack of pain may be attributed to the relief of leaving the battlefield alive. This suggests that perception of pain is influenced by one's circumstances and not only a product of specific stimuli. Another proposal by J.P. Nafe in 1929, called the pattern theory, surmised that nerve fibers were non-specific, and that pain was a product of intense activation of any nerve fiber given the appropriate stimulus (Moayedi & Davis, 2013). Given our current understanding of specific nerve fiber types and their differences, this theory no longer holds.

While a multitude of other theories have been proposed, arguably the most influential, is called the gate control theory (GCT), popularized by Melzack and Wall in 1965 (Melzack & Wall, 1965). This theory postulates that there is a "gate control system" that modulates the communication between PNS and CNS. They identified the substantia gelatinosa (SG) as the area likely to act as this gate keeper (Melzack & Wall, 1965). The SG is between the afferent nerve fibers coming from the periphery and central transmission cells (T) located in the dorsal horn of the spinal cord that transmit to the brain (Melzack & Wall, 1965). The SG opens or closes the "gates", modifying the communication of T cells with the brain (Melzack & Wall, 1965). Opening or closing by the SG is dictated by a variety of inputs. Most important for discussion in this chapter is the belief that external factors play a role altering the effects of the gate control system, which rectifies some of the flaws present in the other theories. The three major factors described are: (1) Activity prior to stimulation, (2) Stimulus-evoked activity, and (3) Balance of fiber types (Melzack & Wall, 1965). Each of these factors regulate the extent to which the gate opens and closes, which in turn, changes how one perceives the stimulus. Activity prior to stimulation refers to an individual's environment and circumstances such as emotional state. This is consistent with the observation that people experience identical stimuli in different ways depending on the situation and past experiences. This also suggests that in addition to peripheral to central transmission of signal, there is modification of signal that is centrally mediated. Melzack and Wall's GCT spurred a change in research focus and solidified the idea that the CNS actively plays a role in pain perception.

As more evidence arose, certain limitations to the GCT revealed themselves and therefore Melzack described the body-self neuromatrix theory of pain (BSNT) in 1999 (Melzack, 2001, 1999). This theory aims to correct the limitations of the GCT in explaining phantom limb pain (PLP), or other chronic pain conditions without peripheral stimulus. Additionally, the theory further elevates the role and importance of the brain in modulating pain perception. Neuromatrix is the term given by Melzack to describe a neural network of neurons connecting the thalamus, cortex, and limbic system (Melzack, 2001, 1999). This network is formed through genetics and an individual's sensory influences, resulting in a personalized neurosignature (Melzack, 2001, 1999). The neuromatrix is influenced by external inputs such as sensory stimuli, but also hormonal imbalances, emotional stress, and psychologic distress (Melzack, 2001, 1999). Overall, the BSNT suggests that the brain plays the central role in pain perception and that a vast array of factors have the potential to modulate its effects.

Mechanisms of VR in Pain

One reason VR has promising potential for treatment of pain is that it can have effects on many of the areas previously mentioned. This differs from a pharmacologic agent that acts on specific signaling pathways. Despite this potential, the current understanding of the mechanisms explaining how VR diminishes pain is not well understood (Gold et al., 2007). The following section discusses the theories and evidence for how VR therapy can impact pain.

A popular theory is that VR decreases perception of pain by acting as a distraction. Studies measuring brain activity showed certain regions of the brain, such as the anterior cingulate cortex (ACC) and periaqueductal gray (PAG), had activity that correlated with performing tasks of distraction and pain perception (Bantick et al., 2002; Hoffman et al., 2006; Valet et al., 2004). The ACC and PAG are believed to communicate with each other and modulate multiple pathways involved with pain perception (Vogt, Sikes, & Vogt, 1993). These could therefore explain some of the effects of VR on pain. Another area that immersive VR can have a powerful effect on is one's emotions. Evidence suggests that emotions play an important role in modulating perception of pain, with certain emotions heightening pain perception while others dull pain perception (Neugebauer, Li, Bird, & Han, 2004). The major area within the brain that controls emotion is the limbic system, specifically the amygdala, and some studies have shown that the ACC and PAG interact with the amygdala (Gold et al., 2007). As described in the BSNT, perception of pain is controlled through an extremely complex network that requires further understanding. Based on our current knowledge, the effects of VR on pain may be, but are not limited to, its effects on attention and emotion. These findings partially explain the acute pain relief found with VR therapy but cannot explain long-term benefits.

The following section outlines potential explanations for sustained pain relief with VR therapy. In the previous paragraph, the power of VR to create a virtual experience was alluded to. Part of what makes this so powerful is the ability to create an illusion of ownership of one's body. To understand body ownership, it is important to define body schema and body image—two concepts that combine to form body ownership. In brief, body schema refers to one's representation of body position while body image refers to one's external representation of the body (Gallagher & Cole, 1995). For example, controlling the movement of one's body during a coordinated dance would rely on body schema while commenting on one's attractiveness would involve body image. An early study that showed how body ownership could be manipulated is now known as the rubber hand illusion (RHI) (Botvinick & Cohen, 1998). In this experiment, researchers were able to fool subjects into thinking a rubber hand was their own hand by simultaneously stroking the subject's hand and the rubber hand (Botvinick & Cohen, 1998). Follow up studies found limitations in how the RHI could be achieved. One study altered the positioning of the rubber hand by turning it either 90 or 180 degrees (Ehrsson, Spence, & Passingham, 2004; Tsakiris & Haggard, 2005). In both instances, this stopped the RHI, demonstrating the importance of body schema on creating these ownership illusions. Another study replaced the rubber hand with inaccurate objects such as the opposite hand (Tsakiris & Haggard, 2005). Again, this modification ended the RHI, showing the importance of body image on forming ownership illusions (Costantini & Haggard, 2007). With further development, researchers have been able to create a full body illusion with virtual reality showing the power of VR in this realm (Slater, Spanlang, Sanchez-Vives, & Blanke, 2010). The power to create these illusions may form the foundation of VR therapies' effect on chronic pain.

One way for chronic changes to occur is adaptive changes of the CNS, also known as neuroplasticity. Traditionally, the CNS is thought of as rigid and unchanging, with distinct regions that perform specific functions (Ramachandran & Altschuler, 2009). Elimination of a distinct region would permanently remove its associated function. While largely true, more recent observations have demonstrated that some ability for neuroplastic change is available. An example is central remapping, which explains the phenomenon that amputees may feel tactile sensation in the phantom limb when touched on the face (Ramachandran, Stewart, & Rogers-Ramachandran, 1992). Normally, the sensory cortex of the brain processes sensory information from differing regions of the body along an organized map called a homunculus. In the sensory homunculus, the face is located adjacent to the upper limb (Ramachandran

& Altschuler, 2009). The concept of remapping suggests that in amputees, there is a neuroplastic change that results in stimuli of the face activating the homunculus at both the face region and the adjacent upper limb region, allowing tactile sensation to be felt at both locations (Ramachandran, 1993; Yang et al., 1994). Similar CNS changes are also believed to play a role in certain chronic pain conditions such as PLP and complex regional pain syndrome (CRPS) (Ramachandran & Rogers-Ramachandran, 2000). Researchers have described this theory as "learned" paralysis or pain (Ramachandran & Altschuler, 2009). For example, patients with PLP often describe a paralyzed feeling of being unable to move a frozen arm. The learned theory explains that this is the brain's adaptive response to repetitive motor commands that do not result in visual arm movement (Ramachandran & Altschuler, 2009). As each additional motor command fails, the brain begins to believe that the amputated arm is indeed "paralyzed" (Ramachandran & Altschuler, 2009). While this malleability has significant clinical impact on patients, it also provides potential in therapy development as, in theory, reversing the maladaptive neuroplastic changes should also be possible (Ramachandran & Altschuler, 2009).

An early application of this phenomenon for chronic pain was in 1992 when Ramachandran described the use of mirror visual feedback or mirror therapy (MT) for PLP (Ramachandran & Altschuler, 2009). For amputees with PLP, MT involves viewing a reflection of one's healthy limb in a mirror, which creates the illusion of having a "normal" amputated limb. Multiple studies have validated the success of this type of therapy for PLP, which helps with both the learned paralysis and pain discussed previously (Chan et al., 2007; Darnall, 2009; Ramachandran, Rogers-Ramachandran, & Cobb, 1995). The concept behind learned pain is that an injury to a body limb leads to extreme sensitivity to pain such that any movement results in pain (Ramachandran & Altschuler, 2009). Overtime, the brain's adaptive response to any sensory stimuli from that area becomes exaggerated pain (Ramachandran & Altschuler, 2009). Therefore, this is very similar to learned paralysis, as a maladaptive neuroplastic response occurs dues to a disconnect between stimulus and expected result. While the mechanism explaining the effects of MT are not fully understood, there are three main mechanisms that likely contribute.

Firstly, MT rectifies the disconnect between stimulus and response. For example, a PLP using MT will see corresponding movement of the reflected limb to motor commands to move the phantom limb. This connects the stimulus (motor command) with the expected response (movement of limb) (Ramachandran & Altschuler, 2009). Similarly, for learned pain, a stimulus of any type causes pain. Using MT, the patient sees the reflection of a freely moving limb unrestricted by pain. Again, this connects the stimulus (movement of limb) with the healthy response (painless movement). In theory, this could result in CNS changes that reverse the maladaptive changes associated with the illness (Ramachandran & Altschuler, 2009). Recent brain imaging studies support this hypothesis as one study of PLP patients treated with MT found significant reversal of cortical dysfunction in the primary somatosensory cortex (Foell, Bekrater-Bodmann, Diers, & Flor, 2014). Secondly, MT may facilitate rehabilitation through stimulation of mirror neurons. First described in 1992, mirror neurons are cells that activate through visualization of a stimulus causing a replicate action within the person (di Pellegrino, Fadiga, Fogassi, Gallese, & Rizzolatti, 1992). For example, seeing a pin violently prick a hand often causes one to pull back his or her own hand in fear of pain despite never being physically touched (Ramachandran & Altschuler, 2009). Therefore, through the visualization done in MT, it may be possible to train mirror neurons and improve rehabilitative efforts (Ramachandran & Altschuler, 2009). In both mechanisms, changes are adaptive and therefore one would expect results to take time. In practice, MT is frequently reported to work instantly therefore another mechanism must be present. One theory suggests that visual confirmation of a normal limb acts as a safeguard against unwarranted pain (Ramachandran & Altschuler, 2009). For example, after an individual undergoes an amputation, he/she is no longer able to visualize the limb and feel phantom pain. Using MT, they can visualize the reflected limb, showing the brain that the limb is intact and pain-free, thereby acting as visual confirmation that the limb is normal (Ramachandran & Altschuler, 2009). This allows the brain to override the sensory information coming from the phantom limb. This process would act acutely as simple visualization would immediately activate the illusion of a healthy limb.

A discussion of MT is relevant to this chapter because of the similarities between VR therapy and MT. Like MT, VR creates a visual environment that results in a type of body transfer illusion (Moseley, Gallace, & Spence, 2012). The net effect of which is likely reversal of maladaptive neuroplastic changes (Ramachandran & Altschuler, 2009; Ramachandran & Rogers-Ramachandran, 2000). Despite similarities, differences may impact the potential efficacy of VR therapy. Two potential advantages of MT are realism of the visual hand and realistic speed of hand movements (Ramachandran & Altschuler, 2009). Currently, it is not known how much these factors impact efficacy of therapy. Potential advantages to VR include increased interaction with the environment, ability to perform more actions/tasks, use for bilaterally affected patients, and personalization with software changes (Ramachandran & Altschuler, 2009). Additional research may help differentiate which factors are most important. In summary, current evidence suggests there are multiple factors contributing to the impact of VR therapy on chronic pain, including distraction and reversal of maladaptive CNS changes.

Use of VR for Chronic Pain

While overall evidence for VR therapy for chronic pain is limited, early findings are promising and warrant further research and application. As alluded to earlier, VR is a computer technology that allows users to experience a simulated virtual environment. The VR devices available are increasingly diverse but two general types of devices are available: non-immersive and immersive VR devices. Non-immersive refers to an external display showing the VR environment. Immersive refers to use of a head mounted display, a device worn over the eyes that displays the virtual environment while completely blocking out the user's surroundings. Evidence for the efficacy of VR in acute pain is relatively abundant compared to chronic pain and immersive VR has been shown to be more efficacious than non-immersive VR for acute pain (Shahrbanian, Ma, Aghaei, Korner-bitensky, & Simmonds, 2012). Advantages of VR therapy such as decreased opioid consumption, minimal adverse effects, simple application, and customizability make it a promising technology for use in chronic pain. Given the broad array of conditions that can manifest with chronic pain, the following section will review the current evidence related to these conditions.

The most common causes of chronic pain are musculoskeletal such as lower back and joint pain. Multiple studies have demonstrated the use of VR therapy for these types of conditions. A pilot study of six patients found significant pain reduction in patients with chronic pain during VR sessions (Wiederhold, Gao, Sulea, & Wiederhold, 2014). Long-term effects were not measured. Based on subjective comments from patients, the authors concluded that the primary effect of VR in pain reduction was distraction from pain that occurred during the VR sessions. Similarly, a study of 30 pain clinic patients demonstrated significant pain reduction following a single VR session. While pain was reduced both during and immediately post-session, pain reduction was greater during the session (60%) than post-session (33%) (Jones, Moore, & Choo, 2016). Another study trialed self-administered VR therapy within the home environment for eight chronic pain patients. Combined findings did not reveal significant quantitative difference in pain scores pre-post sessions. Despite this result, a majority of patients were positive about the experience and reported subjective decrease in pain (Garrett, Taverner, & McDade, 2017). This study highlights the individualized effects of VR on patients as each patient has a unique response and impression of VR therapy.

As previously mentioned, PLP is a chronic pain condition that is common in amputee patients. Pain manifests in the amputated limb—the mechanism of which is not fully understood, but is believed to be due in part to maladaptive CNS neuroplasticity (Ramachandran & Rogers-Ramachandran, 2000). A review of the literature on use of VR therapy for PLP noted multiple studies supporting positive outcomes for patients suffering from PLP (Dunn, Yeo, Moghaddampour, Chau, & Humbert, 2017). Pain reduction, measured both quantitatively or qualitatively, was found across all studies and adverse effects were minimal (Dunn et al., 2017). While these findings are promising, the major limitation is their low quality. All studies were either case studies or case report studies suggesting the need for higher quality studies for better understanding. Additional challenges include differing protocols and prolonged benefit. Increase in technology and software innovation has allowed more limb control and immersion within the VR environment. This limits the ability to standardize protocols across study institutions. Finally, the eight studies identified in the review focused on immediate post-intervention changes in pain (Dunn et al., 2017). Given the chronic nature of PLP, further research to understand the long-term impact of VR is needed.

Some evidence suggests the potential for VR treatment of CRPS, another chronic pain syndrome. Pilot studies on four pediatric patients with CRPS demonstrated feasibility of VR for CRPS patients as well as markedly improved function and pain during VR sessions. Subjective feedback on sessions was positive (Won, Tataru, Cojocaru, Krane, Bailenson, & Niswonger, 2015). Another study involving 10 patients with CRPS trialed a virtual reality body swapping intervention (Jeon, Cho, & Lee, 2014). While there was no significant reduction in pain, patients did report significant improvement of body perception disturbance, a common complaint of CRPS patients (Jeon et al., 2014). Finally, two case reports of traditional treatment refractory CRPS patients treated with VR therapy demonstrated significant pain reduction with sustained benefit for multiple months (Chau, Phelan, Dunn, Yeo, Hata, 2016; Chi, Chau, Phelan, Ta, Hata, 2017). These studies suggest the potential for use of VR in treatment of CRPS. Additionally, current ongoing studies on this condition are active and promising.

In addition to multiple motor, sensory, and functional deficits, spinal cord injury (SCI) patients can present with persistent neuropathic pain. The literature in this area is limited but does suggest the potential for VR in reducing pain associated with SCI. An RCT investigating VR-augmented motor imagery found treatment reduced pain (Soler et al., 2010). Additionally, analgesic effects seen with combined VR and transcranial direct current stimulation treatment suggest a synergistic effect between treatments. This shows the potential for VR to augment other types of treatment. Another example is virtual reality hypnosis used for neuropathic pain in a SCI patient (Oneal, Patterson, Soltani, Teeley, & Jensen, 2008). While promising, more evidence is needed to verify the use of VR therapy in SCI-associated pain.

Another relatively common chronic pain condition, fibromyalgia, predominantly effects women. There are two studies that have assessed the use of VR for this condition. An initial case study found significant pain reduction in a fibromyalgia patient after 15 sessions of MT in conjunction with pain medication. The authors concluded that VR may be a useful adjunct to pharmacotherapy in treating fibromyalgia (Botella et al., 2013). In a 2013 study, VR therapy was used to supplement 10 sessions of group

CBT for six patients suffering from fibromyalgia. Importantly, patients were followed 6-months post-treatment and outcomes including reduction in pain and depression, improved functional status, and increased positive affect persisted (Chirico et al., 2016). These studies suggest a potential role for VR in treatment of fibromyalgia, particularly as adjuncts to more traditional therapies such as medication or CBT.

Researchers have targeted VR for relief of cancer-related discomfort for many years. A patient's experience with cancer can involve chronic pain, chemotherapy side effects, procedural discomfort, and psychologic effects. The strongest evidence for VR in cancer therapy is reduction in side effects from chemotherapy, but literature also supports efficacy in acute pain reduction from cancer-related procedures, and improvement of psychologic symptoms such as anxiety (Chirico et al., 2016). Cancer is also an active area in the private sector with multiple startup companies offering VR for anxiety, pain, and other cancer-related complications.

Use of VR in Pediatrics

Chronic pain is common in pediatric populations, often significantly impacting affected individuals (King et al., 2011). In the last few decades, rates of chronic pain have also increased in children making this an important issue (Bandell-Hoekstra et al., 2001; Sillanpää & Anttila, 1996). The following section addresses the current understanding of chronic pain in children compared to chronic pain in adults. The prevalence of chronic pain in pediatric populations ranges from 15-30% (Palermo, Eccleston, Lewandowski, Williams, & Morley, 2010; Perquin et al., 2000; Roth-Isigkeit, 2005; Stanford, Chambers, Biesanz, & Chen, 2008). Studies have shown that girls have higher rates and greater intensity of pain relative to boys, and in general, rates of chronic pain also rise with increasing age (King et al., 2011). While many conditions can cause chronic pain in children, the most common is headache, followed by abdominal pain, musculoskeletal pain, and a variety of other chronic pain conditions (King et al., 2011). Of these, headache is the most studied although there is growing literature on other chronic pain conditions. As with adults, children suffering from chronic pain experience psychologic effects with evidence suggesting a correlation between chronic pain and depression, anxiety, and decreased self-esteem (Rhee, 2000; Stanford et al., 2008). Additional impacts include negative effects on school performance, and family and social life. There is also evidence of lasting effects in a study which found young adolescents with chronic abdominal pain had significantly higher rates of anxiety as adults (Campo et al., 2001).

One obstacle to better understanding chronic pain in children relates to limitations in the literature on this subject. Studies have typically been focused on a single chronic pain condition (e.g. headache) making it difficult to generalize findings. However, some trends across multiple studies are present. Significant impacts on education include disruption in school attendance and school activity participation (Hershey, Powers, Bentti, & DeGrauw, 2000; Reid, Lang, & McGrath, 1997; Walker, Guite, Duke, Barnard, & Greene, 1998). Additionally, mothers of children with chronic pain reported significant impact on family quality of life, including restrictions on family social life and difficulty of family members to deal with the condition (Hunfeld et al., 2001). Studies looking at functional disability have used indices such as the Functional Disability Inventory, to represent a more complete picture of a child's functional ability (Walker & Greene, 1991). One study of children with chronic pain due to both headache and musculoskeletal causes found the intensity of pain to be highly correlated with functional disability (Kashikar-Zuck, Goldschneider, Powers, Vaught, & Hershey, 2001). Additionally, functional disability was highly correlated with depression (Kashikar-Zuck et al., 2001). These findings suggest that as with adults, chronic pain has significant effects on functionality and mental health in children. Interestingly, intensity of pain was not correlated with depression (Kashikar-Zuck et al., 2001). Therefore, assessing functional disability may be more useful than pain intensity when predicting the psychologic impact of chronic pain on patients. In addition, it highlights the importance of understanding external factors that affect functional disability and response to chronic pain.

One difference between the response of children and adults to chronic pain is the effect of coping mechanisms on functional disability (Kashikar-Zuck et al., 2001; Keefe et al., 2000). Studies of adults have shown that mature coping mechanisms are correlated with improved functionality while catastrophizing is correlated with diminished functionality (Keefe et al., 2000). Alternatively, in pediatric populations, evidence suggests there is no correlation between coping skills and functional disability (Kashikar-Zuck et al., 2001). The reason for this is not understood, but multiple theories have been proposed to explain the difference. One theory is that coping mechanisms mature with age, and therefore catastrophizing by children is simply a reflection of parental reactions to their condition or their limited life exposure (Kashikar-Zuck et al., 2001). A second theory is that the effect of catastrophizing actions requires consistency across a period of time and situations, which requires abstract thinking (Kashikar-Zuck et al., 2001). As children are less developed abstract thinkers, it would follow that the effect of catastrophizing is diminished. The importance of understanding coping mechanisms and other factors that may influence functionality in children with chronic pain lies in its clinical implications. As seen with coping mechanisms, there are differences in response between adult and pediatric populations. Thus, in developing treatment options, it is important to recognize these differences and create pediatric-specific therapies.

Given the psychologic impacts of chronic pain on children, psychotherapies have been used as part of the treatment plan. CBT and behavioral therapies are the most popular methods used (Fisher et al., 2014). A 2014 systematic review and meta-analysis of 35 RCT on the topic found sufficient evidence to support efficacy of psychotherapies on chronic pain, disability, and depression for certain conditions (Fisher et al., 2014). The strongest evidence is for reduction of pain in patients with headache following treatment, in which the number to treat was 2.72 at post-treatment and 2 at follow-up—meaning less than three children needed to be treated for one child to receive benefit (Fisher et al., 2014). Also, children with abdominal pain and musculoskeletal pain had significant improvements in pain and disability following treatment although only those suffering from musculoskeletal pain received reduction in depression (Fisher et al., 2014). When analyzing the entire cohort of chronic pain subjects, there was insufficient evidence to suggest psychologic interventions caused an effect on depression, anxiety, or sleep patterns (Fisher et al., 2014). In summary, current psychologic therapies are effective in reducing pain in children, but evidence is inconclusive in their effect on the psychologic co-morbidities of chronic pain. This emphasizes the need for research to better understand psychologic conditions associated with chronic pain, factors modulating them, and potential therapies.

VR therapy has been successfully used for pain in the pediatric population for almost two decades (Mahrer & Gold, 2009; Malloy & Milling, 2010). In fact, the first study demonstrating use of VR for treating pain was a case study in 2000 of two adolescents receiving burn wound care (Hoffman, Doctor, Patterson, Carrougher, & Furness, 2000). Since that time, while multiple studies of childhood acute pain have been completed, the only study addressing chronic pain is the small trial on CRPS mentioned previously (Won, Tataru, Cojocaru, Krane, Bailenson, & Niswonger, 2015). Evidence supporting use of VR therapy for acute pain in children is relatively strong with studies on both experimental and clinical acute pain. A set of studies assessed use of non-immersive VR to decrease experimenter-mediated cold pressor pain in children. They found that those who received VR therapy experienced greater pain reduction than those who did not (Dahlquist et al., 2007, 2010; Hoffman, Seibel, et al., 2006). Additionally, those treated with interactive VR reported less pain than those treated with non-interactive VR (Dahlquist et al., 2007). In a follow-up study, comparing immersive VR and non-immersive VR, adolescents treated with immersive VR reported greater reduction in pain (Dahlquist et al., 2010). These experimental pain studies provide strong evidence that VR therapy can reduce acute pain, as study conditions can be strictly controlled. However, they are limited, because of the inability to show clinical significance.

A variety of smaller studies have shown decreased pain in pediatric patients undergoing a variety of painful procedures. These include burn wounds dressing changes, intravenous placement, and port access (Gershon, Zimand, Pickering, Rothbaum, & Hodges, 2004; Gold, Kim, Kant, Joseph, & Rizzo, 2006; Gold & Mahrer, 2017; Hunter G. Hoffman et al., 2008; Kokinsky, Enska, Nilsson, & Finnstro, 2009). In summary, current evidence supports use of VR therapy for acute pain in children. As with adults, immersive VR is more effective than non-immersive VR although the benefits are maximized in older children (Won et al., 2017). Overall, the results with acute pain in children and chronic pain in adults illustrate the potential for VR therapy in pediatric chronic pain.

Finally, it is important to consider some of the unique challenges that pertain to use of VR for pediatric populations. While there are many similarities between adults and children with respect to VR, an important difference is the level of presence experienced within virtual environments. Presence refers to a subjective sensation that an individual feels engaged with a virtual world (Won et al., 2017). Children were found to have higher levels of presence using VR than adults, suggesting there is a difference in how people process virtual environments (Baumgartner, 2008; Sharar et al., 2007). Findings from brain imaging studies displayed greater activation in the prefrontal cortex of older adolescents and adults, as compared to young children (Baumgartner, 2008; Jäncke, Cheetham, & Baumgartner, 2009). The prefrontal cortex is known to be an area in the brain where executive functioning occurs and is needed to fully experience VR (Baumgartner, 2008; Jäncke et al., 2009). These findings are consistent with the difference in presence between children and adults, as young children are still developing executive function. Implications of this difference should be considered in studies involving children. For example, to ensure children separate real world from virtual world, more thorough debriefing following VR therapy may be useful (Won et al., 2017).

Another concern pertains to the safety of children using VR. Current evidence suggests that VR therapy has minor adverse effects (Won et al., 2017). Similar to VR use in adults, the primary complaint is motion sickness. Despite this, other potential safety considerations have been discussed. Developmental differences may be a potential concern, as children have more difficulty separating real and virtual as previously mentioned. This may manifest with the virtual environment as well as virtual avatars that possess special abilities (Won et al., 2017). Ensuring that children comprehend the differences may be useful in preventing unwanted effects. While increased immersion and interactivity are correlated with efficacy of VR therapy, they also increase the risk of collisions with surrounding objects (Won et al., 2017). Therefore, proper room setup and supervision should be part of any VR therapy session. Finally, VR devices offer social aspects that may prove beneficial for children suffering from chronic pain as these patients often have school and social disadvantages described earlier (Forgeron et al., 2010). Conversely, as with all social media devices, there is the possibility of social isolation which may be particularly detrimental during developmental years (Won et al., 2017). Despite these concerns, overall evidence suggests that VR therapy should be safe for use in children provided proper precautions are taken.

CONCLUSION

The evidence for use of VR therapy in treatment of chronic pain is growing. VR has been used successfully for a variety of chronic pain conditions as stand-alone or adjunctive treatment. Some findings were consistent across studies and highlight advantages to using VR. For example, adverse effects were rare and limited to motion discomfort. VR was used on a wide range of patients differing in condition, functional status, and age (pediatric and geriatric populations) suggesting its broad applications. Furthermore, VR is relatively easy to use, portable, and is potentially customizable for individual patients. Cost of devices have been significantly decreasing in recent years, making VR an increasingly affordable option. Finally, as an adjunct to pain medications, VR has the potential to help alleviate our dependence on opioid medications. All these factors make VR therapy a promising treatment option for chronic pain and its comorbid psychiatric disorders.

REFERENCES

Akil, H., Mayer, D. J., & Liebeskind, J. C. (1976). Antagonism of stimulation-produced analgesia by naloxone, a narcotic antagonist. *Science*, *191*(4230), 961–962. doi:10.1126cience.1251210 PMID:1251210

Bandell-Hoekstra, I. E. N. G., Abu-Saad, H. H., Passchier, J., Frederiks, C. M. A., Feron, F. J. M., & Knipschild, P. (2001). Prevalence and characteristics of headache in Dutch schoolchildren. *European Journal of Pain (London, England)*, *5*(2), 145–153. doi:10.1053/eujp.2001.0234 PMID:11465980

Bantick, S. J., Wise, R. G., Ploghaus, A., Clare, S., Smith, S. M., & Tracey, I. (2002). Imaging how attention modulates pain in humans using functional MRI. *Brain*, *125*(2), 310–319. doi:10.1093/brain/awf022 PMID:11844731

Baumgartner, T. (2008). Feeling present in arousing virtual reality worlds: Prefrontal brain regions differentially orchestrate presence experience in adults and children. *Frontiers in Human Neuroscience*, *2*. doi:10.3389/neuro.09.008.2008 PMID:18958209

Botella, C., Garcia-Palacios, A., Vizcaíno, Y., Herrero, R., Baños, R. M., & Belmonte, M. A. (2013). Virtual Reality in the Treatment of Fibromyalgia: A Pilot Study. *Cyberpsychology, Behavior, and Social Networking*, *16*(3), 215–223. doi:10.1089/cyber.2012.1572 PMID:23496678

Botvinick, M., & Cohen, J. (1998). Rubber hands "feel" touch that eyes see [8]. *Nature, 391*(6669), 756. doi:10.1038/35784 PMID:9486643

Breivik, H., Collett, B., Ventafridda, V., Cohen, R., & Gallacher, D. (2006). Survey of chronic pain in Europe: Prevalence, impact on daily life, and treatment. *European Journal of Pain (London, England), 10*(4), 287. doi:10.1016/j.ejpain.2005.06.009 PMID:16095934

Campo, J. V., Di Lorenzo, C., Chiappetta, L., Bridge, J., Colborn, D. K., & Gartner, J. C. Jr. … Brent, D. (2001). Adult Outcomes of Pediatric Recurrent Abdominal Pain: Do They Just Grow Out of It? *Pediatrics*. doi:10.1542/peds.108.1.e1

Chan, B. L., Witt, R., Charrow, A. P., Magee, A., Howard, R., & Pasquina, P. F. … Tsao, J. W. (2007). Mirror Therapy for Phantom Limb Pain. *The New England Journal of Medicine*. doi:10.1056/NEJMc071927

Chau, B., Phelan, I., Dunn, J., Yeo, E., & Hata, J. H. S. (2016). *Complex Regional Pain Syndrome: A Case Report*. Academic Press.

Chi, B., Chau, B., Phelan, I., Ta, P., & Hata, J. H. S. (2017). *Successful Complex Regional Pain Syndrome Treatment with Immersive Virtual Reality: Case Report*. Academic Press.

Chirico, A., Lucidi, F., De Laurentiis, M., Milanese, C., Napoli, A., & Giordano, A. (2016). Virtual Reality in Health System: Beyond Entertainment. A Mini-Review on the Efficacy of VR During Cancer Treatment. *Journal of Cellular Physiology, 231*(2), 275–287. doi:10.1002/jcp.25117 PMID:26238976

Choinière, M., Dion, D., Peng, P., Banner, R., Barton, P. M., Boulanger, A., … Ware, M. (2010). The Canadian STOP-PAIN project - Part 1: Who are the patients on the waitlists of multidisciplinary pain treatment facilities? *Canadian Journal of Anaesthesia = Journal Canadien d'anesthésie*. doi:10.100712630-010-9305-5

Costantini, M., & Haggard, P. (2007). The rubber hand illusion: Sensitivity and reference frame for body ownership. *Consciousness and Cognition, 16*(2), 229–240. doi:10.1016/j.concog.2007.01.001 PMID:17317221

Dahlquist, L. M., McKenna, K. D., Jones, K. K., Dillinger, L., Weiss, K. E., & Ackerman, C. S. (2007). Active and Passive Distraction Using a Head-Mounted Display Helmet: Effects on Cold Pressor Pain in Children. *Health Psychology, 26*(6), 794–801. doi:10.1037/0278-6133.26.6.794 PMID:18020853

Dahlquist, L. M., Weiss, K. E., Law, E. F., Sil, S., Herbert, L. J., & Horn, S. B. … Ackerman, C. S. (2010). Effects of videogame distraction and a virtual reality type head-mounted display helmet on cold pressor pain in young elementary school-aged children. *Journal of Pediatric Psychology*. doi:10.1093/jpepsy/jsp082

Darnall, B. D. (2009). Self-Delivered Home-Based Mirror Therapy for Lower Limb Phantom Pain. *American Journal of Physical Medicine & Rehabilitation*, *88*(1), 78–81. doi:10.1097/PHM.0b013e318191105b PMID:19096290

Demyttenaere, K., Bruffaerts, R., Lee, S., Posada-Villa, J. A., Kovess, V., & Angermeyer, M. … Von Korff, M. (2007). Mental disorders among persons with chronic back or neck pain: Results from the World Mental Health Surveys. *Pain*. doi:10.1016/j.pain.2007.01.022

di Pellegrino, G., Fadiga, L., Fogassi, L., Gallese, V., & Rizzolatti, G. (1992). Understanding motor events: A neurophysiological study. *Experimental Brain Research*, *91*(1), 176–180. doi:10.1007/BF00230027 PMID:1301372

Dunn, J., Yeo, E., Moghaddampour, P., Chau, B., & Humbert, S. (2017). Virtual and augmented reality in the treatment of phantom limb pain: A literature review. *NeuroRehabilitation*, *40*(4), 595–601. doi:10.3233/NRE-171447 PMID:28211829

Ehde, D. M., Dillworth, T. M., & Turner, J. A. (2014). Cognitive-Behavioral Therapy for Individuals With Chronic Pain. *The American Psychologist*, *69*(2), 153–166. doi:10.1037/a0035747 PMID:24547801

Ehrsson, H. H., Spence, C., & Passingham, R. E. (2004). That's my hand! Activity in premotor cortex reflects feeling of ownership of a limb. *Science*, *305*(5685), 875–877. doi:10.1126cience.1097011 PMID:15232072

Fisher, E., Heathcote, L., & Palermo, T. M. de C., Williams, A. C., Lau, J., & Eccleston, C. (2014). Systematic Review and Meta-Analysis of Psychological Therapies for Children With Chronic Pain. *Journal of Pediatric Psychology*. doi:10.1093/jpepsy/jsu008

Foell, J., Bekrater-Bodmann, R., Diers, M., & Flor, H. (2014). *Mirror therapy for phantom limb pain: Brain changes and the role of body representation*. European Journal of Pain. doi:10.1002/j.1532-2149.2013.00433.x

Fordyce, W. E., & Company, M. C. V. (1977). Behavioral methods for chronic pain and illness. *Pain*, *3*(3), 291–292. doi:10.1016/0304-3959(77)90029-X

Forgeron, P. A., King, S., Stinson, J. N., McGrath, P. J., MacDonald, A. J., & Chambers, C. T. (2010). Social functioning and peer relationships in children and adolescents with chronic pain: A systematic review. *Pain Research & Management, 15*(1), 27–41. doi:10.1155/2010/820407 PMID:20195556

Gallagher, S., & Cole, J. (1995). Body image and body schema in a deafferented subject. *Journal of Mind and Behavior.*

Garrett, B., Taverner, T., & McDade, P. (2017). Virtual Reality as an Adjunct Home Therapy in Chronic Pain Management: An Exploratory Study. *JMIR Medical Informatics, 5*(2), e11. doi:10.2196/medinform.7271 PMID:28495661

Gatchel, R. J., Peng, Y. B., Peters, M. L., Fuchs, P. N., & Turk, D. C. (2007). The Biopsychosocial Approach to Chronic Pain: Scientific Advances and Future Directions. *Psychological Bulletin, 133*(4), 581–624. doi:10.1037/0033-2909.133.4.581 PMID:17592957

Gershon, J., Zimand, E., Pickering, M., Rothbaum, B. O., & Hodges, L. (2004). A pilot and feasibility study of virtual reality as a distraction for children with cancer. *Journal of the American Academy of Child and Adolescent Psychiatry, 43*(10), 1243–1249. doi:10.1097/01.chi.0000135621.23145.05 PMID:15381891

Gold, J. I., Belmont, K. A., & Thomas, D. A. (2007). The Neurobiology of Virtual Reality Pain Attenuation. *Cyberpsychology & Behavior, 10*(4), 536–544. doi:10.1089/cpb.2007.9993 PMID:17711362

Gold, J. I., Kim, S. H., Kant, A. J., Joseph, M. H., & Rizzo, A. "Skip." (2006). Effectiveness of Virtual Reality for Pediatric Pain Distraction during IV Placement. *Cyberpsychology & Behavior.* doi:10.1089/cpb.2006.9.207

Gold, J. I., & Mahrer, N. E. (2017). Is Virtual Reality Ready for Prime Time in the Medical Space? A Randomized Control Trial of Pediatric Virtual Reality for Acute Procedural Pain Management. *Journal of Pediatric Psychology.* doi:10.1093/jpepsy/jsx129 PMID:29053848

Hassett, A. L., Aquino, J. K., & Ilgen, M. A. (2014). The risk of suicide mortality in chronic pain patients. *Current Pain and Headache Reports, 18*(8), 436. doi:10.100711916-014-0436-1 PMID:24952608

Heppelmann, B., Messlinger, K., Neiss, W. F., & Schmidt, R. F. (1990). Ultrastructural three-dimensional reconstruction of group III and group IV sensory nerve endings ("free nerve endings") in the knee joint capsule of the cat: Evidenence for multiple receptive sites. *The Journal of Comparative Neurology, 292*(1), 103–116. doi:10.1002/cne.902920107 PMID:2312785

Hershey, A. D., Powers, S. W., Bentti, A. L., & DeGrauw, T. J. (2000). Effectiveness of amitriptyline in the prophylactic management of childhood headaches. *Headache*, *40*(7), 539–549. doi:10.1046/j.1526-4610.2000.00085.x PMID:10940092

Hoffman, H. G., Doctor, J. N., Patterson, D. R., Carrougher, G. J., & Furness, T. III. (2000). Virtual reality as an adjunctive pain control during burn wound care in adolescent patients. *Pain*, *85*(1), 305–309. doi:10.1016/S0304-3959(99)00275-4 PMID:10692634

Hoffman, H. G., Patterson, D. R., Seibel, E., Soltani, M., Jewett-Leahy, L., & Sharar, S. R. (2008). Virtual reality pain control during burn wound debridement in the hydrotank. *The Clinical Journal of Pain*, *24*(4), 299–304. doi:10.1097/AJP.0b013e318164d2cc PMID:18427228

Hoffman, H. G., Richards, T. L., Bills, A. R., Van Oostrom, T., Magula, J., Seibel, E. J., & Sharar, S. R. (2006). Using fMRI to study the neural correlates of virtual reality analgesia. *CNS Spectrums*, *11*(01), 45–51. doi:10.1017/S1092852900024202 PMID:16400255

Hoffman, H. G., Seibel, E. J., Richards, T. L., Furness, T. A., Patterson, D. R., & Sharar, S. R. (2006). Virtual Reality Helmet Display Quality Influences the Magnitude of Virtual Reality Analgesia. *The Journal of Pain*, *7*(11), 843–850. doi:10.1016/j.jpain.2006.04.006 PMID:17074626

Hunfeld, J. a, Perquin, C. W., Duivenvoorden, H. J., Hazebroek-Kampschreur, a a, Passchier, J., van Suijlekom-Smit, L. W., & van der Wouden, J. C. (2001). Chronic pain and its impact on quality of life in adolescents and their families. *Journal of Pediatric Psychology*. doi:10.1093/jpepsy/26.3.145

Ilgen, M. A., Kleinberg, F., Ignacio, R. V., Bohnert, A. S. B., Valenstein, M., & McCarthy, J. F. … Katz, I. R. (2013). Noncancer Pain Conditions and Risk of Suicide. *JAMA Psychiatry*. doi:10.1001/jamapsychiatry.2013.908

Jäncke, L., Cheetham, M., & Baumgartner, T. (2009). Virtual reality and the role of the prefrontal cortex in adults and children. *Frontiers in Neuroscience*, *3*(1). doi:10.3389/neuro.01.006.2009 PMID:19753097

Jeon, B., Cho, S., & Lee, J.-H. (2014). Application of Virtual Body Swapping to Patients with Complex Regional Pain Syndrome: A Pilot Study. *Cyberpsychology, Behavior, and Social Networking*, *17*(6), 366–370. doi:10.1089/cyber.2014.0046 PMID:24892199

Jones, T., Moore, T., & Choo, J. (2016). The impact of virtual reality on chronic pain. *PLoS One*, *11*(12), e0167523. doi:10.1371/journal.pone.0167523 PMID:27997539

Kashikar-Zuck, S., Goldschneider, K. R., Powers, S. W., Vaught, M. H., & Hershey, A. D. (2001). Depression and functional disability in chronic pediatric pain. *The Clinical Journal of Pain, 17*(4), 341–349. doi:10.1097/00002508-200112000-00009 PMID:11783815

Katz, J., Rosenbloom, B. N., & Fashler, S. (2015). Chronic pain, psychopathology, and DSM-5 somatic symptom disorder. *Canadian Journal of Psychiatry, 60*(4), 160–167. doi:10.1177/070674371506000402 PMID:26174215

Keefe, F. J., Lefebvre, J. C., Egert, J. R., Affleck, G., Sullivan, M. J., & Caldwell, D. S. (2000). The relationship of gender to pain, pain behavior, and disability in osteoarthritis patients: The role of catastrophizing. *Pain, 87*(3), 325–334. doi:10.1016/S0304-3959(00)00296-7 PMID:10963912

King, S., Chambers, C. T., Huguet, A., MacNevin, R. C., McGrath, P. J., Parker, L., & MacDonald, A. J. (2011). The epidemiology of chronic pain in children and adolescents revisited: A systematic review. *Pain, 152*(12), 2729–2738. doi:10.1016/j.pain.2011.07.016 PMID:22078064

Kokinsky, E., Enska, K., Nilsson, S., & Finnstro, B. (2009). The use of Virtual Reality for needle-related procedural pain and distress in children and adolescents in a paediatric oncology unit. *European Journal of Oncology Nursing, 13*, 102–109. doi:10.1016/j.ejon.2009.01.003

Mahrer, N. E., & Gold, J. I. (2009). The use of virtual reality for pain control: A review. *Current Pain and Headache Reports, 13*(2), 100–109. doi:10.100711916-009-0019-8 PMID:19272275

Malloy, K. M., & Milling, L. S. (2010). The effectiveness of virtual reality distraction for pain reduction: A systematic review. *Clinical Psychology Review, 30*(8), 1011–1018. doi:10.1016/j.cpr.2010.07.001 PMID:20691523

Melzack, R. (1999). From the gate to the neuromatrix. *Pain, 82*, S121–S126. doi:10.1016/S0304-3959(99)00145-1 PMID:10491980

Melzack, R. (2001). Pain and the neuromatrix in the brain. *Journal of Dental Education*. PMID:11780656

Melzack, R., & Wall, P. D. (1965). Pain mechanisms: A new theory. *Science, 150*(3699), 971–978. doi:10.1126cience.150.3699.971 PMID:5320816

Moayedi, M., & Davis, K. D. (2013). Theories of pain: From specificity to gate control. *Journal of Neurophysiology, 109*(1), 5–12. doi:10.1152/jn.00457.2012 PMID:23034364

Moseley, G. L., Gallace, A., & Spence, C. (2012). Bodily illusions in health and disease: Physiological and clinical perspectives and the concept of a cortical "body matrix.". *Neuroscience and Biobehavioral Reviews*, *36*(1), 34–46. doi:10.1016/j.neubiorev.2011.03.013 PMID:21477616

Neugebauer, V., Li, W., Bird, G. C., & Han, J. S. (2004). The amygdala and persistent pain. *The Neuroscientist*, *10*(3), 221–234. doi:10.1177/1073858403261077 PMID:15155061

Oneal, B. J., Patterson, D. R., Soltani, M., Teeley, A., & Jensen, M. P. (2008). Virtual reality hypnosis in the treatment of chronic neuropathic pain: A case report. *The International Journal of Clinical and Experimental Hypnosis*, *56*(4), 451–462. doi:10.1080/00207140802255534 PMID:18726807

Palermo, T. M., Eccleston, C., Lewandowski, A. S., Williams, A. C. de C., & Morley, S. (2010). Randomized controlled trials of psychological therapies for management of chronic pain in children and adolescents: An updated meta-analytic review. *Pain*. doi:10.1016/j.pain.2009.10.004 PMID:19910118

Perquin, C. W., Hazebroek-Kampschreur, A. A. J. M., Hunfeld, J. A. M., Bohnen, A. M., Van Suijlekom-Smit, L. W. A., Passchier, J., & Van Der Wouden, J. C. (2000). Pain in children and adolescents: A common experience. *Pain*, *87*(1), 51–58. doi:10.1016/S0304-3959(00)00269-4 PMID:10863045

Ramachandran, V. S. (1993). Behavioral and magnetoencephalographic correlates of plasticity in the adult human brain. *Proceedings of the National Academy of Sciences*. 10.1073/pnas.90.22.10413

Ramachandran, V. S., & Altschuler, E. L. (2009). The use of visual feedback, in particular mirror visual feedback, in restoring brain function. *Brain*, *132*(7), 1693–1710. doi:10.1093/brain/awp135 PMID:19506071

Ramachandran, V. S., & Rogers-Ramachandran, D. (2000). Phantom Limbs and Neural Plasticity. *Archives of Neurology*, *57*(3), 317. doi:10.1001/archneur.57.3.317 PMID:10714655

Ramachandran, V. S., Rogers-Ramachandran, D., & Cobb, S. (1995). Touching the phantom limb. *Nature*, *377*(6549), 489–490. doi:10.1038/377489a0 PMID:7566144

Ramachandran, V. S., Stewart, M., & Rogers-Ramachandran, D. C. (1992). Perceptual correlates of massive cortical reorganization. *Neuroreport*, *3*(7), 583–586. doi:10.1097/00001756-199207000-00009 PMID:1421112

Reid, G. J., Lang, B. A., & McGrath, P. J. (1997). Primary juvenile fibromyalgia: Psychological adjustment, family functioning, coping, and functional disability. *Arthritis and Rheumatism*, *40*(4), 752–760. doi:10.1002/art.1780400423 PMID:9125260

Rhee, H. (2000). Prevalence and predictors of headaches in US adolescents. *Headache*, *40*(7), 528–538. doi:10.1046/j.1526-4610.2000.00084.x PMID:10940091

Roth-Isigkeit, A. (2005). Pain Among Children and Adolescents: Restrictions in Daily Living and Triggering Factors. *Pediatrics*, *115*(2), e152–e162. doi:10.1542/peds.2004-0682 PMID:15687423

Shahrbanian, S., Ma, X., Aghaei, N., Korner-bitensky, N., & Simmonds, M. J. (2012). Use of virtual reality (immersive vs. non immersive) for pain management in children and adults: A systematic review of evidence from randomized controlled trials. *European Journal of Experimental Biology*.

Sharar, S. R., Carrougher, G. J., Nakamura, D., Hoffman, H. G., Blough, D. K., & Patterson, D. R. (2007). Factors Influencing the Efficacy of Virtual Reality Distraction Analgesia During Postburn Physical Therapy: Preliminary Results from 3 Ongoing Studies. *Archives of Physical Medicine and Rehabilitation*, *88*(12), S43–S49. doi:10.1016/j.apmr.2007.09.004 PMID:18036981

Sillanpää, M., & Anttila, P. (1996). Increasing prevalence of headache in 7-year-old schoolchildren. *Headache*, *36*(8), 466–470. doi:10.1046/j.1526-4610.1996.3608466.x PMID:8824000

Slater, M., Spanlang, B., Sanchez-Vives, M. V., & Blanke, O. (2010). First person experience of body transfer in virtual reality. *PLoS One*, *5*(5), e10564. doi:10.1371/journal.pone.0010564 PMID:20485681

Soler, M. D., Kumru, H., Pelayo, R., Vidal, J., Tormos, J. M., Fregni, F., ... Pascual-Leone, A. (2010). Effectiveness of transcranial direct current stimulation and visual illusion on neuropathic pain in spinal cord injury. *Brain*, *133*(9), 2565–2577. doi:10.1093/brain/awq184 PMID:20685806

Songer, D. (2005). Psychotherapeutic Approaches in the Treatment of Pain. *Psychiatry*. PMID:21152145

Stanford, E. A., Chambers, C. T., Biesanz, J. C., & Chen, E. (2008). The frequency, trajectories and predictors of adolescent recurrent pain: A population-based approach. *Pain*, *138*(1), 11–21. doi:10.1016/j.pain.2007.10.032 PMID:18093737

Tsakiris, M., & Haggard, P. (2005). The rubber hand illusion revisited: Visuotactile integration and self-attribution. *Journal of Experimental Psychology. Human Perception and Performance*, *31*(1), 80–91. doi:10.1037/0096-1523.31.1.80 PMID:15709864

Turk, D. C., & Okifuji, A. (2002). Psychological factors in chronic pain: Evolution and revolution. *Journal of Consulting and Clinical Psychology*, *70*(3), 678–690. doi:10.1037/0022-006X.70.3.678 PMID:12090376

Turk, D. C., Swanson, K. S., & Tunks, E. R. (2008). Psychological approaches in the treatment of chronic pain patients - When pills, scalpels, and needles are not enough. *Canadian Journal of Psychiatry*, *53*(4), 213–223. doi:10.1177/070674370805300402 PMID:18478824

Valet, M., Sprenger, T., Boecker, H., Willoch, F., Rummeny, E., & Conrad, B., ... Tolle, T. R. (2004). Distraction modulates connectivity of the cingulo-frontal cortex and the midbrain during pain - An fMRI analysis. *Pain*. doi:10.1016/j.pain.2004.02.033

Vogt, B. A., Sikes, R. W., & Vogt, L. J. (1993). Anterior Cingulate Cortex and the Medial Pain System. In Neurobiology of Cingulate Cortex and Limbic Thalamus: A Comprehensive Handbook. Academic Press. doi:10.1007/978-1-4899-6704-6_11

Von Korff, M., Crane, P., Lane, M., Miglioretti, D. L., Simon, G., & Saunders, K. ... Kessler, R. (2005). Chronic spinal pain and physical-mental comorbidity in the United States: Results from the national comorbidity survey replication. *Pain*. doi:10.1016/j.pain.2004.11.010

Walker, L. S., & Greene, J. W. (1991). The functional disability inventory: Measuring a neglected dimension of child health status. *Journal of Pediatric Psychology*, *16*(1), 39–58. doi:10.1093/jpepsy/16.1.39 PMID:1826329

Walker, L. S., Guite, J. W., Duke, M., Barnard, J. A., & Greene, J. W. (1998). Recurrent abdominal pain: A potential precursor of irritable bowel syndrome in adolescents and young adults. *The Journal of Pediatrics*, *132*(6), 1010–1015. doi:10.1016/S0022-3476(98)70400-7 PMID:9627595

Wiederhold, B. K., Gao, K., Sulea, C., & Wiederhold, M. D. (2014). Virtual Reality as a Distraction Technique in Chronic Pain Patients. *Cyberpsychology, Behavior, and Social Networking*, *17*(6), 346–352. doi:10.1089/cyber.2014.0207 PMID:24892196

Williams, A., Eccleston, C., & Morley, S. (2012). Psychological therapies for the management of chronic pain (excluding headache) in adults. *Cochrane Database of Systematic Reviews*. doi:10.1002/14651858.CD007407.pub3 PMID:23152245

Won, A., Bailey, J., Bailenson, J., Tataru, C., Yoon, I., & Golianu, B. (2017). Immersive Virtual Reality for Pediatric Pain. *Children, 4*(7), 52. doi:10.3390/children4070052 PMID:28644422

Won, A. S., Bailey, J., Bailenson, J., Tataru, C., Yoon, I. A., & Golianu, B. (2017). Immersive Virtual Reality for Pediatric Pain. *Children, 4*(52), 1–15. doi:10.3390/children4070052 PMID:28644422

Won, A. S., Tataru, C. A., Cojocaru, C. M., Krane, E. J., Bailenson, J. N., Niswonger, S. G. B., & Golianu, B. (2015). Two Virtual Reality Pilot Studies for the Treatment of Pediatric CRPS. *Pain Medicine, 16*(8), 1644–1647. doi:10.1111/pme.12755 PMID:25930099

Yang, T. T., Gallen, C., Schwartz, B., Bloom, F. E., Ramachandran, V. S., & Cobb, S. (1994). Sensory maps in the human brain. *Nature, 368*(6472), 592–593. doi:10.1038/368592b0 PMID:8145842

ADDITIONAL READING

Bohil, C. J., Alicea, B., & Biocca, F. A. (2011). Virtual reality in neuroscience research and therapy. *Nature Reviews. Neuroscience, 12*(12), 752–762. doi:10.1038/nrn3122 PMID:22048061

Gold, J. I., Belmont, K. A., & Thomas, D. A. (2007). The Neurobiology of Virtual Reality Pain Attenuation. *Cyberpsychology & Behavior, 10*(4), 536–544. doi:10.1089/cpb.2007.9993 PMID:17711362

Gujjar, K. R., van Wijk, A., Sharma, R., & de Jongh, A. (2017). Virtual Reality Exposure Therapy for the Treatment of Dental Phobia: A Controlled Feasibility Study. *Behavioural and Cognitive Psychotherapy*. doi:10.1017/S1352465817000534 PMID:28903790

Li, L., Yu, F., Shi, D., Shi, J., Tian, Z., & Yang, J. … Jiang, Q. (2017). Application of virtual reality technology in clinical medicine. *American Journal of Translational Research*. doi:10.3969/j.issn.1673-8225.2011.30.036

Pozeg, P., Palluel, E., Ronchi, R., Solcà, M., Al-Khodairy, A. W., & Jordan, X. … Blanke, O. (2017). Virtual reality improves embodiment and neuropathic pain caused by spinal cord injury. *Neurology*. doi:10.1212/WNL.0000000000004585

Raghav, K., Van Wijk, A. J., Abdullah, F., Islam, M. N., Bernatchez, M., & De Jongh, A. (2016). Efficacy of virtual reality exposure therapy for treatment of dental phobia: A randomized control trial. *BMC Oral Health*, *16*(1), 25. doi:10.118612903-016-0186-z PMID:26920573

Ramachandran, V. S., & Altschuler, E. L. (2009). The use of visual feedback, in particular mirror visual feedback, in restoring brain function. *Brain*, *132*(7), 1693–1710. doi:10.1093/brain/awp135 PMID:19506071

Sharar, S. R., Alamdari, A., Hoffer, C., Hoffman, H. G., Jensen, M. P., & Patterson, D. R. (2016). Circumplex Model of Affect: A Measure of Pleasure and Arousal During Virtual Reality Distraction Analgesia. *Games for Health Journal*, *5*(3), 197–202. doi:10.1089/g4h.2015.0046 PMID:27171578

KEY TERMS AND DEFINITIONS

Biopsychosocial: A model or approach that recognizes biologic, psychologic, and social effects.

Chronic Pain: Persistent pain, typically lasting three or more months.

Cortical Reorganization: A change in the original mapping pattern of the brain so that stimuli activate different parts of the cortex.

Immersive Virtual Reality: A type of virtual reality where the user is fully immersed in the virtual environment, most often achieved using a head-mounted display.

Neuroplasticity: The ability of the brain to adapt to the environment.

Perception: The conscious result of the brain's interpretation of sensory information.

Sensation: The physiologic detection of a stimuli through peripheral receptors.

This research was previously published in Virtual and Augmented Reality in Mental Health Treatment edited by Giuliana Guazzaroni, pages 221-240, copyright year 2019 by Medical Information Science Reference (an imprint of IGI Global).

Chapter 14
Videogames as Therapy:
An Updated Selective Review of the Medical and Psychological Literature

Mark D. Griffiths
Nottingham Trent University, UK

Daria J. Kuss
Nottingham Trent University, UK

Angelica B. Ortiz de Gortari
Nottingham Trent University, UK & University of Liège, Belgium

ABSTRACT

There is a long history of using videogames in a therapeutic capacity including rehabilitation for stroke patients, people with traumatic brain injuries, burns victims, wheelchair users, Erb's palsy sufferers, children undergoing chemotherapy, children with muscular dystrophy, autistic children and individuals looking to overcome real-life challenges (including symptoms of depression) and boost their wellbeing (including boosting life satisfaction, self-efficacy and social support). This paper briefly and selectively examines a number of areas including: (1) videogames as physiotherapy and occupational therapy, (2) videogames as distractors in the role of pain management, (3) videogames and cognitive rehabilitation, (4) videogames and the development of social and communication skills among the learning disabled, (5) videogames and impulsivity/attention deficit disorders, (6) videogames and therapeutic benefits in the elderly, (7) videogames in psychotherapeutic settings, (8) videogames and health care, (9) videogames and anxiety disorders, and (10) videogames and psychological wellbeing. It is concluded that there has been considerable success when games are specifically designed to address a specific problem or to teach a certain skill. However, generalizability outside the game-playing situation remains an important consideration.

DOI: 10.4018/978-1-7998-1680-5.ch014

INTRODUCTION

The most reported effects of videogames typically report the alleged negative consequences. These include videogame addiction (e.g., Griffiths, 2008a, 2008b), increased aggressiveness (e.g., Anderson & Bushman, 2001), and the various medical and psychosocial effects (Griffiths, 2005). However, there are abundant references to the positive benefits of videogames in the literature including various review papers (Griffiths, 2004; Kato, 2010; Lawrence, 1986; Rauterberg, 2004; Wiemeyer, 2010). Despite research into the more negative effects, for over 25 years, researchers have been using videogames as a means of researching individuals. Videogames may be useful in therapy in different ways including:

- **Videogames as a Therapeutic Setting:** Videogames allow participants to experience novelty and challenge when engaging in fictional activities without real life consequences (Washburn & Gulledge, 1995). Playing videogames has also been used to establish an effective patient-therapist relationship, particularly with young people (Ceranoglu, 2010b). Furthermore, psychotherapy has been conducted exclusively in videogame settings (Coyle, Matthews, Sharry, Nisbet, & Doherty, 2005). For instance, through game immersion, anxious patients can be presented with aversive stimuli via a videogame to progressively eliminate their anxiety. Adopting fictional roles has also been used for encouraging the practice of healthy behaviors and developing social skills (Brown et al., 1997; Lieberman, 2001).
- **Videogames as a Therapeutic or Intervention Tool:** Playing videogames makes it easier to achieve and maintain a person's undivided attention for long periods of time (Donchin, 1995). For this reason, videogames can be used as a cognitive distractor task helping patients in pain to learn relaxation techniques and/or to achieve the relaxation and ease that can be essential for successful experimentation. Furthermore, videogames' immersive nature may facilitate the suspension of reality that can be used in order to access different states of consciousness helping people regress to childhood play. Moreover, videogame playing has been proposed as a visuospatial task for interfering with the elaboration of sensory imagery that leads to the indulgence of cravings crucial to addictions, or sensory imagery from traumatic events that are stressful (Holmes, James, Coode-Bate, & Deeprose, 2009; Skorka-Brown, Andrade, Whalley, & May, 2015).

- **Videogames as a Measurement Tool:** Videogames can allow measuring of performance on a very wide variety of tasks, and they can be easily adapted, standardized, and understood. Also, videogames can be used to observe individual behavior or performance and examine individual characteristics such as self-esteem, self-concept, goal-setting, and individual differences.
- **Videogames as a Motivating Tool:** Videogames are fun and stimulating, so they can be used to assist patients in setting goals, ensuring goal rehearsal, providing feedback, reinforcement, and maintaining records of behavioral change (Ceranoglu, 2010b).
- **Videogames as a Clinical Research Tool:** Videogames can provide a large spectrum of people's profiles and diversity in study cases since videogames' diversity can attract participation of individuals across many demographic boundaries (e.g., age, gender, ethnicity, educational status) (Washburn & Gulledge, 1995), especially with the implementations of online videogames in clinical settings that may facilitate access to individuals situated in different physical locations and/or to provide therapy to the ones that have difficulties to attend health care services.
- **Videogames to Increase Knowledge:** Videogames have been successfully used to increase knowledge regarding academia, health and society (Donohue, 2015). A meta-analysis (Wouters, van Nimwegen, van Oostendorp, & van der Spek, 2013) revealed that videogames using student-centered learning were significantly better than more conventional learning in terms of learning and retention. However, it has been suggested that guidelines for using videogames in the school context need to be developed to ensure that all learners benefit from using videogames in educational contexts (Baranowski et al., 2016).
- **Videogames to Change Behavior:** Videogames have been used in order to change the players' behavior regarding health in a positive way (Baranowski, et al., 2016). A meta-analysis (DeSmet et al., 2014) using research on 64 different videogames targeting improvements in lifestyle indicated that using games had beneficial consequences for health. These beneficial outcomes include effects on diabetes (DeShazo, Harris, & Pratt, 2010), obesity prevention (Lu, Kharrazi, Gharghabi, & Thompson, 2013), as well as health and safety behaviors in young individuals aged 18 years and under (Hieftje, Edelman, Camenga, & Fiellin, 2013).
- **Videogames as Physical Activity:** Videogames are also used in the context of exergaming – using games as physical exercise (Baranowski, et al., 2016). Research regarding exergaming is mixed, with some naturalistic research (Baranowski et al., 2012) suggesting little effects on physical activity intensity and duration, whereas other research shows that exergaming can decrease body mass index (BMI) and weight (Trost, Sundal, Foster, Lent, &

Vojta, 2014). It has been suggested that exergaming should be implemented in everyday school routines of children and adolescents given the primarily sedentary nature of school education (Baranowski, et al., 2016).

- **Videogames to Influence Health Precursors:** Videogames have been successfully used to impact on health precursors (such as anxiety) in the context of health outcomes following hospital stays (Yip, Middleton, Cyna, & Carlyle, 2009). Beneficial outcomes have been observed regarding chemotherapy (Cole, Yoo, & Knutson, 2012) and enhancing resilience and health in clinical populations (Govender, Bowen, German, Bulaj, & Bruggers, 2015) suggesting videogames can be powerful tools in various physical-health related circumstances (Baranowski, et al., 2016).

Research dating right back to the early 1980s has consistently shown that playing computer games (irrespective of genre) produces increases in reaction times, improved hand-eye co-ordination, and raises players' self-esteem. What's more, curiosity, fun and the nature of the challenge also appear to add to a game's therapeutic potential. Commonly, videogames developed specifically for therapeutic interventions or health care (often referred to as 'good games' or 'serious games') have been used in therapy. However, some commercial videogames have also been adapted and used for therapeutic purposes.

This paper focuses on some of the reported therapeutic benefits of videogame playing. Some evidence suggests that important skills may be built or reinforced by videogames. For example, spatial visualization ability (i.e., mentally, rotating and manipulating two- and three-dimensional objects) can be improved through videogame playing (Green & Bavelier, 2006; Subrahmanyam & Greenfield, 1994). However, videogames were more effective for children who started out with relatively poor skills. It was therefore suggested that videogames may be useful in equalizing individual differences in spatial skill performance.

Many people seem surprised that videogames have been used in a wide variety of therapeutic and medical contexts. As we shall see during the course of this paper, "videogame therapy" has been used successfully in rehabilitation for stroke patients, people with traumatic brain injuries, burns victims, wheelchair users, Erb's palsy sufferers, children undergoing chemotherapy, children with muscular dystrophy, and autistic children. This paper briefly examines a number of areas including: (1) videogames as physiotherapy and occupational therapy, (2) videogames as distractors in the role of pain management, (3) videogames and cognitive rehabilitation, (4) videogames and the development of social and communication skills among the learning disabled, (5) videogames and impulsivity/attention deficit disorders, (6) videogames and therapeutic benefits in the elderly, (7) videogames in psychotherapeutic settings, (8) videogames and health care, and (9) videogames and anxiety disorders.

Videogames as Physiotherapy and Occupational Therapy

Videogames have been used as a form of physiotherapy and/or occupational therapy in many different groups of people (e.g., those who are physically handicapped, learning disabled, emotionally disturbed, etc.). Much has been written about how boring and repetitive exercises are if someone is attempting to recover from or cope with a physical problem. The introduction of videogames into this context can be of huge therapeutic benefit. As we shall see, the same appears to be true for more complex psychological abnormalities.

Videogames have been used innovatively as a form of physiotherapy for arm injuries (Szer, 1983), in training the movements of a 13-year old child with Erb's palsy (Krichevets, Sirotkina, Yevsevicheva, & Zeldin, 1994), cerebral palsy (Huber et al., 2010; Hurkmans, van den Berg-Emons, & Stam, 2010; Jannink et al., 2008; Weightman et al., 2010), finger and hand function (Szturm, Peters, Otto, Kapadia, & Desai, 2008), chronic severe hemiparesis (Housman, Scott, & Reinkensmeyer, 2009), rheumatology (McCormack et al., 2009), postural stability and balance (Fitzgerald, Trakarnratanakul, Smyth, & Caulfield, 2010), and as a form of occupational therapy to increase hand strength (King, 1993). For instance, King (1993) showed that videogames could be used in an occupational therapy setting to increase hand strength among patients with just three-minute "exercise" periods on computer games. Videogames have also been used as therapeutic interventions to promote and increase arm reach in persons with traumatic brain injury (Sietsema, Nelson, Mulder, Mervau-Scheidel, & White, 1993). This paper reported the use of a computer game (described as an occupationally embedded intervention) to promote and increase arm reach in persons with traumatic brain injury. The study showed that the game produced significantly more range of motion in all of their 20 participants. Moreover, interactive games have been successfully used to improve balance, mobility, and gait after brain injury (Lange, Flynn, Proffitt, Chang, & Rizzo, 2010).

Therapeutic benefits have also been reported for wheelchair users (Synofzik et al., 2013), burns victims (Sharar et al., 2008), and muscular dystrophy sufferers. More specifically, some wheelchair users find regular exercise programs too difficult physically or psychologically, and many find that using standard arm crank or roller systems is monotonous. O'Connor, Cooper, Fitzgerald, Dvorznak, Boninger, VanSickle and Glass (2000) looked for ways that individuals with spinal cord injuries would be motivated to exercise on a regular basis. As a consequence, they developed an interactive videogame system (*Gamewheels*) that provided an interface between a portable roller system and a computer. This system enabled wheelchair users to play commercially available videogames and their results demonstrated improved physical fitness in a sample of people with spinal cord injuries, spinal cord diseases, amputations, nerve diseases, and multiple sclerosis. Most of their participants (86%) reported that they would like a *Gamewheels* system for their home.

Adriaenssens, Eggermont, Pyck, Boeckx and Gilles (1988) reported the use of videogame playing as an exercise program to facilitate the rehabilitation of upper-limb burn victims (using a variety of large to smaller joysticks). This technique not only helped overcome initial therapy resistance but also encouraged and shaped movement of the hand wrist and elbow by providing feedback for the desired performance while also offering a distraction from pain. Moreover, in another study (Fung et al., 2010), occupational therapists and physiotherapists advocated the use of videogame systems for burn- and nonburn patients for similar reasons. Additionally, videogames were also used as a respiratory muscle training aid for young patients with Duchenne Muscular Dystrophy (Vilozni, Bar-Yishay, Shapira, Meyer, & Godfrey, 1994).

Joei Mioto and Goncalves Ribas (2014) furthermore found that using virtual reality games appears beneficial in the physical rehabilitation of individuals with Down's syndrome, a genetic disease that has negative impacts on basic motor skills, including gross and fine motor skills. The commercially available *Nintendo Wii* and *Wii Sports* CDs have been used with five volunteers with Down's syndrome, and *Wii* games including tennis, bowling, boxing, baseball and golf games were used for 30 minutes twice weekly. Results indicated that these games increased motivation to engage in physical rehabilitation in a playful manner. Moreover, it was suggested to replicate and extend these results beyond this small population to increase external validity.

The use of videogames in almost all these differing contexts capitalizes on a number of inter-related factors. One of the most important is the person's motivation to succeed. Furthermore, videogames have advantages over traditional therapeutic methods that rely on passive, repetitive movements and painful limb manipulation (i.e., they focus attention away from potential discomfort).

Videogames as Distractors in the Role of Pain Management

Studies have shown that cognitive/attentional distraction may block the perception of pain (Wohlheiter & Dahlquist, 2012). The reasoning is that distractor tasks consume some degree of the attentional capacity that would otherwise be devoted to pain perception. Videogame playing offers an ideal way to analyze the role of distraction in symptom control in pediatric patients. Redd et al. (1987) argued that the main reasons for this are that:

1. Videogames are likely to engage much of a person's individual active attention because of the cognitive and motor activity required.
2. Videogames allow the possibility to achieve sustained achievement because of the level of difficulty (i.e., challenge) of most games during extended play.
3. Videogames appear to appeal most to adolescents.

Videogames have also been used in a number of studies as "distractor tasks". For instance, one study (Phillips, 1991) reported the case of using a handheld videogame (*Nintendo Game Boy*) to stop an 8-year old boy picking at his face. The child had neurodermatitis and scarring due to continual picking at his upper lip. Previous treatments (e.g., behavior modification program with food rewards for periods free of picking and the application of a bitter tasting product to the child's fingers) had failed so a handheld videogame was used to keep the boy's hands occupied. After two weeks, the affected area had healed.

Another creative use of videogames has been to help increase sitting tolerance for people with lower back pain (Butler, 1985). Furthermore, a study (Leibovici, Magora, Cohen, & Ingber, 2009) reported that virtual reality immersion (VRI) helped patients suffering from pruritus to distract them from the pain they felt. Moreover, it decreased scratching before and after playing. Functional magnetic resonance imaging indicated that the brain activity associated with the pain experience was significantly reduced.

There are also a number of studies (e.g., Kato, Cole, Bradlyn, & Pollock, 2008; Kolko & Rickard-Figueroa, 1985; Redd, et al., 1987; Reichlin et al., 2011; Vasterling, Jenkins, Tope, & Burish, 1993) that have demonstrated that videogames can provide cognitive distraction during cancer chemotherapy in children, adolescents and adults. All these studies have reported that distracted patients report less nausea prior to chemotherapy and lower systolic pressure after treatment (when compared with controls). Such distraction tasks also reduce the amount of painkillers needed. There are many practical advantages for using videogame therapy for patients during chemotherapy treatment. Redd et al. (1987) argue that:

1. Videogame playing can be easily integrated with most chemotherapy administration procedures.
2. Videogames represent a more cost-effective intervention than many traditional behavioral procedures such as hypnosis and relaxation.
3. Videogames can be played without medical supervision.

To date there has been no long-term follow-up to such interventions and it is unclear whether patients eventually tire of such games. Therefore, factors need to be explored such as novelty, game preference, and relative level of challenge. This pain management technique utilizing videogames has also been applied successfully to children undergoing treatment for sickle cell disease (Pegelow, 1992). As mentioned in the previous section, the studies by Adriaenssens et al. (1988) and O'Connor et al. (2000) on burns victims and wheelchair users claimed that success was in part due to the distraction from pain.

Finally, in this section it is worth noting that one report alerted doctors that children may mistake patient-controlled analgesia (PCA) devices for videogame consoles. Blunt, Hastie and Stephens (1998) reported the case of a seven-year old boy with Ollier's disease undergoing an operation whose pain was managed via a PCA pump. On the third day following his operation the boy's PCA usage escalated from zero to a total of 74 demands during a four-hour period. Upon questioning it became clear that on the night in question the boy had been playing a videogame and he had mistakenly been pressing his PCA pump as if it had been a videogame!

Videogames and Cognitive Rehabilitation

One way in which videogames have been used is as a rehabilitation aid among various groups of people. Fisher (1986) argued that computers (including videogames) have the potential to aid cognitive remediation. Areas that can be helped include perceptual disorders, conceptual thinking, attention, concentration, memory, spatial cognition, mental rotation, creativity computation, visual plasticity, executive functioning, processing speed, attention, fluid intelligence, and subjective cognitive performance, and difficulties with language (Achtman, Green, & Bavelier, 2008; Chandrasekharan, Mazalek, Nitsche, Chen, & Ranjan, 2010; Eow, Ali, Mahmud, & Baki, 2010; Leng, Ali, Mahmud, & Baki, 2010; Miller & Robertson, 2010; Reijnders, van Heugten, & van Boxtel, 2013). These ideas have been studied empirically by a number of researchers.

For instance, Larose, Gagnon, Ferland and Pepin (1989) carried out a study to test the hypothesis that computer games may be an efficient therapeutic tool in a cognitive rehabilitation program. Sixty participants who showed attention difficulties with or without cerebral dysfunctions participated in a 12-hour training program based on intensive use of a videogame. Analyses showed improvement for the experimental group on scanning and tracking variables, notwithstanding the nature of their particular dysfunctions. Other studies have successfully used videogames in rehabilitation programs to improve sustained attention in patients with craniocerebral trauma (Funk, Germann, & Buchman, 1997; Lawrence, 1986), and as a training and rehabilitation aid to cognitive and perceptual-motor disorders in stroke patients (Broeren, Claesson, Goude, Rydmark, & Sunnerhagen, 2008; Joo et al., 2010; Lynch, 1983; Yavuzer, Senel, Atay, & Stam, 2008), and other motor deficits (Cameirao, Bermúdez i Badia, Duarte Oller, Zimmerli, & Verschure, 2007).

Other authors have advocated the use of videogames as a cognitive rehabilitation aid (attention, perceptual spatial abilities, reasoning, memory) to assist patients who have had brain damage to regain lost function (Lawrence, 1986; Skilbeck, 1991). Videogames have also been used to increase spatial visualization (Dorval & Pepin, 1986). However, more recent research by Subrahmanyam and Greenfield (1994) has suggested that spatial skills are only improved in those whose skills were very weak to begin with but unlikely to improve skills for those with average or above-average spatial abilities.

Videogames and the Development of Social and Communication Skills Among the Learning Disabled

Videogames have also been used in comprehensive programs to help develop social skills in children and adolescents who have learning disabilities, such as dyslexia (Bavelier, Green, & Seidenberg, 2013), are severely retarded, or who have severe developmental problems like autism (Gaylord-Ross, Haring, Breen, & Pitts-Conway, 1984; Sedlak, Doyle, & Schloss, 1982; Tanaka et al., 2010). Case studies such as those by Demarest (2000) are persuasive. Demarest's account of her own autistic seven-year old son reported that although he had serious deficiencies in language and understanding, and social and emotional difficulties, videogame playing was one activity he was able to excel. This was ego-boosting for him and also had a self-calming effect. Videogames provided the visual patterns, speed, and storyline that help children's basic skills development. Some of the therapeutic benefits Demarest (2000) outlined were language skills, mathematics and reading skills, and social skills.

Horn, Jones and Hamlett (1991) used videogames to train three children with multiple handicaps (e.g., severely limited vocal speech acquisition) to make scan and selection responses. These skills were later transferred to a communication device. Other researchers have used videogames to help learning disabled children in their development of spatial abilities (Masendorf, 1993), problem-solving exercises (Hollingsworth & Woodward, 1993), and mathematical ability (Okolo, 1992a). Other researchers have offered critiques on how best to use computer technology for improved achievement and enhanced motivation among the learning disabled (e.g., Blechman, Rabin, & McEnroe, 1986; Okolo, 1992b).

Videogames and Impulsivity/Attention Deficit Disorders

There are now a few studies that have examined whether videogames might be able to help in the treatment of children with impulsive and attentional difficulties. Kappes and Thompson (1985) tried to reduce impulsivity in incarcerated juveniles (ages 15- to 18-years) by providing either biofeedback or experience with a videogame.

Impulsivity scores improved for both conditions. Improvement was also noted in negative self-attributions and in internal locus of control. The authors concluded that the most likely explanation for the improvement in both experimental conditions was the immediate feedback. Clarke and Schoech (1994) also used videogames to help adolescents learn impulse control. A videogame was used for four weeks with four subjects (11-to 17-years) diagnosed with impulse control problems. After the experimental trial, the participants became more enthusiastic and co-operative about treatment.

Unpublished research (Wright, 2001) suggests videogames linked to brain-wave biofeedback may help children with attention deficit disorders. Biofeedback teaches patients to control normally involuntary body functions such as heart rate by providing real-time monitors of those responses. With the aid of a computer display, attention-deficit patients can learn to modulate brain waves associated with focusing. With enough training, changes become automatic and lead to improvements in grades, sociability, and organizational skills. Following on from research involving pilot attentiveness during long flights, a similar principle has been developed to help attention-deficit children stay focused by rewarding an attentive state of mind. This has been done by linking biofeedback to commercial videogames. In their trial, Pope and Palsson (2001; cited in Wright, 2001) selected half a dozen *Sony PlayStation* games and tested 22 girls and boys between the ages of 9 and 13 years who had attention deficit disorder. Half the group got traditional biofeedback training and the other half played the modified videogames. After 40 one-hour sessions, both groups showed substantial improvements in everyday brain-wave patterns as well as in tests of attention span, impulsiveness, and hyperactivity. Parents in both groups also reported that their children were doing better in school. The difference between the two groups was motivation. The video-game group showed fewer no-shows and no dropouts. The researchers do warn that the 'wrong kinds of videogame' may be detrimental to children with attention disorders. For instance, 'shoot 'em up' games may have a negative effect on children who already have a tendency toward short attention and impulsivity. They also state that the technique is an adjunct to drug therapy and not a replacement for it.

Finally, Lim et al. (2010) used a brain-computer interface program to improve inattention in ten children diagnosed with attention deficit hyperactivity disorder. They found that compared to a control group which received no treatment, inattention symptoms had significantly decreased. Although these findings appear promising, the researchers call for larger-scale studies to improve the generalizability of results.

Videogames and Therapeutic Benefits in the Elderly

It could perhaps be argued that videogame manufacturers have done very little to target older persons as prospective videogame users. This might be different if they were aware that there is a growing body of evidence that videogames may have beneficial therapeutic effects for the elderly. Given that videogame playing involves concentration, attention, hand-eye co-ordination, memory, decision-making, and speed reactions, the activity may be of great benefit to this particular cohort. Researchers working in this area have postulated that the intellectual decline which is part of the natural aging process may be slowed (and perhaps counteracted) by getting the elderly involved as active users of technology (Farris, Bates, Resnick, & Stabler, 1994).

For instance, a game as simple as *Tetris*, can engage the mind in an enjoyable problem solving exercise. The same enjoyable pleasures that occur when any of us master a new computer skill may have therapeutic value to both young and old. Learning something new on the computer results in a sense of accomplishment and satisfaction that invariably creates a feeling of wellbeing. Technology with the aged can therefore foster greater independence and can be put to therapeutic use. Dustman, Emmerson, Laurel and Shearer (1992) showed that videogames could increase reaction times among the elderly after an 11-week period of videogame playing

For instance, McGuire (1984, 1986) examined the effectiveness of videogames in improving self-esteem among elderly long-term care residents. In one wing of the institution, videogames were made available for an eight-week period. Residents of a second wing did not have the opportunity to play them and were used as a control group. Results showed that the videogame group exhibited significant improvement in self-esteem. Similar results have been found by other researchers. For instance, Goldstein, Cajko, Oosterbroek, Michielsen, van Houten and Salverda (1997) reported that elderly (non-institutionalized) people increased reaction times, self-esteem, and positive sense of wellbeing, as a result of playing videogames for five hours a week for five weeks. However, there was little improvement in cognitive performance compared with controls. Riddick, Spector and Drogin (1986) examined the impact of videogame play on the emotional states and affiliative behavior of elderly nursing home residents. The experimental group had an opportunity to play videogames three times per week for up to three hours per session, over a six-week period. In comparison to the control group, the experimental group underwent significant changes in their arousal state and affiliative behavior.

Weisman (1983) suggested that videogames may have a role to play in meeting clients' needs for fun and mental stimulation and in enhancing self-esteem. He reported that moderate mental and physical impairments did not prevent 50 nursing home residents from participating in four videogames which were especially adapted for this population. Further research by Weisman (1994) on the institutionalized elderly found that computer and videogame use was found to be a valuable learning and diagnostic tool. The author urged practitioners to investigate the possibilities of using videogames in their work with the elderly.

Farris et al. (1994) suggested that older adults can benefit significantly from ongoing education, and that computers can be valuable tools in this process. They advocate the use of computers for long- and short-term memory functioning memory skills. They reported a study using the videogame *Memory of Goblins*. This game was developed primarily for use in the assessment of working memory but can also be used for the training of working memory. Conclusions were difficult to draw from this particular study, but there is evidence to suggest that the impact of computer use among the elderly population can be profound. Ryan (1994) also used the Memory for Goblins videogame to assess memory skills among various groups. Preliminary results with older users suggested they find it novel and interesting although there appeared to be little effect on improvement of working memory.

Hollander and Plummer (1986) reported the use of a hands-on microcomputer experience in 41 senior adults. Over a three-week period, videogames served as a therapeutic and rehabilitative tool, as well as a form of social and educational enrichment. Results indicated that thought-provoking games (*Trivia* and *Hangperson*) held the participants' highest level of attention, and were perceived as exciting and stimulating. Schueren (1986) also analyzed the value of videogames as an activity program for geriatric populations in skilled nursing home facilities. It was concluded that videogame playing may be a successful small group recreational activity for those residents with adequate eye-hand coordination, vision and mental functioning. Suggestions were also proposed for equipment adaptations to correct problems of poor visual clarity and awkward manipulation of controls. Such findings have also been reported in more recent studies (Gamberini et al., 2008). In addition to this, videogames have been found useful regarding home-based step training for older people in terms of choice stepping reaction time (and consequent decreased risk of falling down), better physical assessment scores, and postural sway compared to controls (Schoene et al., 2013).

Given this small but growing body of evidence, there is clearly a need for more research on videogame use among this particular group of people. There are many areas that need to be explored in more detail including elderly use of technology in general, the use of computers and videogames to develop and strengthen memory skills, intergenerational computing projects (teaming seniors with school aged students), and the use of computers and videogames to assess cognitive functions, etc. Many older adults may be receptive to using technology if introduced to it in a comfortable environment. If introduced in the right way, technology (including videogames) may become a major hobby and interest in the lives of the elderly, and may also be of therapeutic value.

Videogames in Psychotherapeutic Settings

Therapists working with children have long used games in therapy and games for therapy in sessions with their young patients (Ceranoglu, 2010a, 2010b; Gardner, 1991). Play has been a feature in therapy since the work of Anna Freud (1928) and Melanie Klein (1932) and has been used to promote fantasy expression and the ventilation of feeling. The recent technological explosion has brought a proliferation of new games which some therapists claim to be an excellent ice-breaker and rapport builder with children in therapy and behavior management (e.g., Gardner, 1991; Spence, 1988). Research in the mid-1980s had already suggested that videogames may actually facilitate co-operative behavior and reinforcement in more educational settings (e.g., Salend & Santora, 1985; Strein & Kochman, 1984).

Lawrence (1986) advocates that videogames can be used in the treatment of psychological problems during therapy. In an overview, he reported that there had been approximately two dozen efforts in the published literature to deliver counseling or other psychological intervention services by computer. Although not concentrating on videogames specifically, he did refer to games, computer-aided instruction, biofeedback, and behavior therapy. He concluded that computers (including games) could make meaningful contributions to the treatment of psychological problems.

Gardner (1991) claimed that the use of videogames in his psychotherapy sessions provided common ground between himself and his child clients, and provided excellent behavioral observation opportunities. According to Gardner such observations allowed him to observe:

1. The child's repertoire of problem solving strategies
2. The child's ability to perceive and recall subtle cues as well as foresee consequences of behavior and act on past consequences
3. Eye-hand co-ordination
4. The release of aggression and control
5. The ability to deal with appropriate methods of dealing with the joys of victory and frustrations of defeat in a more sports oriented arena
6. The satisfaction of cognitive activity in the involvement of the recall of bits of basic information
7. The enjoyment of mutually co-ordinating one's activities with another in the spirit of co-operation

Gardner went on to describe four particular case studies where videogames were used to support psychotherapy. Although other techniques were used as an adjunct in therapy (e.g., story telling, drawing, other games etc.), Gardner claimed it was the videogames that were the most useful factors in the improvement during therapy. It is

Gardner's contention that clinical techniques tend to change as a function of the trends of the times, though the goals remain the same. Slower paced and more traditional activities like those outlined above may lengthen the time it takes to form a therapeutic relationship as the child may perceive the therapist not to be 'cool' or 'with it'.

Spence (1988) is another advocate of the therapeutic value of videogames and has incorporated them into his repertoire of behavior management techniques. Spence believes that videogames can be used instrumentally to bring about changes in a number of areas and provided case study examples for each of these changes. These are briefly outlined below.

1. **Development of Relationships:** Used videogames to provide the basis to develop a therapeutic relationship. The videogames gave an acceptable "middle ground" for both parties to "meet" which provided an enjoyable experience that could be shared. Relationships become close and trusting.
2. **Motivation:** Used videogames as "bargaining counters" to motivate children to do things. This simply involved negotiating with an individual for a set period of work time or tasks in return for a set period of time playing videogames.
3. **Co-operative Behavior:** Used videogames to develop social skills and co-operation in individuals by making them share a computer with peers. Through the medium of videogames, individuals developed friendships that fostered co-operation.
4. **Aggressive Behavior:** Used videogames to "take the heat out of situations", i.e., individuals played videogames when they were angry so that the "damage" was inflicted on the videogames' characters rather than human beings.
5. **Self-Esteem:** Used videogames as a measure of achievement to raise self-esteem. Since videogames are skill based and provide scores, they can be compared and provide a basis for future goals. Beating personal high scores raised self-esteem in the individual.

As can be seen from Spence's brief summaries, the benefits outlined are similar to those outlined by Gardner (1991). Similar techniques have also been advocated for behavioral management of exceptional children (Buckalew & Buckalew, 1983). Brezinka (2008) has argued that therapeutic games can help therapists to structure therapy sessions and reports that psychotherapeutic computer games translated into foreign languages can form a useful tool in the treatment of migrant children. For instance, *Treasure Hunt*, a game based on principles of cognitive behavior modification, was developed for eight to twelve-year-old children who are in cognitive-behavioral treatment for various disorders. Brezinka claimed reactions of children and therapists to experimental versions of the game are positive and that serious games might prove a useful tool to support psychotherapeutic treatment of children.

Coyle, Matthews, Sharry, et al. (2005) reported their use of the *Personal Investigator* (*PI*), a 3D computer game specifically designed to help adolescents overcome mental health problems such as depression and help them engage more easily with professional mental health care services. Their model had its theoretical foundations in play therapy and therapeutic storytelling and applied current research on the educational use of computer gaming and interactive narrative. The *PI* incorporated a goal-oriented, strength-based model of psychotherapy called Solution Focused Therapy (SFT). By engaging adolescents, in a client-centerd way, it aimed to build stronger therapeutic relationships between therapists and adolescents. Results of trials of *PI* with four adolescents, referred to clinics for issues including anxiety and behavior problems, attempted suicide, and social skills difficulties, were presented and argued to be effective.

Olsen-Rando (1994) reported on the development and initial assessment of a videogame version of the *Talking, Feeling, and Doing Game*. The game was developed by Dr. Richard Gardner in order to facilitate the therapeutic process for those children who are inhibited, constrained, or resistive or as an alternative therapeutic tool for children who are not characterized as resistive and thus freely reveal information. The game provides children an opportunity to talk about themselves in a way that is less anxiety provoking than traditional methods of eliciting information about their underlying psychodynamics. Unfortunately, this was a descriptive account only and contained no evaluation. Similarly, Kokish (1994) described the use of a personal computer loaded with various videogames to aid play therapy with children. Case studies were outlined and reference was made to the fact that learning to use the computer as a play therapy tool was more difficult and slower than expected.

Favelle (1994) also described some therapeutic applications of computer software and videogames in work with both individuals and groups. The applications described were used with adolescents at a psychiatric treatment center and involved using commercially available software and videogames. An adventure-fantasy game and a role-playing game were described as helpful in work with individuals. This is because the importance and utilization of fantasy in play was expressed. A mystery computer game was presented as useful when working with groups. The author concluded that videogames have useful therapeutic value if applied by skilled professionals. It was suggested that further research would result in improvements to computer-assisted therapy.

Sherer (1994) described the development and application of a computerized therapeutic simulation game for the purpose of raising the moral level of youth in distress. The effects of the videogame on moral development were determined by a moral development measure. The level of moral development of a research group (n=13) and a control group (n=14) were measured before and after exposure to the therapeutic videogame. A total of five indices of moral development were used. Two of these, Moral stage and Punishment revealed a positive effect on the participants.

There is some research suggesting that videogames can be useful when evaluating schizophrenics in their attitudes and responses (Samoilovich, Riccitelli, Scheil, & Siedi, 1992). To do this, Samoilovich et al. (1992) investigated the initial attitude of ten chronic, defected schizophrenic patients to a computer videogame session. Six of them enjoyed the experience and wanted to repeat it. Cooperation and performance were compared by means of videogames and a standard psychometric test (Wechsler Adult Intelligence Scale). Videogame performance correlated with the execution test IQ more than with the verbal test IQ. The authors also claimed that videogames can be used for psychological testing, motivation and reward, and can be used to evaluate psychomotor activity.

More recent research (Ducharme et al., 2012) reported the case of a 16-year-old girl who underwent Acceptance and Commitment Therapy (ACT) using a RAGE-Control intervention designed to increase emotion control abilities by monitoring and controlling physiological arousal whilst faced with stress in a virtual reality environment. This treatment used five CBT techniques together with a videogame using active biofeedback. The aim was to improve the individual's self-regulation, and was implemented on a daily basis over five consecutive days. The results of this study showed that the patient's state and trait anger scores decreased significantly following treatment, suggesting both her anger and aggression levels benefitted from this videogame therapy element. Additional benefits included increased control over physiological arousal (i.e., heart rate). Although this study only provides evidence from one person, the results showed promise regarding reductions of both anger and aggression and increases in self-control, and should be replicated in larger samples.

It has also been suggested that some psychiatric patients who are socially undisciplined may be reachable with computers and videogames (Matthews, De Santi, Callahan, Koblenz-Sulcov, & Werden, 1987). Studies were reported that explored the usefulness of computers with chronic psychiatric patients. In one study, videogames were made available to patients and one half showed an active interest. The second study showed a neutral relationship between patients' social communication skills and their involvement with videogames. Thus, some patients who were socially intractable may be reachable with computers. It was argued that the computer can be used effectively to automate many tasks normally undertaken by clinicians and that the computer may have special advantages over the clinician for some purposes.

Videogames and Health Care

In randomized clinical trials, it has been reported that children and adolescents improved their self-care and significantly reduced their use of emergency clinical services after playing health education and disease management videogames (Brown, et al., 1997; Lieberman, 2001). Three games have been investigated. *Bronkie the Bronchiasaurus* for asthma self-management; *Packy & Marlon* for diabetes self-management; and *Rex Ronan* for smoking prevention. In these interactive videogames, children and adolescents assume the role of a main character who also has their chronic condition or is battling the effects of smoking and nicotine addiction. Children who used them for one week (smoking prevention) to 6 months (diabetes self-care) increased their resolve not to smoke, markedly improved their ability to manage their asthma or diabetes, and reduced by as much as 77 percent, on average, their urgent or emergency care visits related to their illness.

Electronic games have also been used to enhance adolescents' perceived self-efficacy in HIV/AIDS prevention programs (Cahill, 1994; Thomas, Cahill, & Santilli, 1997). Using a time travel adventure videogame format, information and opportunities for practice discussing prevention practices were provided to high-risk adolescents. Videogame playing resulted in significant gains in factual information about safe sex practices, and in the participants' perceptions of their ability to successfully negotiate and implement such practices with a potential partner.

Videogames and simulations have been used extensively in a comprehensive health promotion for adolescents. For instance, Bosworth (1994) used these strategies to attract adolescents to BARN (Body Awareness Resource Network), as well as helping to hold interest. In each of the six topic areas (AIDS, Alcohol and Other Drugs, Body Management, Human Sexuality, Smoking and Stress Management) videogame quizzes challenged users to test their knowledge on a topic. Simulations challenged users to apply health information in hypothetical situations. Videogames were a more important factor in the selection of BARN for younger users than for older users. BARN game users were not more likely than non-game users to be users of other computer or videogames, nor did game users engage in more risk-taking behaviors (e.g., alcohol and other drugs) than non-game users. Similar types of health promotion videogames have been used successfully for cystic fibrosis (Davis, Quittner, Stack, & Young, 2004), drug use (Oakley, 1994), alcohol (Resnick, 1994a), marijuana use (Henningson, Gold, & Duncan, 1986), sexual behavior (Starn & Paperny, 1990), life choices (D. L. Thomas, 1994), and anti-social behavior (Resnick, 1994b). One of the major problems with this area is that reported positive effects from videogames in a health promotion context is that almost all of the videogames evaluated were specially designed rather than those that were already commercially available. This does raise questions about the utility of generally commercial games in helping health promotion activities.

Finally, Murphy, Carson, Neal, Baylis, Donley and Yeater (2009) reported that music and rhythm videogames (usually referred to as 'exergaming') used with overweight children have a positive effect. *Dance Dance Revolution* (DDR), a game that requires players to move their feet in co-ordination with arrows scrolling across the screen was used in the study with 35 overweight children. The results showed that after 12 weeks of playing, the children improved their flow-mediated dilation, aerobics fitness, and mean arterial pressure without changes in inflammatory markers or nitric oxide production. However, a review by Daley (2009) stressed caution on this topic and asserted that active gaming was no substitute for real sports and activities. She also stressed the need for high-quality randomized, controlled trials to evaluate the effectiveness and sustainability of active gaming.

Videogames and Anxiety Disorders

Therapeutic uses of videogames to reduce stress, anxiety, and specific anxiety disorders have taken place in different ways. Potential benefits of videogame playing have been reported as a way of reducing preoperative anxiety among children (Patel, et al., 2006). There is also evidence which suggests that playing puzzle games, specifically the game *Tetris*, can mitigate flashbacks of traumatic experiences (Holmes, et al., 2009; James et al., 2015).

There is also evidence suggesting that videogame playing by military personnel has a protective mechanism versus nightmares (Gackenbach, Ellerman, & Hall, 2011). However, it seems that the therapeutic effects of videogames depends largely on what context, with what intensity and who is playing. In a qualitative study done by Ortiz de Gortari, Aronsson and Griffiths (2011), high frequency players reported disturbing, intrusive and stereotypical after images after playing games like *Tetris*. Also, in an experimental study with normal and amnesic volunteers playing *Tetris*, the participants experienced visual images from the game at sleep onset (Stickgold, Malia, Maguire, Roddenberry, & O'Connor, 2000).

Videogames have also been used, not only in a palliative context but also as a more structured form of therapy via the use of simulation videogames for the treatment of clinical disorders. Specifically, virtual reality exposure therapy (VRET) has been applied to target anxiety disorders. It has been efficiently used in the treatment of acrophobia (Krijn et al., 2004), claustrophobia (Botella, Banos, Villa, Perpina, & Garcia-Palacios, 2000), panic disorder with agoraphobia (Vincelli et al., 2003), fear of flying (Rothbaum, Hodges, Smith, Lee, & Price, 2000), driving phobia (Wald & Taylor, 2000), spider phobia (Garcia-Palacios, Hoffman, Carlin, Furness, & Botella, 2002), and post-traumatic stress disorder (Holmes, et al., 2009; James, et al., 2015; Rothbaum, Hodges, Ready, Graap, & Alarcon, 2001; Wiederhold & Wiederhold, 2010).

In VRET, therapy does not take place *in vivo*, but via a virtual game-like simulation. VRET can be delineated as an intermediary between in vivo and imaginal cognitive behavioral therapy (CBT). In VRET, virtual environments (VEs) are made use of, by means of which anxiety-provoking situations are not merely imagined, but virtually *reconstructed*. In fact, reality is reconstructed in such a way so as to make the patient feel present in the VE (Krijn, Emmelkamp, Olafsson, & Biemond, 2004). Presence, in this respect, can be defined as a

...psychological state or subjective perception in which even though part of or all of an individual's current experience is generated by and/or filtered through human-made technology, part or all of the individual's perception fails to accurately acknowledge the role of the technology in the experience (International Society for Presence Research, 2000).

Therefore, even though the experience in VRET is entirely mediated, it feels as if it was real for the patient. They immerse in the VE so that the experience becomes seemingly de-mediated.

There are two ways in which a virtual experience can be created. On the one hand, there is the possibility to use a head-mounted display (HMD), a technical apparatus attached to the patient's head, which consists of glasses and speakers. The VE will be projected inside the glasses. Attached sensors are connected to a computer. The patient can follow the movements of the virtual scenery by means of moving his head. His experience is closely monitored by the therapist, who views the VE which the patient is confronted with on his own computer screen (Krijn, Emmelkamp, Olafsson et al., 2004).

The second technological equipment that can be used is the computer automatic virtual environment (CAVE). It allows for the synchronous attendance of both the patient and the therapist, who experience the VE in a four-to-six sides cubicle, which projects the virtual scenario. Utilizing an electromagnetic tracking system, the CAVE enables the patient to move freely in the VE (Krijn, Emmelkamp, Olafsson, et al., 2004). As such, the CAVE offers the option for a more immersive experience in such a way that the patient is entirely surrounded by the VE.

VRET works by exposing the patient to threat-provoking situations, while the level of threat is increased gradually. To describe but one instance of a therapy session, Roy, Klinger, Légeron, Lauer, Chemin and Nugues (2003) made use of a particular VRET, in which they created four treatment environments associated with real social situations that provoke fear in social phobics, namely performance, intimacy, scrutiny, and assertiveness environments, respectively. Using the most common instance in which anxiety would be provoked, namely the performance situation, the patient was asked to speak in public. This was achieved through the VE, which reconstructed a meeting room, in which seven people were present. The patient was asked to take a seat, introduce himself, and present a project. For the patient, this situation provoked anxiety since he saw himself confronted with strangers, whom he was asked to interact with publicly. In fact, he was directly exposed to his fear.

By means of repetition of the treatment, that was gradually modified to provoke more fear (e.g., the number of persons in the audience was increased), the patient learned to cope with his fears and the anxietal response diminished. In this particular study, patients drew attention to the fact that they experienced the situation in a way comparable to *in vivo* procedures (Roy, et al., 2003).

In fact, in another study the fear-provoking quality of VEs for patients suffering from fear of public speaking as compared to a non-phobic control group has been proven. The fear response in the experimental group was provoked when the participants were asked to hold a speech in front of a virtual audience, whereas this scenario instigated lessened degrees of anxiety in the control group as measured by questionnaires quantifying levels of anxiety and heart rate. This result leads to the conclusion that in fact, the study participants experienced presence during the experimental conditions, which testifies to the real effectiveness of the treatment (Slater, Pertaub, Barker, & Clark, 2006).

The meta-analysis of VRETs for anxiety disorders conducted by Powers and Emmelkamp (2008), in which they compared 13 studies, offers highly positive results with regards to the efficacy and efficiency of VRET for treating anxiety disorders. The measures of between-group effect sizes (measured by Cohen's *d*) comparing the effects of VRET treatment for specific phobias, social phobia, PTSD and panic disorder to control conditions (Cohen's $d = 1.1$) and/or in vivo therapies (Cohen's $d = 0.35$) revealed that VRET is highly efficient in treating anxiety disorders and even outperforms the golden standard of therapy, *in vivo* procedures, in efficacy (Powers & Emmelkamp, 2008).

Overall, there appear a number of advantages involved in making use of VRET for the purpose of treating anxiety disorders. First, the therapist has complete control over the therapy. Therapists not only monitor the therapy, but they also ensure that the patient is gradually exposed to his or her individual anxieties. Second, VRET is entirely private and confidential and it includes low risk of the patient to be embarrassed in front of others. Patients receive therapy by themselves and do not have to interact with other patients seeking help. Moreover, he does not have to fear their disapproval, as is the case with group CBT. Therefore, VRET is very appealing to patients. This might seem a hindrance at first sight because a therapist would want to expose the patient to their feared situation. However, this takes place in VRET by means of the virtual environment which functions as a realistic simulation of the real world.

Third, the anxietal response is provoked easily, for the VE is constructed so as to expose the patient directly to the fearful situations. Fourth, there are certain economic considerations involved as well. Administering VRET to a patient requires relatively low costs. Still, instruments such as the HMD and especially the CAVE as well as the development of effective software involve significant costs. A second drawback is the fact that VRET is a new therapy and thus both researchers as well as therapists are rather unacquainted with it heretofore (Bush, 2008). Still, the problem of high costs of the technological equipment can be overcome.

Tichon and Banks (2006) found that both 150-degree screens (semi-immersive interfaces) as well as regular desktop PCs incorporating VEs designed to treat schizophrenia can provide patients with a sense of presence. In their study, this was measured by a presence questionnaire (PQ), which asked for causal factors of the experience of presence, such as control, distraction, sensory, and realism factors, as well as an introspective group presence questionnaire (IGPQ), by means of which individual presence experiences were recorded. In both conditions, the experience of being present in the VE was reported by the study's participants (Tichon & Banks, 2006). Consequently, high-end technological devices, such as the HMD and CAVE do not necessarily have to be included in VRET in order to produce experiences of presence. Nevertheless, current scientific knowledge is in need for a controlled study that compares VRET utilizing HMD and CAVE with one another as well as with more cost-efficient technological devices, such as regular desktop PCs. The utilization of the latter is in fact an appealing idea not only because it saves costs, but also because the computer has become a popular and familiar device for most people nowadays. Today, the computer cannot be assumed away of everyday life. Therefore, VRET including computers could very soon gain significant popularity among the patient population.

Videogames and Psychological Wellbeing

It also needs to be noted that videogames are now being used with new platforms, including smartphones, making them accessible on the move. One game that has recently been developed to function via both the Internet and smartphones is *SuperBetter*. *SuperBetter* has been designed to improve any individuals' resilience, to foster personal growth, and to be better able to cope with life's challenges (McGonigal, 2015). Following a traumatic head trauma that left her depressed and suicidal, the game developer decided she wanted to get better and developed simple but effective strategies to overcome her difficult condition. These included recruiting allies (family and friends), engaging in low-level physical activity (e.g., walking around the block), and creating happy emotions (e.g., cuddling her dog). These strategies quickly lifted her out of her miserable state and allowed her to cope effectively with her difficult condition.

Given her professional interest in game design, she decided to design a game that can be used by individuals in a similar position, suffering from some form of physical, mental, emotional or other ailments – *SuperBetter* emerged. *SuperBetter* uses game-mechanisms and play to confront difficulties in life, harnessing characteristics of the game player (i.e., optimism, creativity, courage, resilience, and willpower). It asks players to engage in various tasks, including physical, mental, emotional and social challenges to reach personally identified goals (e.g., overcoming depression). Whilst playing, players are encouraged to activate power-ups (i.e., bonuses that make them stronger). Examples may include anything that creates moments of happiness, strength, and connection, such as a song that increases the player's strength, particular food that provides energy, or a short activity that creates calm. Playing *SuperBetter* resulted in positive outcomes for psychological wellbeing, self-efficacy, and success in life (McGonigal, 2015).

In order to test the effectiveness of *SuperBetter,* Roepke and colleagues (2015) recruited 283 adult *iPhone* users who had clinically significant depression scores as based on self-reports including the Center for Epidemiological Studies Depression (CES-D) questionnaire (Radloff, 1977) to participate in a randomized controlled trial (RCT). Participants were randomly allocated to one of three groups. The first group played a version of *SuperBetter* that included cognitive behavioral therapy elements and positive psychotherapy strategies to alleviate depression (CBT-PPT SB). The second group used a general version of *SuperBetter* that was aimed to increase self-esteem and acceptance (general SB). The third group was a waiting list (WL) control group. Each of the group members were asked to play *SuperBetter* for the period of ten minutes over one month, and were asked to fill in self-report questionnaires online that assessed psychological distress and wellbeing every two weeks.

Results indicated that playing *SuperBetter* resulted in decreased self-reported depression scores, and that CBT-PPT SB and general SB were similarly effective to decrease depression symptoms, in comparison to the WL group. In addition to this, similar effects were observed with regards to decreases in anxiety, improvements in life satisfaction, self-efficacy, and social support, where both SB groups faired similarly significantly better than the WL group (Roepke, et al., 2015). Using a sophisticated RCT methodology, this study was able to show the significant benefits of using general *SuperBetter* (which is freely available via the Internet and downloadable using app stores on both *iPhone* and *Android* smartphones) regarding decreasing negative mental symptoms (including anxiety and depression) whilst at the same time boosting positive outcomes for psychological wellbeing (such as life satisfaction, self-efficacy, and social support). Future studies should attempt to replicate these results, possibly including samples of clinically diagnosed patients suffering from various mental ailments to ascertain the viability of serious games for psychological wellbeing, such as *SuperBetter*. Nevertheless, it seems safe to state that *SuperBetter* can be used by anybody for real-life everyday challenges.

Videogame Playing for Interfering with Distressful Imagery

Treatments for post-traumatic stress disorder and addiction are well established, but there are scarcely any effective early interventions and management strategies. Playing videogames such as the tile puzzle game *Tetris* has been proposed as a visuospatial task to compete with the working memory resources required for the formation of sensory imagery in post-traumatic stress disorder and addiction (Holmes, et al., 2009; James, et al., 2015; Skorka-Brown, et al., 2015). The use of videogame playing as an interfering task is still being investigated, although the use of videogames in this context appears to have potential as previous findings have suggested. Holmes and colleagues (2009) demonstrated the benefits of playing *Tetris* under laboratory settings for interfering with the consolidation of traumatic memories that manifested as flashbacks of scenes of a traumatic film. Also, Skorka-Brown and colleagues showed that participants that played *Tetris* in a laboratory setting (2014) or in day-to-day contexts (2015) experienced reduction in cravings for various substances and behaviors. According to Ortiz de Gortari and Griffiths (2016), videogames are both, a useful exercise combining visual and spatial memory, and game content (including videogame elements, sensory perception) remains active upon discontinuation of playing (also referred to as *Game Transfer Phenomena*). This can potentially provide further advantages to overcoming unwelcome intrusions.

FUTURE RESEARCH DIRECTIONS

Clearly there are potentially interesting areas or future research and development in this area is disparate in terms of positive therapeutic consequences. To advance the field there is also a need to closely examine the factors that facilitate therapeutic benefits in the first place. This is because benefits (such as educational learning) depend on other factors than the nature of the videogame itself. For instance, psychologists have shown that working in-group co-operatively can speed up the time taken to do problem-solving tasks but it can also slow down the speed when the tasks are done competitively. Also, psychologists have found that girls who do problem-solving tasks together with other girls tend to co-operate whereas boys compete against each other. For those videogames reliant on strategy and problem solving, such findings may have implications for therapeutic potential.

One unexplored area in videogame research is people's attitudes towards playing. How a person thinks about a particular game - or videogame playing in general - may actually affect the therapeutic value. For instance, it could be speculated that when it comes to videogames there are three different types of people. The first are the technophobes who think that videogames are (literally) a complete waste of time and want nothing to do with them whatsoever. They would probably take every opportunity to be critical about them on a matter of principle and therefore gain little therapeutically. The second are the techno-sceptics who use and enjoy the technology but are not convinced that it is a vital therapeutic tool although there may be some therapeutic uses in some circumstances. The third are the techno-romantics who raise people's expectations about the capabilities and potential of computer games, and who sing their praises at every available opportunity. It is these individuals who may benefit most therapeutically from videogames.

The use of commercial videogames in therapy may be controversial since these games were not created for therapeutic purposes and lack the carefully standardized conditions of therapeutic games. However, it appears important to investigate their uses in therapy as some current videogames allow the personalization of the videogames' settings and content such as modifying the character appearance, and even integration of real life elements into the game. This may provide new avenues for clinicians to explore the therapeutic use of videogames at a low-cost compared to specialized and expensive videogames platforms. Particularly, the recent commercialization of virtual reality head-sets which enhance the sense of presence in the virtual world making gaming a more realistic experience has opened a world of opportunities for therapy.

Moreover, the advance in artificial intelligence (through the use of more receptive videogame characters that simulate understanding and that respond to players' behaviors) may facilitate the use of videogame characters as companions. This may be of therapeutic help to specific sub-groups (e.g., autistic children or those with learning difficulties).

Also, control devices in some of the latest videogames offer new possibilities to explore videogames' physiotherapeutic qualities since some control devices require physical challenge. For example, the use of motion sensing controls that track acceleration and movement allows users to operate the videogames by pointing at the screen that is different from gamepads based only on pushing buttons. It is also possible to use peripheral platforms where players stand while playing, controlling the game with body movements such as the *Wii* balance board, or (perhaps even better) to use videogames for treatment of patients incapable of using videogame controls via natural user interfaces where gestures, movements and spoken commands can be used to control the game. Moreover, haptic technology provides tactile feedback with vibration enhancing videogame playing experiences that may result positively in the treatment of certain patients.

Even involuntary phenomena provoked by playing videogames such as spontaneous visualization of videogame images or recurrently hearing music from the game after stopping playing can potentially be used with therapeutic means if used properly (Ortiz de Gortari & Griffiths, 2016).

Lastly, it has been suggested that design choices, specific effects and working mechanisms in videogames and their impact on behavior change need to be investigated further, particularly with regards to the games' effectiveness on the one hand and the reduction of potentially disadvantageous consequences of playing videogames for children and adolescents. It has furthermore been stated that a number of of individuals and organizations should be involved in creating videogames to make them more effective. These include policymakers, the gamers, the gamers' families, scientists, game designers, retailers, and publishers, and supported by appropriate funding bodies (Baranowski, et al., 2016).

CONCLUSION

It is clear from the preceding overview that in the right context, videogames can have a positive therapeutic benefit to a large range of different sub-groups. Videogames have been shown to help children undergoing chemotherapy, children undergoing psychotherapy, children with particular emotional and behavioral problems (ADD, impulsivity, autism), individuals with medical and health problems (such as Erb's palsy, muscular dystrophy, burns, strokes, movement impaired), patients suffering from a variety of anxiety disorders, groups such as the elderly, and individuals looking to overcome real-life challenges (including symptoms of depression) and boost their wellbeing (including boosting life satisfaction, self-efficacy and social support). In terms of videogames being distractor tasks, it seems likely that the effects can be attributed to most commercially available videogames. However, as with the literature on videogames aiding health promotion, one of the major problems is that reported positive effects in some of these other instances were from specially designed videogames rather than those that were already commercially available. It is therefore hard to evaluate the therapeutic value of videogames as a whole. As with research into the more negative effects, it may well be the case that some videogames are particularly beneficial whereas others have little or no therapeutic benefit whatsoever. What is clear from the empirical literature is that the negative consequences of videogame playing almost always involve people who are excessive users. It is probably fair to say that therapeutic benefits (including such things as self-esteem) can be gained from moderate videogame playing.

Videogames do seem to have great positive therapeutic potential in addition to their entertainment value. Many positive applications in education and health care have been developed. There has been considerable success when games are specifically designed to address a specific problem or to teach a certain skill. However, generalizability outside the game-playing situation remains an important consideration.

REFERENCES

Achtman, R. L., Green, C. S., & Bavelier, D. (2008). Video games as a tool to train visual skills. *Restorative Neurology and Neuroscience*, *26*(4-5), 435–446. PMID:18997318

Adriaenssens, E. E., Eggermont, E., Pyck, K., Boeckx, W., & Gilles, B. (1988). The video invasion of rehabilitation. *Burns*, *14*(5), 417–419. doi:10.1016/0305-4179(88)90015-0 PMID:3228700

Anderson, C. A., & Bushman, B. J. (2001). Effects of violent games on aggressive behavior, aggressive cognition, aggressive affect, physiological arousal, and prosocial behavior: A meta-analytic review of the scientific literatures. *Psychological Science*, *12*(5), 353–359. doi:10.1111/1467-9280.00366 PMID:11554666

Baranowski, T., Abdelsamad, D., Baranowski, J., OConnor, T. M., Thompson, D., Barnett, A., ... Chen, T.-A. (2012). Impact of an active video game on healthy childrens physical activity. *Pediatrics*, *129*(3), e636–e642. doi:10.1542/peds.2011-2050 PMID:22371457

Baranowski, T., Blumberg, F., Buday, R., DeSmet, A., Fiellin, L. E., Green, C. S., ... Young, K. (2016). Games for health for children - Current status and needed research. *Games for Health Journal*, *5*(1), 1–12. doi:10.1089/g4h.2015.0026 PMID:26262772

Bavelier, D., Green, C. S., & Seidenberg, M. S. (2013). Cognitive development: Gaming your way out of dyslexia? *Current Biology*, *23*(7), R282–R283. doi:10.1016/j.cub.2013.02.051 PMID:23578877

Blechman, E. A., Rabin, C., & McEnroe, M. J. (1986). Family communication and problem solving with boardgames and computer games. In C. E. Schaefer & S. E. Reid (Eds.), *Game play: Therapeutic use of childhood games* (pp. 129–145). New York, NY: John Wiley & Sons.

Blunt, D., Hastie, C., & Stephens, P. (1998). More than he Nintended? *Anaesthesia and Intensive Care*, *26*, 330–331. PMID:9619237

Bosworth, K. (1994). Computer games as tools to reach and engage adolescents in health promotion activities. *Computers in Human Services*, *11*, 109–119.

Botella, C., Banos, R. M., Villa, H., Perpina, C., & Garcia-Palacios, A. (2000). Virtual reality in the treatment of claustrophobic fear: A controlled, multiple-baseline design. *Behavior Therapy*, *31*(3), 583–595. doi:10.1016/S0005-7894(00)80032-5

Brezinka, V. (2008). Treasure hunt - A serious game to support psychotherapeutic treatment of children. In S. K. Anderson (Ed.), *eHealth beyond the horizon* (pp. 71–76). IOS Press.

Broeren, J., Claesson, L., Goude, D., Rydmark, M., & Sunnerhagen, K. S. (2008). Virtual rehabilitation in an activity centre for community-dwelling persons with stroke - The possibilities of 3-dimensional computer games. *Cerebrovascular Diseases (Basel, Switzerland)*, *26*(3), 289–296. doi:10.1159/000149576 PMID:18667809

Brown, S. J., Lieberman, D. A., Germeny, B. A., Fan, Y. C., Wilson, D. M., & Pasta, D. J. (1997). Educational video game for juvenile diabetes: Results of a controlled trial. *Medical Informatics*, *22*(1), 77–89. doi:10.3109/14639239709089835 PMID:9183781

Buckalew, L. W., & Buckalew, P. B. (1983). Behavioral management of exceptional children using video games as reward. *Perceptual and Motor Skills*, *56*(2), 580. doi:10.2466/pms.1983.56.2.580 PMID:6866667

Bush, J. (2008). Viability of virtual reality exposure therapy as a treatment alternative. *Computers in Human Behavior*, *24*(3), 1032–1040. doi:10.1016/j.chb.2007.03.006

Butler, C. (1985). Utilizing video games to increase sitting tolerance. *Archives of Physical Medicine and Rehabilitation*, *66*(8), 527–527.

Cahill, J. M. (1994). Health works: Interactive AIDS education videogames. *Computers in Human Services*, *11*(1-2), 159–176.

Cameirao, M. S., Bermúdez i Badia, S., Duarte Oller, E., Zimmerli, L., & Verschure, P. F. M. J. (2007, September 27-29). The Rehabilitation Gaming System: A virtual reality based system for the evaluation and rehabilitation of motor deficits. *Paper presented at the Proceedings of Virtual Rehabilitation*, Venice, Italy. 10.1109/ICVR.2007.4362125

Ceranoglu, T. A. (2010a). Star Wars in psychotherapy: Video games in the office. *Academic Psychiatry*, *34*(3), 233–236. doi:10.1176/appi.ap.34.3.233 PMID:20431107

Ceranoglu, T. A. (2010b). Video games in psychotherapy. *Review of General Psychology*, *14*(2), 141–146. doi:10.1037/a0019439 PMID:20431107

Chandrasekharan, S., Mazalek, A., Nitsche, M., Chen, Y. F., & Ranjan, A. (2010). Ideomotor design using common coding theory to derive novel video game interactions. *Pragmatics & Cognition*, *18*(2), 313–339. doi:10.1075/pc.18.2.04cha

Clarke, B., & Schoech, D. (1994). A computer-assisted game for adolescents: Initial development and comments. *Computers in Human Services*, *11*(1-2), 121–140.

Cole, S. W., Yoo, D. J., & Knutson, B. (2012). Interactivity and reward-related neural activation during a serious videogame. *PLoS ONE*, *7*(3), e33909. doi:10.1371/journal.pone.0033909 PMID:22442733

Coyle, D., Matthews, M., Sharry, J., Nisbet, A., & Doherty, G. (2005). Personal investigator: A therapeutic 3D game for adolescent psychotherapy. *Interactive Technology and Smart Education*, *2*(2), 73–88. doi:10.1108/17415650580000034

Demarest, K. (2000). Video games - What are they good for? Retrieved 9.03.2011, from http://www.lessontutor.com/kd3.html

DeShazo, J., Harris, L., & Pratt, W. (2010). Effective intervention or childs play? A review of video games for diabetes education. *Diabetes Technology & Therapeutics*, *12*(10), 815–822. doi:10.1089/dia.2010.0030 PMID:20807119

DeSmet, A., Van Ryckeghem, D., Compernolle, S., Baranowski, T., Thompson, D., Crombez, G., ... De Bourdeaudhuij, I. (2014). A meta-analysis of serious digital games for healthy lifestyle promotion. *Preventive Medicine*, *69*, 95–107. doi:10.1016/j.ypmed.2014.08.026 PMID:25172024

Donchin, E. (1995). Video games as research tools: The Space Fortress game. *Behavior Research Methods, Instruments, & Computers*, *27*(2), 217–223. doi:10.3758/BF03204735

Donohue, C. (Ed.). (2015). *Technology and digital media in the early years: Tools for teaching and learning*. New York: Routledge.

Dorval, M., & Pepin, M. (1986). Effect of playing video game on a measure of spatial visualization. *Perceptual and Motor Skills*, *62*(1), 159–162. doi:10.2466/pms.1986.62.1.159 PMID:3960656

Ducharme, P., Wharff, E., Hutchinson, E., Kahn, J., Logan, G., & Gonzalez-Heydrich, J. (2012). Videogame assisted emotional regulation training: An ACT with RAGE-control case illustration. *Clinical Social Work Journal*, *40*(1), 75–84. doi:10.100710615-011-0363-0

Dustman, R. E., Emmerson, R. Y., Laurel, A., Shearer, D., & .... (1992). The effects of videogame playing on neuropsychological performance of elderly individuals. *Journal of Gerontology*, *47*(3), 168–171. doi:10.1093/geronj/47.3.P168 PMID:1573200

Eow, Y. L., Ali, W. Z. B., Mahmud, R. B., & Baki, R. (2010). Computer games development and appreciative learning approach in enhancing students creative perception. *Computers & Education*, *54*(1), 146–161. doi:10.1016/j.compedu.2009.07.019

Farris, M., Bates, R., Resnick, H., & Stabler, N. (1994). Evaluation of computer games' impact upon cognitively impaired frail elderly. *Computers in Human Services, 11*(1-2), 219–228.

Favelle, G. K. (1994). Therapeutic applications of commercially available computer software. *Computers in Human Services, 11*(1-2), 151–158.

Fisher, S. (1986). Use of computers following brain injury. *Activities, Adaptation and Aging, 8*(1), 81–93. doi:10.1300/J016v08n01_10

Fitzgerald, D., Trakarnratanakul, N., Smyth, B., & Caulfield, B. (2010). Effects of a wobble board-based therapeutic exergaming system for balance training on dynamic postural stability and intrinsic motivation levels. *The Journal of Orthopaedic and Sports Physical Therapy, 40*(1), 11–19. doi:10.2519/jospt.2010.3121 PMID:20044704

Freud, A. (1928). *Introduction to the technique of child analysis*. New York, NY: Nervous and Mental Disease Publishing.

Fung, V., So, K., Park, E., Ho, A., Shaffer, J., Chan, E., & Gomez, M. (2010). The utility of a video game system in rehabilitation of burn and nonburn patients: A survey among occupational therapy and physiotherapy Practitioners. *Journal of Burn Care & Research; Official Publication of the American Burn Association, 31*(5), 768–775. doi:10.1097/BCR.0b013e3181eed23c PMID:20628305

Funk, J. B., Germann, J. N., & Buchman, D. D. (1997). Children and electronic games in the United States. *Trends in Communication, 2*, 111–126.

Gamberini, L., Alcaniz, M., Barresi, G., Fabregat, M., Prontu, L., & Seraglia, B. (2008). Playing for a real bonus: Videogames to empower elderly people. *Journal of Cyber Therapy and Rehabilitation, 1*(1), 37–48.

Garcia-Palacios, A., Hoffman, H., Carlin, A., Furness, T. A. III, & Botella, C. (2002). Virtual reality in the treatment of spider phobia: A controlled study. *Behaviour Research and Therapy, 40*(9), 983–993. doi:10.1016/S0005-7967(01)00068-7 PMID:12296495

Gardner, J. E. (1991). Can the Mario Bros. help? Nintendo games as an adjunct in psychotherapy with children. *Psychotherapy (Chicago, Ill.), 28*(4), 667–670. doi:10.1037/0033-3204.28.4.667

Gaylord-Ross, R. J., Haring, T. G., Breen, C., & Pitts-Conway, V. (1984). The training and generalization of social interaction skills with autistic youth. *Journal of Applied Behavior Analysis, 17*(2), 229–247. doi:10.1901/jaba.1984.17-229 PMID:6735954

Goldstein, J., Cajko, L., Oosterbroek, M., Michielsen, M., van Houten, O., & Salverda, F. (1997). Video games and the elderly. *Social Behavior and Personality, 25*(4), 345–352. doi:10.2224bp.1997.25.4.345

Govender, M., Bowen, R. C., German, M. L., Bulaj, G., & Bruggers, C. S. (2015). Clinical and neurobiological perspectives of empowering pediatric cancer patients using videogames. *Games for Health Journal, 4*(5), 362–374. doi:10.1089/g4h.2015.0014 PMID:26287927

Green, C. S., & Bavelier, D. (2006). Effect of action video games on the spatial distribution of visuospatial attention. *Journal of Experimental Psychology, 32*, 1465–1478. PMID:17154785

Griffiths, M. D. (2004). Can videogames be good for your health? *Journal of Health Psychology, 9*(3), 339–344. doi:10.1177/1359105304042344 PMID:15117533

Griffiths, M. D. (2008a). Diagnosis and management of video game addiction. *New Directions in Addiction Treatment and Prevention, 12*, 27–41.

Griffiths, M. D. (2008b). Videogame addiction: Fact or fiction? In T. Willoughby & E. Wood (Eds.), *Children's learning in a digital world* (pp. 85–103). Oxford: Blackwell.

Henningson, K. A., Gold, R. S., & Duncan, D. F. (1986). A computerized marijuana decision maze: Expert opinion regarding its use in health education. *Journal of Drug Education, 16*(3), 243–261. doi:10.2190/NAQ3-4XQC-93FU-G8ME PMID:3534206

Hieftje, K., Edelman, E. J., Camenga, D. R., & Fiellin, L. E. (2013). Electronic media-based health interventions promoting behavior change in youth: A systematic review. *JAMA Pediatrics, 167*(6), 574–580. doi:10.1001/jamapediatrics.2013.1095 PMID:23568703

Hollander, E. K., & Plummer, H. R. (1986). An innovative therapy and enrichment program for senior adults utilizing the personal computer. *Activities, Adaptation and Aging, 8*(1), 59–68. doi:10.1300/J016v08n01_08

Hollingsworth, M., & Woodward, J. (1993). Integrated learning: Explicit strategies and their role in problem solving instruction for students with learning disabilities. *Exceptional Children, 59*, 444–445. PMID:8440301

Holmes, E. A., James, E. L., Coode-Bate, T., & Deeprose, C. (2009). Can playing the computer game "Tetris'' reduce the build-up of flashbacks for trauma? A proposal from cognitive science. *Plos One, 4*(1). doi:10.1371/journal.pone.0004153

Horn, E., Jones, H. A., & Hamlett, C. (1991). An investigation of the feasibility of a video game system for developing scanning and selection skills. *Journal for the Association for People with Severe Handicaps*, *16*, 108–115.

Housman, S. J., Scott, K. M., & Reinkensmeyer, D. J. (2009). A randomized controlled trial of gravity-supported, computer-enhanced arm exercise for individuals with severe hemiparesis. *Neurorehabilitation and Neural Repair*, *23*(5), 505–514. doi:10.1177/1545968308331148 PMID:19237734

Huber, M., Rabin, B., Docan, C., Burdea, G. C., AbdelBaky, M., & Golomb, M. R. (2010). Feasibility of modified remotely monitored in-home gaming technology for improving hand function in adolescents with cerebral palsy. *IEEE Transactions on Information Technology in Biomedicine*, *14*(2), 526–534. doi:10.1109/TITB.2009.2038995 PMID:20071262

Hurkmans, H. L., van den Berg-Emons, R. J., & Stam, H. J. (2010). Energy expenditure in adults with cerebral palsy playing Wii Sports. *Archives of Physical Medicine and Rehabilitation*, *91*(10), 1577–1581. doi:10.1016/j.apmr.2010.07.216 PMID:20875517

International Society for Presence Research. (2000). The concept of presence: Explication statement. Retrieved 17.06.2015, from http://ispr.info/about-presence-2/about-presence/

James, E. L., Bonsall, M. B., Hoppitt, L., Tunbridge, E. M., Geddes, J. R., Milton, A. L., & Holmes, E. A. (2015). Computer game play reduces intrusive memories of experimental trauma via reconsolidation-update mechanisms. *Psychological Science*, *26*(8), 1201–1215. doi:10.1177/0956797615583071 PMID:26133572

Jannink, M. J. A., Van Der Wilden, G. J., Navis, D. W., Visser, G., Gussinklo, J., & Ijzerman, M. (2008). A low-cost video game applied for training of upper extremity function in children with cerebral palsy: A pilot study. *Cyberpsychology & Behavior*, *11*(1), 27–32. doi:10.1089/cpb.2007.0014 PMID:18275309

Joei Mioto, B. B., & Goncalves Ribas, C. (2014). The usage of videogames as a psychotherapeutic intervention in individuals with Down Syndrome. *Open Access Library Journal*, *1*, 1–9.

Joo, L. Y., Yin, T. S., Xu, D., Thia, E., Chia, P. F., Kuah, C. W. K., & He, K. K. (2010). A feasibility study using interactive commercial off-the-shelf computer gaming - Gaming in upper limb rehabilitation patients after stroke. *Journal of Rehabilitation Medicine*, *42*(5), 437–441. doi:10.2340/16501977-0528 PMID:20544153

Kappes, B. M., & Thompson, D. L. (1985). Biofeedback vs. video games: Effects on impulsivity, locus of control and self-concept with incarcerated individuals. *Journal of Clinical Psychology*, *41*(5), 698–706. doi:10.1002/1097-4679(198509)41:5<698::AID-JCLP2270410520>3.0.CO;2-Q PMID:4044854

Kato, P. M. (2010). Video games in health care: Closing the gap. *Review of General Psychology*, *14*(2), 113–121. doi:10.1037/a0019441

Kato, P. M., Cole, S. W., Bradlyn, A. S., & Pollock, B. H. (2008). A video game improves behavioral outcomes in adolescents and young adults with cancer: A randomized trial. *Pediatrics*, *122*(2), E305–E317. doi:10.1542/peds.2007-3134 PMID:18676516

King, T. I. (1993). Hand strengthening with a computer for purposeful activity. *The American Journal of Occupational Therapy*, *47*(7), 635–637. doi:10.5014/ajot.47.7.635 PMID:8322884

Klein, M. (1932). *The psychoanalysis of children*. London: Hogarth.

Kokish, R. (1994). Experiences using a PC in play therapy with children. *Computers in Human Services*, *11*(1-2), 141–150.

Kolko, D. J., & Rickard-Figueroa, J. L. (1985). Effects of video games on the adverse corollaries of chemotherapy in pediatric oncology patients. *Journal of Consulting and Clinical Psychology*, *53*(2), 223–228. doi:10.1037/0022-006X.53.2.223 PMID:3858296

Krichevets, A. N., Sirotkina, E. B., Yevsevicheva, I. V., & Zeldin, L. M. (1994). Computer games as a means of movement rehabilitation. *Disability and Rehabilitation: An International Multidisciplinary Journal*, *17*(2), 100–105. doi:10.3109/09638289509166635 PMID:7795259

Krijn, M., Emmelkamp, P. M. G., Biemond, R., de Ligny, C. D., Schuemie, M. J., & van der Mast, C. (2004). Treatment of acrophobia in virtual reality: The role of immersion and presence. *Behaviour Research and Therapy*, *42*(2), 229–239. doi:10.1016/S0005-7967(03)00139-6 PMID:14975783

Krijn, M., Emmelkamp, P. M. G., Olafsson, R. P., & Biemond, R. (2004). Virtual reality exposure therapy of anxiety disorders: A review. *Clinical Psychology Review*, *24*(3), 259–281. doi:10.1016/j.cpr.2004.04.001 PMID:15245832

Lange, B., Flynn, S., Proffitt, R., Chang, C. Y., & Rizzo, A. (2010). Development of an interactive game-based rehabilitation tool for dynamic balance training. *Topics in Stroke Rehabilitation*, *17*(5), 345–352. doi:10.1310/tsr1705-345 PMID:21131259

Larose, S., Gagnon, S., Ferland, C., & Pepin, M. (1989). Psychology of computers: XIV. Cognitive rehabilitation through computer games. *Perceptual and Motor Skills*, *69*(3), 851–858. doi:10.2466/pms.1989.69.3.851 PMID:2608401

Lawrence, G. H. (1986). Using computers for the treatment of psychological problems. *Computers in Human Behavior*, *2*(1), 43–62. doi:10.1016/0747-5632(86)90021-X

Leibovici, V., Magora, F., Cohen, S., & Ingber, A. (2009). Effects of virtual reality immersion and audiovisual distraction techniques for patients with pruritus. *Pain Research & Management*, *14*(4), 283–286. doi:10.1155/2009/178751 PMID:19714267

Leng, E. Y., Ali, W., Mahmud, R. B., & Baki, R. (2010). Computer games development experience and appreciative learning approach for creative process enhancement. *Computers & Education*, *55*(3), 1131–1144. doi:10.1016/j.compedu.2010.05.011

Lieberman, D. A. (2001). Management of chronic pediatric diseases with interactive health games: Theory and research findings. *The Journal of Ambulatory Care Management*, *24*(1), 26–38. doi:10.1097/00004479-200101000-00004 PMID:11189794

Lim, C. G., Lee, T. S., Guan, C. T., Fung, D. S. S., Cheung, Y. B., Teng, S. S. W., ... Krishnan, K. R. (2010). Effectiveness of a brain-computer interface based programme for the treatment of ADHD: A pilot study. *Psychopharmacology Bulletin*, *43*(1), 73–82. PMID:20581801

Lu, A. S., Kharrazi, H., Gharghabi, F., & Thompson, D. (2013). A Systematic Review of Health Videogames on Childhood Obesity Prevention and Intervention. *Games for Health Journal*, *2*(3), 131–141. doi:10.1089/g4h.2013.0025 PMID:24353906

Lynch, W. J. (1983). Cognitive retraining using microcomputer games and commercially available software. *Paper presented at the Meeting of the International Neuropsychological Society*, Mexico City.

Masendorf, F. (1993). Training of learning disabled children's spatial abilities by computer games. *Zeitschrift fur Padagogische Psychologie*, *7*, 209–213.

Matthews, T. J., De Santi, S. M., Callahan, D., Koblenz-Sulcov, C. J., & Werden, J. I. (1987). The microcomputer as an agent of intervention with psychiatric patients: Preliminary studies. *Computers in Human Behavior*, *3*(1), 37–47. doi:10.1016/0747-5632(87)90009-4

McCormack, K., Fitzgerald, D., Fitzgerald, O., Caulfield, B., O'Huiginn, B., & Smyth, B. (2009). A comparison of a computer game-based exercise system with conventional approaches of exercise therapy in rheumatology patients. *Rheumatology*, *48*, I29–I29.

McGonigal, J. (2015). *SuperBetter: A revolutionary approach to getting stronger, happier, braver, and resilient - Powered by the science of games*. London: Penguin.

McGuire, F. A. (1984). Improving quality of life for residents of long term care facilities through video games. *Activities, Adaptation and Aging*, *6*(1), 1–7. doi:10.1300/J016v06n01_01

McGuire, F. A. (1986). *Computer technology and the aged: Implications and applications for activity programs*. New York, NY: Haworth.

Miller, D. J., & Robertson, D. P. (2010). Using a games console in the primary classroom: Effects of Brain Training programme on computation and self-esteem. *British Journal of Educational Technology*, *41*(2), 242–255. doi:10.1111/j.1467-8535.2008.00918.x

Oakley, C. (1994). SMACK: A computer driven game for at-risk teens. *Computers in Human Services*, *11*(1-2), 97–99.

OConnor, T. J., Cooper, R. A., Fitzgerald, S. G., Dvorznak, M. J., Boninger, M. L., VanSickle, D. P., & Glass, L. (2000). Evaluation of a manual wheelchair interface to computer games. *Neurorehabilitation and Neural Repair*, *14*(1), 21–31. doi:10.1177/154596830001400103 PMID:11228946

Okolo, C. (1992a). The effect of computer-assisted instruction format and initial attitude on the arithmetic facts proficiency and continuing motivation of students with learning disabilities. *Exceptionality*, *3*(4), 195–211. doi:10.1080/09362839209524815

Okolo, C. (1992b). Reflections on the effect of computer-assisted instruction format and initial attitude on the arithmetic facts proficiency and continuing motivation of students with learning disabilities. *Exceptionality*, *3*(4), 255–258. doi:10.1080/09362839209524818

Olsen-Rando, R. A. (1994). Proposal for development of a computerized version of talking, feeling and doing game. *Computers in Human Services*, *11*(1-2), 69–80.

Ortiz de Gortari, A. B., Aronsson, K., & Griffiths, M. D. (2011). Game Transfer Phenomena in video game playing: A qualitative interview study. *International Journal of Cyber Behavior, Psychology and Learning*, *1*(3), 15–33. doi:10.4018/ijcbpl.2011070102

Ortiz de Gortari, A. B., & Griffiths, M. D. (2016). Commentary: Playing the computer game tetris prior to viewing traumatic film material and subsequent intrusive memories: Examining proactive interference. *Frontiers in Psychology*, *7*, 260. doi:10.3389/fpsyg.2016.00260 PMID:26941702

Pegelow, C. H. (1992). Survey of pain management therapy provided for children with sickle cell disease. *Clinical Pediatrics*, *31*(4), 211–214. doi:10.1177/000992289203100404 PMID:1373356

Phillips, W. R. (1991). Video game therapy. *The New England Journal of Medicine*, *325*, 1056–1057. PMID:1922219

Powers, M. B., & Emmelkamp, P. M. G. (2008). Virtual reality exposure therapy for anxiety disorders: A meta-analysis. *Journal of Anxiety Disorders*, *22*(3), 561–569. doi:10.1016/j.janxdis.2007.04.006 PMID:17544252

Radloff, L. S. (1977). The CES-D Scale: A self-report depression scale for research in the general population. *Applied Psychological Measurement*, *1*(3), 385–401. doi:10.1177/014662167700100306

Rauterberg, M. (2004). Positive effects of entertainment technology on human behaviour. In R. Jaquart (Ed.), *Building the information society* (pp. 51–58). Kluwer. doi:10.1007/978-1-4020-8157-6_8

Redd, W. H., Jacobsen, P. B., Die-Trill, M., Dermatis, H., McEvoy, M., & Holland, J. C. (1987). Cognitive-attentional distraction in the control of conditioned nausea in pediatric cancer patients receiving chemotherapy. *Journal of Consulting and Clinical Psychology*, *55*(3), 391–395. doi:10.1037/0022-006X.55.3.391 PMID:3597954

Reichlin, L., Mani, N., McArthur, K., Harris, A. M., Rajan, N., & Dacso, C. C. (2011). Assessing the acceptability and usability of an interactive serious game in aiding treatment decisions for patients with localized prostate cancer. *Journal of Medical Internet Research, 13*(1), 188-201. doi:10.2196/jmir.1519

Reijnders, J., van Heugten, C., & van Boxtel, M. (2013). Cognitive interventions in healthy older adults and people with mild cognitive impairment: A systematic review. *Ageing Research Reviews*, *12*(1), 263–275. doi:10.1016/j.arr.2012.07.003 PMID:22841936

Resnick, H. (1994a). Ben's Grille. *Computers in Human Services*, *11*(1-2), 203–211.

Resnick, H. (1994b). Electronic technology and rehabilitation: A computerised simulation game for youthful offenders. *Computers in Human Services*, *11*(1-2), 61–67.

Riddick, C. C., Spector, S. G., & Drogin, E. B. (1986). The effects of videogame play on the emotional states and affiliative behavior of nursing home residents. *Activities, Adaptation and Aging*, *8*(1), 95–107. doi:10.1300/J016v08n01_11

Roepke, A. M., Jaffee, S. R., Riffle, O. M., McGonigal, J., Broome, R., & Maxwell, B. (2015). Randomized controlled trial of SuperBetter, a smartphone-based/Internet-based self-help tool to reduce depressive symptoms. *Games for Health Journal*, *4*(3), 235–246. doi:10.1089/g4h.2014.0046 PMID:26182069

Rothbaum, B. O., Hodges, L., Smith, S., Lee, J. H., & Price, L. (2000). A controlled study of virtual reality exposure therapy for the fear of flying. *Journal of Consulting and Clinical Psychology*, *68*(6), 1020–1026. doi:10.1037/0022-006X.68.6.1020 PMID:11142535

Rothbaum, B. O., Hodges, L. F., Ready, D., Graap, K., & Alarcon, R. D. (2001). Virtual reality exposure therapy for Vietnam veterans with posttraumatic stress disorder. *The Journal of Clinical Psychiatry*, *62*(8), 617–622. doi:10.4088/JCP.v62n0808 PMID:11561934

Roy, S., Klinger, E., Legeron, P., Lauer, F., Chemin, I., & Nugues, P. (2003). Definition of a VR-based protocol to treat social phobia. *Cyberpsychology & Behavior*, *6*(4), 411–420. doi:10.1089/109493103322278808 PMID:14511454

Ryan, E. B. (1994). Memory for Goblins: A computer game for assessing and training working memory skill. *Computers in Human Services*, *11*(1-2), 213–217.

Salend, S., & Santora, D. (1985). Employing access to the computer as a reinforcer for secondary students. *Behavioral Disorders*.

Samoilovich, S., Riccitelli, C., Scheil, A., & Siedi, A. (1992). Attitude of schizophrenics to computer videogames. *Psychopathology*, *25*(3), 117–119. doi:10.1159/000284761 PMID:1448536

Schoene, D., Lord, S. R., Delbaere, K., Severino, C., Davies, T. A., & Smith, S. T. (2013). A randomised controlled pilot study of home-based step training in older people using videogame technology. *PLoS ONE*, *8*(3), e57734. doi:10.1371/journal.pone.0057734 PMID:23472104

Schueren, B. (1986). Video games: An exploration of their potential as recreational activity programs in nursing homes. *Activities, Adaptation and Aging*, *8*(1), 49–58. doi:10.1300/J016v08n01_07

Sedlak, R. A., Doyle, M., & Schloss, P. (1982). Video games - A training and generalization demonstration with severely retarded adolescents. *Education and Training in Mental Retardation and Developmental Disabilities*, *17*(4), 332–336.

Sharar, S. R., Miller, W., Teeley, A., Soltani, M., Hoffman, H. G., Jensen, M. P., & Patterson, D. R. (2008). Applications of virtual reality for pain management in burn-injured patients. *Expert Review of Neurotherapeutics*, *8*(11), 1667–1674. doi:10.1586/14737175.8.11.1667 PMID:18986237

Sherer, M. (1994). The effect of computerized simulation games on the moral development of youth in distress. *Computers in Human Services*, *11*(1-2), 81–95.

Sietsema, J. M., Nelson, D. L., Mulder, R. M., Mervau-Scheidel, D., & White, B. E. (1993). The use of a game to promote arm reach in persons with traumatic brain injury. *The American Journal of Occupational Therapy*, *47*(1), 19–24. doi:10.5014/ajot.47.1.19 PMID:8418672

Skilbeck, C. (1991). Microcomputer-based cognitive rehabilitation. In A. Ager (Ed.), *Microcomputers and clinical psychology: Issues, applications and Future Developments* (pp. 95–118). Chichester: Wiley.

Skorka-Brown, J., Andrade, J., & May, J. (2014). Playing Tetris reduces the strength, frequency and vividness of naturally occurring cravings. *Appetite*, *76*, 161–165. doi:10.1016/j.appet.2014.01.073 PMID:24508486

Skorka-Brown, J., Andrade, J., Whalley, B., & May, J. (2015). Playing Tetris decreases drug and other cravings in real world settings. *Addictive Behaviors*, *51*, 165–170. doi:10.1016/j.addbeh.2015.07.020 PMID:26275843

Slater, M., Pertaub, D. P., Barker, C., & Clark, D. M. (2006). An experimental study on fear of public speaking using a virtual environment. *Cyberpsychology & Behavior*, *9*(5), 627–633. doi:10.1089/cpb.2006.9.627 PMID:17034333

Spence, J. (1988). The use of computer arcade games in behaviour management. *Maladjustment and Therapeutic Education*, *6*, 64–68.

Starn, J., & Paperny, D. M. (1990). Computer games to enhance adolescent sex education. *Journal of Maternal Child Nursing*, *15*(4), 250–253. PMID:2115955

Strein, W., & Kochman, W. (1984). Effects of computer games on children's co-operative behaviour. *Journal of Research and Development in Education*, *18*(1).

Subrahmanyam, K., & Greenfield, P. (1994). Effect of video game practice on spatial skills in boys and girls. *Journal of Applied Developmental Psychology*, *15*(1), 13–32. doi:10.1016/0193-3973(94)90004-3

Synofzik, M., Schatton, C., Giese, M., Wolf, J., Schols, L., & Ilg, W. (2013). Videogame-based coordinative training can improve advanced, multisystemic early-onset ataxia. *Journal of Neurology, 260*(10), 2656–2658. doi:10.100700415-013-7087-8 PMID:23989345

Szer, J. (1983). Video games as physiotherapy. *The Medical Journal of Australia, 1*, 401–402. PMID:6835150

Szturm, T., Peters, J. F., Otto, C., Kapadia, N., & Desai, A. (2008). Task-specific rehabilitation of finger-hand function using interactive computer gaming. *Archives of Physical Medicine and Rehabilitation, 89*(11), 2213–2217. doi:10.1016/j.apmr.2008.04.021 PMID:18996252

Tanaka, J. W., Wolf, J. M., Klaiman, C., Koenig, K., Cockburn, J., Herlihy, L., ... Schultz, R. T. (2010). Using computerized games to teach face recognition skills to children with autism spectrum disorder: The Lets Face It! program. *Journal of Child Psychology and Psychiatry, and Allied Disciplines, 51*(8), 944–952. doi:10.1111/j.1469-7610.2010.02258.x PMID:20646129

Thomas, D. L. (1994). LIFE CHOICES: The program and its users. *Computers in Human Services, 11*(1-2), 189–202.

Thomas, R., Cahill, J., & Santilli, L. (1997). Using an interactive computer game to increase skill and self-efficacy regarding safer sex negotiation: Field test results. *Health Education & Behavior, 24*(1), 71–86. doi:10.1177/109019819702400108 PMID:9112099

Tichon, J., & Banks, J. (2006). Virtual reality exposure therapy: 150-degree screen to desktop PC. *Cyberpsychology & Behavior, 9*(4), 480–488. doi:10.1089/cpb.2006.9.480 PMID:16901251

Trost, S. G., Sundal, D., Foster, G. D., Lent, M. R., & Vojta, D. (2014). Effects of a pediatric weight management program with and without active video games - A randomized trial. *JAMA Pediatrics, 168*(5), 407–413. doi:10.1001/jamapediatrics.2013.3436 PMID:24589566

Vasterling, J., Jenkins, R. A., Tope, D. M., & Burish, T. G. (1993). Cognitive distraction and relaxation training for the control of side effects due to cancer chemotherapy. *Journal of Behavioral Medicine, 16*(1), 65–80. doi:10.1007/BF00844755 PMID:8433358

Vilozni, D., Bar-Yishay, E., Shapira, Y., Meyer, S., & Godfrey, S. (1994). Computerized respiratory muscle training in children with Duchenne Muscular Dystrophy. *Neuromuscular Disorders*, *4*(3), 249–255. doi:10.1016/0960-8966(94)90026-4 PMID:7919973

Vincelli, F., Anolli, L., Bouchard, S., Wiederhold, B. K., Zurloni, V., & Riva, G. (2003). Experiential cognitive therapy in the treatment of panic disorders with agoraphobia: A controlled study. *Cyberpsychology & Behavior*, *6*(3), 321–328. doi:10.1089/109493103322011632 PMID:12855090

Wald, J., & Taylor, S. (2000). Efficacy of virtual reality exposure therapy to treat driving phobia: A case report. *Journal of Behavior Therapy and Experimental Psychiatry*, *31*(3-4), 249–257. doi:10.1016/S0005-7916(01)00009-X PMID:11494960

Weightman, A. P. H., Preston, N., Holt, R., Allsop, M., Levesley, M., & Bhakta, B. (2010). Engaging children in healthcare technology design: Developing rehabilitation technology for children with cerebral palsy. *Journal of Engineering Design*, *21*(5), 579–600. doi:10.1080/09544820802441092

Weisman, S. (1983). Computer games for the frail elderly. *The Gerontologist*, *23*(4), 361–363. doi:10.1093/geront/23.4.361 PMID:6618244

Weisman, S. (1994). Computer games for the frail elderly. *Computers in Human Services*, *11*(1-2), 229–234.

Wiederhold, B. K., & Wiederhold, M. D. (2010). Virtual reality treatment of Posttraumatic Stress Disorder due to motor vehicle accident. *Cyberpsychology, Behavior, and Social Networking*, *13*(1), 21–27. doi:10.1089/cyber.2009.0394 PMID:20528289

Wiemeyer, J. (2010). Gaming for health - Serious games in prevention and rehabilitation. *Deutsche Zeitschrift fur Sportmedizin*, *61*(11), 252–257.

Wohlheiter, K. A., & Dahlquist, L. M. (2012). Interactive versus passive distraction for acute pain management in young children: The role of selective attention and development. *Journal of Pediatric Psychology*, *38*(2), 202–212. doi:10.1093/jpepsy/jss108 PMID:23092971

Wouters, P., van Nimwegen, C., van Oostendorp, H., & van der Spek, E. D. (2013). A meta-analysis of the cognitive and motivational effects of serious games. *Journal of Educational Psychology*, *105*(2), 249–265. doi:10.1037/a0031311

Wright, K. (2001). Winning brain waves: Can custom-made video games help kids with attention deficit disorder? *Discover*, 22.

Yavuzer, G., Senel, A., Atay, M. B., & Stam, H. J. (2008). "PlayStation Eyetoy games" improve upper extremity-related motor functioning in subacute stroke: A randomized controlled clinical trial. *European Journal of Physical and Rehabilitation Medicine*, *44*(3), 237–244. PMID:18469735

Yip, P., Middleton, P., Cyna, A. M., & Carlyle, A. V. (2009). Non-pharmacological interventions for assisting the induction of anaesthesia in children. *Cochrane Database of Systematic Reviews*, *8*(3), CD006447. PMID:19588390

This research was previously published in the International Journal of Privacy and Health Information Management (IJPHIM), 5(2); edited by Francesco Longo and Letizia Nicoletti (CAL-TEK, Italy), pages 71-96, copyright year 2017 by IGI Publishing (an imprint of IGI Global).

Chapter 15
Look of Life:
The Wonder Therapy

Vittoria Sichi
ANT Foundation, Italy

Giacomo Ercolani
ANT Foundation, Italy

Luca Franchini
ANT Foundation, Italy

Luca Golfari
ANT Foundation, Italy

Silvia Varani
ANT Foundation, Italy

Daniela Rizzoli
ANT Foundation, Italy

Raffaella Pannuti
ANT Foundation, Italy

Daniele Roganti
ANT Foundation, Italy

ABSTRACT

The use of virtual reality (VR) shows promising results in improving the emotional wellbeing of cancer patients, reducing anxiety, depression, and pain symptoms. No data exist concerning the use of VR in cancer patients assisted at home. The ANT Foundation decided to conduct a pilot study to test the use of VR in cancer patients assisted at home. Fifty-eight ANT patients were randomized and assigned to a control group that didn't use VR devices and to an experimental group that used them. The primary objective of the pilot study was to determine whether VR device could be a viable instrument in homecare patients. Furthermore, the aim of the study was to discover if VR could have beneficial effects on patients' quality of life as well as discover which kind of videos were more effective. The innovative aspect of this study was to test the use of VR directly at home of patients, proposing a use of VR that is compatible with the needs and the daily rhythms of families, and investigating its effectiveness through appropriate validated psychometric questionnaires and semi-structured interviews.

DOI: 10.4018/978-1-7998-1680-5.ch015

INTRODUCTION

The experience of a cancer diagnosis and progression of the disease in its different phases can lead to psychological distress, relationship problems, cognitive limitations and numerous physical symptoms of a strong emotional impact. Besides compromising the physical health of the patient, cancer often causes psychological discomfort characterized by anxious and depressive symptoms that may be clinically significant in some cases. These factors can seriously affect the quality of life of the person and his family environment, hampering the adherence to treatment, the efficacy of therapies and deteriorating the clinical prognosis. Cancer greatly interferes with all aspects of daily life of the person affected, from family and personal relationships to business and financial areas. Numerous studies confirm that a high number of cancer patients experience severe levels of psychological distress such as depression and anxiety, with a percentage people affected respectively of 20% and 10% (Pitman et al., 2018). Contrary to expectations, percentages of people suffering of depression and anxiety in end-of-life phase do not differ significantly from those of patients in non-palliative care settings (Mitchell et al., 2011). In addition to the emotional distress related to the anguish of confronting death, advanced stages of the disease very often imply a progressive loss of functional autonomy. This puts the patient in a state of deprivation and forced isolation from a relational and social aspect that was hitherto part of their life. This state of psychological distress naturally adds to the burden of the physical symptoms caused by the disease and/or invasive therapies, above pain. The reduction of the opportunities in which it is possible to experience positive emotions and meaningful social interactions often corresponds to an intensification of the concerns and the obsessive thoughts, which in turn increase stress and connect to further negative emotional experiences. This vicious circle, in absence of rapid and effective intervention, risks to worsen patients' quality of life. Beyond pharmacological approach, complementary psychological techniques aiming to deflect patient's attention from unpleasant symptoms have been employed (e.g. muscular progressive relaxation, mindfulness, guided imagery). By moving attention towards neutral or positive emotions and sensations, these techniques may help patients to manage distress and pain.

BACKGROUND

Alongside traditional interventions, in recent years several studies have tested the effectiveness of the use of immersive audiovisual technologies, which are able to emotionally involve the person, capture his attention and directing it to new stimuli (Nichols & Patel 2002; Spagnolli et al., 2003; Spagnolli & Gamberini, 2005; Scozzari

& Gamberini, 2011; Gamberini & Spagnolli, 2015). Moreover, such a technology offers the significant advantage of being used in low mobility conditions and without specific and complicated training. In recent years, Virtual Reality (VR) has been employed with great success to manage anxiety in different anxiety disorders – through the Virtual Reality Exposure Therapy – chronic pain and acute pain in patients undergoing routine and invasive medical interventions (Li et al., 2011; Morina et al., 2015). Indeed, use of VR has shown promising results in reducing emotional and physical discomfort among cancer patients. A common disturbing experience relating to cancer is definitely pain: chronic cancer pain often involves persistent pain – which may last all day – and breakthrough pain–a brief flare-up of severe pain occurring even while patient is regularly taking pain medication. Cancer-related pain affects about 70% of patients and recent data suggest that it may be inadequately controlled in up to 50% of patients (Neufeld et al. 2017). VR has gained recognition as means of attenuating pain in several medical procedure, such as burn care procedures (Morris et al., 2009; Malloy & Milling, 2010). Scientific rationale behind the employment of this technology refers to Melzack and Wall's Gate Control Theory (1968) and to the observation of McCaul and Malot (1984) about role of attention and effect of distraction on the perception of painful stimuli. From a neurobiological point of view VR likely act differently from other known pain interventions. In particular, VR may affect the pain modulation system of body by acting directly and not on pain perception and signaling through senses, attention, memory and emotions: indeed, both attention and emotions are able to affect significantly pain perception via the descending pain-control system (Gold et al. 2007). Authors who have investigated feasibility and effectiveness of VR in cancer patients have applied this tool to pediatric settings certainly because of its playful character. In addition, several studies have investigated feasibility and effectiveness of VR as a tool for supporting and monitoring treatments in cancer adult patients by influencing their psychological and physiological functions (Chirico et al., 2016). As early as the late 1990's, Oyama (1997) already explored potential of VR for cancer patients in palliative care: the author argued that VR could enhance possibilities of communication both by creating a medical cyberspace to provide mental care and by allowing patients and relatives to communicate and support each other – reducing as a result loneliness and despair. Even though attention of research is currently concentrating on symptoms management, it is possible that these applications could be future directions of investigations on integration of technology in health system. Although this research field is steadily increasing – also because of the ongoing technological innovation –there is a lack of robust data concerning the use of VR in cancer patients assisted at home. It will be interesting testing the use of VR in this particular setting for two main reasons: first of all, nowadays VR is accessible almost to everyone, due to its partial low-cost; secondly, there is a growing interest in home care in term of cost and benefits for patients and his relatives. Therefore, the ANT Italian Foundation in collaboration with the Human Inspired Technology Research Centre (HIT) of University of Padova and with the cultural association MenoMale, decided to conduct a pilot exploratory study to test the feasibility of VR in cancer patients assisted at home.

ANT ITALIA FOUNDATION

ANT is one of the leading organization, working in Italy in the field of palliative home care and pain management. ANT provides free social-health assistance at home to cancer sufferers and, depending on the resources available in the local area, runs free of charge cancer prevention initiatives. ANT's philosophy can be summed up by the term *Eubiosia* (from ancient Greek 'good life'), meaning overall quality to guarantee a dignified life right up until one's last breath. Since 1985, ANT has assisted more than 110.000 sufferers, completely free of charge, in 20home oncology clinics (ODO-ANT) in 9 Italian regions. There are currently 4.000patients receiving care throughout Italy every day. ANT offers specialized care provided by 433 healthcare professionals, including physicians, nurses, psychologists, nutritionists, physiotherapists, social-health workers, pharmacists who are able to provide patients with round the clock care, 365 days of the year.

AIM

The primary objective of the pilot study was to determine whether VR device could be a viable instrument in home care patients. Furthermore, the aim of the study was to discover if VR could have beneficial effects on patient's quality of life as well as discover which kind of videos were more effective. The innovative aspect of this study was to test the use of VR directly at home of patients, proposing a use of VR that is compatible with the needs and the daily rhythms of families, and investigating its effectiveness through appropriate validated psychometric questionnaires and semi-structured interviews.

VIRTUAL REALITY HEAD-MOUNTED DISPLAY

The VR device employed in the study is the Samsung Gear VR headset, a portable VR viewer developed from Samsung Electronics in collaboration with Oculus. The device is used in combination with Samsung Galaxy S6 Edge Plus, which performs the function of VR display. The Gear VR contains a sensor capable of perceiving the movement and rotation of the head and able to modulate the image according to the movement of the subject, giving the illusion of being immersed in a three-dimensional scenario. In this way Oculus reproduces 3D environments of everyday life giving you the feeling of actually being immersed in a virtual environment. There are twenty infrared sensors positioned on the viewer, which, when combined with a camera placed in front of the user, are able to detect any shifts in movement in 3 directions, thus allowing the users to be able to move in a 3D environment. The model also integrates the control box in the head-mounted display, a small box containing the control board that acts as a link between the screen and the device. It has a 7-inch LCD screen with a colour depth of 24 bits per pixel and is 3D stereoscopic enabled. The field of vision is of more than 90 degrees horizontally (110 degrees diagonal), which is more than double when compared to other competing devices. The resolution is 1280x800 (16:10 aspect ratio), i.e. 640 × 800 per eye (4: 5 aspect ratio).The viewer can be calibrated to compensate for visual disturbances such as myopia, thanks to a wheel on the front of the viewer that adjusts the focal distance of the lenses. The Gear VR used by the authors was released in November 2015 and it is one of the first devices for virtual reality to be used by a significant number of users.

SAFETY PRECAUTIONS

The scientific literature has reported the possibility of some episodes of nausea during the exposure to VR, especially with the first types of devices, with particular contents and in predisposed subjects. However, in the case of the specific technology used by the authors (Samsung Gear VR), adverse effects have been reported only in very few cases, as demonstrated by the study of Mosadeghi et al. (2016), in which there was a single subject who experience nausea and therefore interrupted the vision. Video used in *The Look Of Life* have been selected because they contain the least possible amount of stimuli that can hinder motion sickness or emotional distress. At the same time, videos should provide audiovisual experiences considered pleasant and comfortable by the vast majority of users, according to reviews on the appropriate Samsung Gear VR market.All the videos have been specifically selected for content and duration by the scientific committee of the ANT Research Department in collaboration with the interdepartmental research center 'Human Inspired Technologies research center-HIT' of the University of Padova, headed by Professor Luciano Gamberini.

SANITARY AND HYGIENIC PRECAUTIONS

Regarding the hygiene measures, authors followed the guidelines of the Health and Social Agency of Emilia-Romagna (Mongardi et al., 2011), concerning the disinfection of medical devices and equipment. Prior to each use by the subjects the viewer was disinfected with special disposable wipes (Clorox Disinfectant Wipes - Clorox Germicidal Wipes) and the lenses were cleaned with specific cloths based on alcohol. As an additional measure of safety, the viewer has not been placed directly in contact with the head and face of the subjects, but special disposable sterilized cloths have been used in order to minimize any direct contact with the device.

SAMPLE

The study involved 58 ANT patients in the metropolitan area of Bologna. Exclusion criteria were: age> 18; presence of brain cancer or brain metastases; epilepsy; had a heart attack in the last year; suffering from a severe psychopathology (e.g. bipolar disorder, schizophrenia); inability to speak and read the Italian language. After the recruitment phase, the participants were randomized and assigned to a control group which didn't use VR device and to an intervention group that used it. Overall, the sample was composed by 32 females and 26 males and the average age was 50 years (between 25 and 60 years old) and most of participants were married or cohabited with partners (67%). As for occupation, 43% of sample worked at the time of the study whereas 39% were retired or in sick leave. Average Karnofsky Performance Status (KPS) score – a measure of functional impairment which allows physicians to assess how a patient's disease is progressing– was 72 ($\sigma = 15$). Average KPS did not differ significantly between control and intervention groups – respectively 72 and 73. Intervention group was composed by 14 females and 15 males and 76% of them were involved with someone and cohabited with their spouses or partners whereas 17% lived alone. As for level of education, half the group had high school diploma and 20% had a university degree or a postgraduate degree. Almost all of participants within intervention group were familiar with PC and smartphone, however none of them has reported to use virtual reality devices usually.

PROCEDURE

ANT psychologists, adequately trained, met each patient in the experimental group four times in a week and during each meeting patients had the opportunity to see an immersive video. Videos shown to patients were selected on the basis of two focus groups conducted in October 2016 with groups of cancer patients followed by ANT. During the first and last meetings, intervention group also completed (before watching the first video and after watching the last video) a personal data card and two questionnaires: the Hospital Anxiety and Depression Scale (HADS) and the Brief Pain Inventory (BPI). During second and third meeting, before and after watching the videos, Edmonton Symptom Assessment Scale (ESAS), a visual-analogue scale for the assessment of symptoms in patients receiving palliative care, has been administered. The evaluated symptoms concerned pain, fatigue, nausea, depression, anxiety, drowsiness, loss of appetite, discomfort and difficulty in breathing. On the fourth day the patients of the experimental group were asked some questions about the frequency with which they would use the VR if they had the device at home. Patients were requested to describe the VR experience just ended: the purpose of the recorded audio interview was to investigate the opinions of the respondents about the effects experienced with VR and preferences for a hypothetical video specifically created for them. Answers to the questions were audio recorded and then categorized. As for patients in the control group, they only met the psychologist twice in a week for filling in the personal registry form and answering the same questionnaire of the experimental group, except for ESAS, which they did not complete. The quantitative data,related to the questionnaires compiled by the two groups, were statistically analyzed using the SPSS software. The authors conducted a qualitative analysis of the frequencies for the answers of the interviews. In particular, the answers were grouped into four thematic or macro-category areas (VR effects, attitude towards VR, preference for interactive videos, comfort) and each of them contained a different number of categories. This chapter will treat exclusively the qualitative results of the study.

MEASURES

Acute and chronic pain. Acute and chronic pain were assessed using four items taken from the Italian version of Brief Pain Inventory - Short Form (Bonezzi et al., 2002), an easy-to-use pain assessment questionnaire which quantify the intensity of pain. It is characterized by a series of questions (descriptors) concerning the intensity of pain. Besides the intensity of current pain, levels of pain investigated are the maximum, minimum and average during the 24 hours before the test.

Anxiety and depression. Mood status, in particular anxiety and depression, was assessed through the Hospital Anxiety and Depression Scale - HADS (Zigmond & Snaith, 1983). This is a very simple scale consisting of 14 items which explore both anxiety and depression symptoms, keeping the two scores divided. The main characteristic of the scale is that it excludes the somatic symptomatology from the evaluation. The scale instead focuses, especially for depression, on the reduction of hedonic capacity, considering it among the most sensitive indicators in the diagnosis of this disorder.

Other symptoms. Other various symptoms were assessed through the ESAS (Edmonton Symptom Assessment Scale), which represents a scale composed by nine visual analog scales (VAS) that investigate specific symptoms such as pain, general activity, nausea, depression, anxiety, drowsiness, appetite, general well-being and shortness of breath.The patient attributes a severity score on a 100 mm line for each of these symptoms.

RESULTS

From the qualitative analysis of the interviews, it appears that most of patients in the experimental group(73%) said they would like to have the instrument at home and that they would use it for a total daily duration ranging from 10 to 60 minutes. The experience of VR, has been defined as "pleasant" (term reported by 16 patients) and "innovative" (reported by 6).

It was definitely a very good experience! After each use I'd go to speak, extremely enthusiastic, with my mother and sister and I told them "you know, I saw that thing and I tried to take it with my hands...wow!". Yes, it was a very impactful experience (Maria 25 years old)

It is something new (VR)... [..] Well it is something funny and innovative to do (Matteo 59 years old)

Relaxation (reported by 10) and distraction (reported by 8) were the most commonly reported effects, followed by reassurance, amusement and amazement (reported by 4).

mh... actually it helps to detach your mind from what you are doing and it casts you in something different... so it calms you down

If a video could be created specifically for them all the patients said they would like to see natural scenarios. In addition, eleven patients (36%) said they preferred interactive videos while ten (33%) wanted to see videos in which they were more aloof as simple observers. All patients, even those who have openly declared themselves unfamiliar with technology, have found the viewer comfortable and easy to use. On the basis of the interviews and focus groups, ANT produced a video of the concert of the Oscar-winning composer Nicola Piovani, a video shot inside the Sigurtà garden park and one at Arte Sella, a contemporary art exhibition inserted in a natural context.These immersive videos were made through the use of complex equipment consisting of 14 cameras recording two spherical videos, one for the left hemisphere and one for the right hemisphere, able to faithfully reproduce the environment where the experience took place.

CONCLUSION

The objective of this pilot study was to evaluate the home use of an innovative technology which has shown to have the potential to alleviate and improve some particular clinical and psychological conditions linked to disabling cancer diseases (Chirico et al., 2016).The VR device has also been appreciated by older patients and this suggests that its use could be extended to subjects with advanced age. More unambiguous and specific conclusions about effects of VR on psychological and physical state of patients can be drawn after that quantitative data will be analyzed. Of course, preliminary data are encouraging. Indeed, employment of VR among patients assisted by ANT seems to have brought positive effects in terms of physical sensations and emotions. Relaxation is definitely the most reported physical effect although short-lived and mild unpleasant physical sensations have been found in rare cases (e.g. mild lightheadedness during the use of device). However, it is reassuring to note that an extremely involving and potentially effective technology such as VR does not cause particular side effects in patients living a condition of frailty and sufferance. The study carried out by ANT Foundation is showing the great potential of VR with respect to the management of particular mood states such as anxiety, boredom and discomfort due to cancer disease and related therapies. Moreover, most of interviews conducted suggest that some experiences can generate positive emotions such as happiness and wonder, which have the potential to balance the empty often caused by being compelled at home and limited in daily activities and relationships.

REFERENCES

Bonezzi, C., Nava, A., Barbieri, M., Demartini, L., Miotti, D., & Paulin, D. (2002). Validazione della versione italiana del Brief Pain Inventory nei pazienti con dolore cronico. *Minerva Anestesiologica*, *68*(7-8), 607–611. PMID:12244292

Chirico, A., Lucidi, F., De Laurentiis, M., Milanese, C., Napoli, A., & Giordano, A. (2016). Virtual Reality in health system: Beyond entertainment. A mini-review on the efficacy of VR during cancer treatment. *Journal of Cellular Physiology*, *231*(2), 275–287. doi:10.1002/jcp.25117 PMID:26238976

Gamberini, L., & Spagnolli, A. (2015). An Action-Based Approach to Presence: Foundations and Methods. In M. Lombard, F. Biocca, J. Freeman, W. IJsselsteijn, & R. Schaevitz (Eds.), *Immersed in Media: Telepresence Theory, Measurement & Technology* (pp. 101–114). Cham: Springer. doi:10.1007/978-3-319-10190-3_6

Gold, J. I., Belmont, K. A., & Thomas, D. A. (2007). The neurobiology of virtual reality pain attenuation. *Cyberpsychology & Behavior*, *10*(4), 536–544. doi:10.1089/cpb.2007.9993 PMID:17711362

Li, A., Montaño, Z., Chen, V. J., & Gold, J. L. (2011). Virtual reality and pain management: Current trends and future directions. *Pain Management*, *1*(2), 147–157. doi:10.2217/pmt.10.15 PMID:21779307

Malloy, K. M., & Milling, L. S. (2010). The effectiveness of virtual reality distraction for pain reduction: A systematic review. *Clinical Psychology Review*, *30*(8), 1011–1018. doi:10.1016/j.cpr.2010.07.001 PMID:20691523

McCaul, K. D., & Malott, J. M. (1984). Distraction and coping with pain. *Psychological Bulletin*, *95*(3), 516–533. doi:10.1037/0033-2909.95.3.516 PMID:6399756

Melzack, R., & Wall, P. D. (1965). Pain mechanisms: A new theory. *Science*, *150*(3699), 971–979. doi:10.1126cience.150.3699.971 PMID:5320816

Mitchell, A. J., Chan, M., Bhatti, H., Halton, M., Grassi, L., Johansen, C., & Meader, N. (2011). Prevalence of depression, anxiety, and adjustment disorder in oncological, haematological, and palliative-care settings: A meta-analysis of 94 interview-based studies. *The Lancet Oncology*, *12*(2), 160–174. doi:10.1016/S1470-2045(11)70002-X PMID:21251875

Morina, N., Ijntema, H., Meyerbröker, K., & Emmelkamp, P. M. (2015). Can virtual reality exposure therapy gains be generalized to real-life? A meta-analysis of studies applying behavioral assessments. *Behaviour Research and Therapy*, *74*, 18–24. doi:10.1016/j.brat.2015.08.010 PMID:26355646

Morris, L. D., Louw, Q. A., & Grimmer-Somers, K. (2009). The effectiveness of virtual reality on reducing pain and anxiety in burn injury patients: A systematic review. *The Clinical Journal of Pain*, *25*(9), 815–826. doi:10.1097/AJP.0b013e3181aaa909 PMID:19851164

Neufeld, N. J., Elnahal, S. M., & Alvarez, R. H. (2017). Cancer pain: A review of epidemiology, clinical quality and value impact. *Future Oncology (London, England), 13*(9), 833–841. doi:10.2217/fon-2016-0423 PMID:27875910

Nichols, S., & Patel, H. (2002). Health and safety implications of virtual reality: A review of empirical evidence. *Applied Ergonomics, 33*(3), 251–271. doi:10.1016/S0003-6870(02)00020-0 PMID:12164509

Oyama, H. (1998). Virtual reality for the palliative care of cancer. *Studies in Health Technology and Informatics, 58*, 140–150. PMID:10350914

Scozzari, S., & Gamberini, L. (2011). Virtual Reality as a Tool for Cognitive Behavioral Therapy: A Review. In S. Brahnam & L. C. Jain (Eds.), *Advanced Computational Intelligence Paradigms in Healthcare 6. Virtual Reality in Psychotherapy, Rehabilitation, and Assessment. Studies in Computational Intelligence* (Vol. 337). Berlin: Springer. doi:10.1007/978-3-642-17824-5_5

Spagnolli, A., & Gamberini, L. (2005). A Place for presence. Understanding the human involvement in mediated interactive environments. *PsychNology Journal, 3*(1), 6–15. PMID:16190023

Spagnolli, A., Gamberini, L., Cottone, P., & Mantovani, G. (2003). Ergonomics of virtual environments for clinical use. *Studies in Health Technology and Informatics, 99*, 217–230. PMID:15295153

Zigmond, A. S., & Snaith, R. P. (1983). The hospital anxiety and depression scale. *Acta Psychiatrica Scandinavica, 67*(6), 361–370. doi:10.1111/j.1600-0447.1983.tb09716.x PMID:6880820

KEY TERMS AND DEFINITIONS

Breakthrough Cancer Pain (BTcP): Transient exacerbation of pain occurring in a patient with otherwise stable, persistent pain. Breakthrough pain is relatively common among cancer patients, particularly those with moderate to severe background pain, and is one of the most difficult pain syndromes to treat.

End-of-Life Care: Care given to people who are near the end of life and have stopped treatment to cure or control their disease. End-of-life care includes physical, emotional, social, and spiritual support for patients and their families.

Home Oncological Clinic: ANT oncological home care service.

Mindfulness: The psychological process of bringing one's attention to the internal and external experiences occurring in the present moment, which can be developed through the practice of meditation and other training.

Palliative Care (PC): Palliative care is an approach that improves the quality of life of patients and their families facing the problem associated with life-threatening illness, through the prevention and relief of suffering by identification, assessment and treatment of pain and other problems, physical, psychosocial, and spiritual.

Psychological Distress (Distress): Is a general term used to describe unpleasant feelings or emotions that impact your level of functioning. Sadness, anxiety, distraction, and symptoms of mental illness are manifestations of psychological distress.

Virtual Reality (VR): The possibility to immerse in a completely virtual world using a device to visualize computer graphics or computer sound.

This research was previously published in Virtual and Augmented Reality in Mental Health Treatment edited by Giuliana Guazzaroni, pages 262-270, copyright year 2019 by Medical Information Science Reference (an imprint of IGI Global).

Related Readings

To continue IGI Global's long-standing tradition of advancing innovation through emerging research, please find below a compiled list of recommended IGI Global book chapters and journal articles in the areas of pain management, alternative medicine, and chronic pain. These related readings will provide additional information and guidance to further enrich your knowledge and assist you with your own research.

Ababio, G. K. (2018). Nutraceuticals: The Dose Makes the Difference – It's All in the Dose. In A. Verma, K. Srivastava, S. Singh, & H. Singh (Eds.), *Nutraceuticals and Innovative Food Products for Healthy Living and Preventive Care* (pp. 24–47). Hershey, PA: IGI Global. doi:10.4018/978-1-5225-2970-5.ch002

Akhter, M. (2018). Herbal Drug Interactions. In M. Tangkiatkumjai, A. Casarin, L. Chen, & D. Walker (Eds.), *Complementary and Alternative Medicine and Kidney Health* (pp. 201–231). Hershey, PA: IGI Global. doi:10.4018/978-1-5225-2882-1.ch008

Alhaj, O. A. (2017). Functional Properties of Camel Milk. In H. Shekhar, Z. Howlader, & Y. Kabir (Eds.), *Exploring the Nutrition and Health Benefits of Functional Foods* (pp. 147–164). Hershey, PA: IGI Global. doi:10.4018/978-1-5225-0591-4.ch007

Anand, A., Pannu, V., Bhalla, A., Singh, G., & Singh, S. (2018). Can Yoga Bring Molecular Changes in Brain and Body: Gaps and Trends. In S. Telles & N. Singh (Eds.), *Research-Based Perspectives on the Psychophysiology of Yoga* (pp. 86–102). Hershey, PA: IGI Global. doi:10.4018/978-1-5225-2788-6.ch006

Basu, A., Sarkar, A., & Basak, P. (2018). Nutraceuticals for Human Health and Hypersensitivity Reaction. In A. Verma, K. Srivastava, S. Singh, & H. Singh (Eds.), *Nutraceuticals and Innovative Food Products for Healthy Living and Preventive Care* (pp. 323–341). Hershey, PA: IGI Global. doi:10.4018/978-1-5225-2970-5.ch015

Bhavanani, A. B., & Ramanathan, M. (2018). Psychophysiology of Yoga Postures: Ancient and Modern Perspectives of Asanas. In S. Telles & N. Singh (Eds.), *Research-Based Perspectives on the Psychophysiology of Yoga* (pp. 1–16). Hershey, PA: IGI Global. doi:10.4018/978-1-5225-2788-6.ch001

Bohra, M., & Visen, A. (2018). Nutraceutical Properties in Flowers. In A. Verma, K. Srivastava, S. Singh, & H. Singh (Eds.), *Nutraceuticals and Innovative Food Products for Healthy Living and Preventive Care* (pp. 217–235). Hershey, PA: IGI Global. doi:10.4018/978-1-5225-2970-5.ch010

Buffo, R. (2017). Yerba Mate: Chemistry, Technology, and Biological Properties. In H. Shekhar, Z. Howlader, & Y. Kabir (Eds.), *Exploring the Nutrition and Health Benefits of Functional Foods* (pp. 185–194). Hershey, PA: IGI Global. doi:10.4018/978-1-5225-0591-4.ch009

Casarin, A. (2018). CAM Recommended by Standard Guidelines for Chronic Illnesses. In M. Tangkiatkumjai, A. Casarin, L. Chen, & D. Walker (Eds.), *Complementary and Alternative Medicine and Kidney Health* (pp. 124–155). Hershey, PA: IGI Global. doi:10.4018/978-1-5225-2882-1.ch006

Casarin, A., Tangkiatkumjai, M., & Walker, D. (2018). An Overview of Complementary and Alternative Medicine. In M. Tangkiatkumjai, A. Casarin, L. Chen, & D. Walker (Eds.), *Complementary and Alternative Medicine and Kidney Health* (pp. 1–23). Hershey, PA: IGI Global. doi:10.4018/978-1-5225-2882-1.ch001

Cascella, M., Muzio, M. R., Bimonte, S., & Cuomo, A. (2018). Nutraceuticals for Prevention of Chemotherapy-Induced Peripheral Neuropathy. In A. Verma, K. Srivastava, S. Singh, & H. Singh (Eds.), *Nutraceuticals and Innovative Food Products for Healthy Living and Preventive Care* (pp. 236–259). Hershey, PA: IGI Global. doi:10.4018/978-1-5225-2970-5.ch011

Chen, L., & Tangkiatkumjai, M. (2018). Economic Evaluation of CAM Use. In M. Tangkiatkumjai, A. Casarin, L. Chen, & D. Walker (Eds.), *Complementary and Alternative Medicine and Kidney Health* (pp. 232–271). Hershey, PA: IGI Global. doi:10.4018/978-1-5225-2882-1.ch009

Dahiya, K., & Dhankhar, R. (2018). Role of Nutraceuticals in Cancer. In A. Verma, K. Srivastava, S. Singh, & H. Singh (Eds.), *Nutraceuticals and Innovative Food Products for Healthy Living and Preventive Care* (pp. 176–194). Hershey, PA: IGI Global. doi:10.4018/978-1-5225-2970-5.ch008

Eshiet, E. R., & Smith, E. E. (2017). Herbal Benefits of Tea. In H. Shekhar, Z. Howlader, & Y. Kabir (Eds.), *Exploring the Nutrition and Health Benefits of Functional Foods* (pp. 117–146). Hershey, PA: IGI Global. doi:10.4018/978-1-5225-0591-4.ch006

Faris, M. A., & Attlee, A. (2017). Lentils (Lens culinaris, L.): A Novel Functional Food. In H. Shekhar, Z. Howlader, & Y. Kabir (Eds.), *Exploring the Nutrition and Health Benefits of Functional Foods* (pp. 42–72). Hershey, PA: IGI Global. doi:10.4018/978-1-5225-0591-4.ch003

Garner, G. (2018). Foundations for Yoga Practice in Rehabilitation. In S. Telles & N. Singh (Eds.), *Research-Based Perspectives on the Psychophysiology of Yoga* (pp. 263–307). Hershey, PA: IGI Global. doi:10.4018/978-1-5225-2788-6.ch015

Gharote, M. (2018). Common Features Between Findings in Traditional Texts and Contemporary Science: Yoga Texts and Contemporary Science. In S. Telles & N. Singh (Eds.), *Research-Based Perspectives on the Psychophysiology of Yoga* (pp. 309–315). Hershey, PA: IGI Global. doi:10.4018/978-1-5225-2788-6.ch016

Griffiths, M. D., Kuss, D. J., & Ortiz de Gortari, A. B. (2017). Videogames as Therapy: An Updated Selective Review of the Medical and Psychological Literature. *International Journal of Privacy and Health Information Management, 5*(2), 71–96. doi:10.4018/IJPHIM.2017070105

Gupta, A. (2017). Functional Foods in Hypertension: Functional Foods in Cardiovascular Diseases. In H. Shekhar, Z. Howlader, & Y. Kabir (Eds.), *Exploring the Nutrition and Health Benefits of Functional Foods* (pp. 376–396). Hershey, PA: IGI Global. doi:10.4018/978-1-5225-0591-4.ch017

Gupta, C., Pacheco, C., & Prakash, D. (2018). Anti-Inflammatory Functional Foods. In A. Verma, K. Srivastava, S. Singh, & H. Singh (Eds.), *Nutraceuticals and Innovative Food Products for Healthy Living and Preventive Care* (pp. 48–78). Hershey, PA: IGI Global. doi:10.4018/978-1-5225-2970-5.ch003

Gupta, S. K., Chaudhary, K. K., & Mishra, N. (2017). Bioinformatics and Its Therapeutic Applications. In R. Keservani, A. Sharma, & R. Kesharwani (Eds.), *Recent Advances in Drug Delivery Technology* (pp. 125–158). Hershey, PA: IGI Global. doi:10.4018/978-1-5225-0754-3.ch005

Hagen, I., Kofoed, S., & Nayar, U. (2018). Yoga for Psychological Wellbeing in Modern Life and Contexts. In S. Telles & N. Singh (Eds.), *Research-Based Perspectives on the Psychophysiology of Yoga* (pp. 316–334). Hershey, PA: IGI Global. doi:10.4018/978-1-5225-2788-6.ch017

Hankey, A. (2018). Yoga and The Physics of Higher States of Consciousness. In S. Telles & N. Singh (Eds.), *Research-Based Perspectives on the Psychophysiology of Yoga* (pp. 335–358). Hershey, PA: IGI Global. doi:10.4018/978-1-5225-2788-6.ch018

Hartfiel, N., & Edwards, R. T. (2018). Research-Based Applied Psychophysiology: Yoga for Occupational Stress and Health. In S. Telles & N. Singh (Eds.), *Research-Based Perspectives on the Psychophysiology of Yoga* (pp. 175–183). Hershey, PA: IGI Global. doi:10.4018/978-1-5225-2788-6.ch010

Hemansi, V. R. K., Shukla, R., Gupta, R., & Saini, J. K. (2018). Food Grade Microorganisms for Nutraceutical Production for Industrial Applications. In A. Verma, K. Srivastava, S. Singh, & H. Singh (Eds.), Nutraceuticals and Innovative Food Products for Healthy Living and Preventive Care (pp. 342-367). Hershey, PA: IGI Global. doi:10.4018/978-1-5225-2970-5.ch016

Hernández-Ceruelos, A., Muñoz-Juarez, S., & Vázquez-Alvarado, P. (2017). Phytoparmaceuticals and Its Applications in Therapy. In R. Keservani, A. Sharma, & R. Kesharwani (Eds.), *Recent Advances in Drug Delivery Technology* (pp. 202–228). Hershey, PA: IGI Global. doi:10.4018/978-1-5225-0754-3.ch007

Howlader, M. Z., & Shekhar, H. U. (2017). Health Benefits and Risks of Rice. In H. Shekhar, Z. Howlader, & Y. Kabir (Eds.), *Exploring the Nutrition and Health Benefits of Functional Foods* (pp. 195–222). Hershey, PA: IGI Global. doi:10.4018/978-1-5225-0591-4.ch010

Ismail, T., Akhtar, S., & Riaz, M. (2017). Pomegranate Peel and Fruit Extracts: A Novel Approach to Avert Degenerative Disorders – Pomegranate and Degenerative Diseases. In H. Shekhar, Z. Howlader, & Y. Kabir (Eds.), *Exploring the Nutrition and Health Benefits of Functional Foods* (pp. 165–184). Hershey, PA: IGI Global. doi:10.4018/978-1-5225-0591-4.ch008

Jain, A., & Rani, V. (2017). Food and Cardiac Health: Protective Effects of Food on Cardiovascular System. In H. Shekhar, Z. Howlader, & Y. Kabir (Eds.), *Exploring the Nutrition and Health Benefits of Functional Foods* (pp. 1–15). Hershey, PA: IGI Global. doi:10.4018/978-1-5225-0591-4.ch001

Jarouliya, U., & Keservani, R. K. (2017). Genomics and Proteomic Approach in the Treatment of Various Human Diseases: Applications of Genomics and Proteomics. In R. Keservani, A. Sharma, & R. Kesharwani (Eds.), *Recent Advances in Drug Delivery Technology* (pp. 97–123). Hershey, PA: IGI Global. doi:10.4018/978-1-5225-0754-3.ch004

Joshi, R. K. (2017). A Perspective on the Phytopharmaceuticals Responsible for the Therapeutic Applications. In R. Keservani, A. Sharma, & R. Kesharwani (Eds.), *Recent Advances in Drug Delivery Technology* (pp. 229–262). Hershey, PA: IGI Global. doi:10.4018/978-1-5225-0754-3.ch008

Ju, K. H., & Eung-Soo, H. (2017). Health Promoting Effects of Kimchi. In H. Shekhar, Z. Howlader, & Y. Kabir (Eds.), *Exploring the Nutrition and Health Benefits of Functional Foods* (pp. 73–98). Hershey, PA: IGI Global. doi:10.4018/978-1-5225-0591-4.ch004

Kasemsap, K. (2018). Nutrition and Functional Foods: Current Trends and Issues. In A. Verma, K. Srivastava, S. Singh, & H. Singh (Eds.), *Nutraceuticals and Innovative Food Products for Healthy Living and Preventive Care* (pp. 158–175). Hershey, PA: IGI Global. doi:10.4018/978-1-5225-2970-5.ch007

Keservani, R. K., Sharma, A. K., & Kesharwani, R. K. (2017). An Overview and Therapeutic Applications of Nutraceutical and Functional Foods. In R. Keservani, A. Sharma, & R. Kesharwani (Eds.), *Recent Advances in Drug Delivery Technology* (pp. 160–201). Hershey, PA: IGI Global. doi:10.4018/978-1-5225-0754-3.ch006

Kondylakis, H., Hors-Fraile, S., Koumakis, L., Kouroubali, A., Notas, G., Rivero-Rodriguez, A., ... Katehakis, D. G. (2019). An Innovative, Information and Communication Technology Supported Approach, Towards Effective Chronic Pain Management. *International Journal of Reliable and Quality E-Healthcare*, *8*(1), 23–39. doi:10.4018/IJRQEH.2019010103

Kumar, B., Singh, S., Srivastava, K., & Wani, K. A. (2018). New Product Development and Regulatory Challenges in Nutraceutical Industry. In A. Verma, K. Srivastava, S. Singh, & H. Singh (Eds.), *Nutraceuticals and Innovative Food Products for Healthy Living and Preventive Care* (pp. 280–303). Hershey, PA: IGI Global. doi:10.4018/978-1-5225-2970-5.ch013

Lee, C. (2017). Application of the Dietary Processed Sulfur Supplementation for Enhancing Nutritional and Functional Properties of Meat Products. In H. Shekhar, Z. Howlader, & Y. Kabir (Eds.), *Exploring the Nutrition and Health Benefits of Functional Foods* (pp. 254–264). Hershey, PA: IGI Global. doi:10.4018/978-1-5225-0591-4.ch012

Manchanda, S., & Madan, K. (2018). Psychophysiological Rationale for Use of Yoga in Heart Disease. In S. Telles & N. Singh (Eds.), *Research-Based Perspectives on the Psychophysiology of Yoga* (pp. 203–217). Hershey, PA: IGI Global. doi:10.4018/978-1-5225-2788-6.ch012

Mayo, B., Guadamuro, L., Flórez, A. B., & Delgado, S. (2017). Soy and Soy Products, Isoflavones, Equol, and Health. In H. Shekhar, Z. Howlader, & Y. Kabir (Eds.), *Exploring the Nutrition and Health Benefits of Functional Foods* (pp. 223–253). Hershey, PA: IGI Global. doi:10.4018/978-1-5225-0591-4.ch011

Ming, L. C., Ang, W. C., Yang, Q., Thitilertdecha, P., Wong, T. W., & Khan, T. M. (2017). Cosmeceuticals: Safety, Efficacy and Potential Benefits. In R. Keservani, A. Sharma, & R. Kesharwani (Eds.), *Recent Advances in Drug Delivery Technology* (pp. 287–308). Hershey, PA: IGI Global. doi:10.4018/978-1-5225-0754-3.ch010

Mishra, A., Chaudhari, D. D., Patel, H. K., & Patel, B. D. (2018). Nutraceutical Properties of Important Weeds in India. In A. Verma, K. Srivastava, S. Singh, & H. Singh (Eds.), *Nutraceuticals and Innovative Food Products for Healthy Living and Preventive Care* (pp. 304–322). Hershey, PA: IGI Global. doi:10.4018/978-1-5225-2970-5.ch014

Mitra, S., & Khandelwal, S. (2017). Health Benefits of Tea: Beneficial Effects of Tea on Human Health. In H. Shekhar, Z. Howlader, & Y. Kabir (Eds.), *Exploring the Nutrition and Health Benefits of Functional Foods* (pp. 99–116). Hershey, PA: IGI Global. doi:10.4018/978-1-5225-0591-4.ch005

Mocenni, C., Montefrancesco, G., & Tiezzi, S. (2019). A Model of Spontaneous Remission From Addiction. *International Journal of Applied Behavioral Economics*, *8*(1), 21–48. doi:10.4018/IJABE.2019010102

Mudila, H., Prasher, P., Khati, B., Kumar, S., & Punetha, H. (2018). Nutraceuticals for Healthy Sporting. In A. Verma, K. Srivastava, S. Singh, & H. Singh (Eds.), *Nutraceuticals and Innovative Food Products for Healthy Living and Preventive Care* (pp. 79–107). Hershey, PA: IGI Global. doi:10.4018/978-1-5225-2970-5.ch004

Mukherjee, S. K., Kumar, J., Jha, A. K., & Rani, J. R. (2019). Role of Social Media Promotion of Prescription Drugs on Patient Belief-system and Behaviour. *International Journal of e-Collaboration*, *15*(2), 23–43. doi:10.4018/IJeC.2019040102

Muyonga, J. H., Nansereko, S., Steenkamp, I., Manley, M., & Okoth, J. K. (2017). Traditional African Foods and Their Potential to Contribute to Health and Nutrition: Traditional African Foods. In H. Shekhar, Z. Howlader, & Y. Kabir (Eds.), *Exploring the Nutrition and Health Benefits of Functional Foods* (pp. 320–346). Hershey, PA: IGI Global. doi:10.4018/978-1-5225-0591-4.ch015

Nagarathna, R., & Chaku, R. (2018). Research-Based Applied Psychophysiology: Yoga for Women's Health. In S. Telles & N. Singh (Eds.), *Research-Based Perspectives on the Psychophysiology of Yoga* (pp. 121–150). Hershey, PA: IGI Global. doi:10.4018/978-1-5225-2788-6.ch008

Narahari, S., Aggithaya, M. G., & Ryan, T. J. (2018). Research-Based Applied Psychophysiology: Yoga as a Therapy for Lymphedema. In S. Telles & N. Singh (Eds.), *Research-Based Perspectives on the Psychophysiology of Yoga* (pp. 241–262). Hershey, PA: IGI Global. doi:10.4018/978-1-5225-2788-6.ch014

Olsen, E. H. (2018). Yoga in the Treatment of Trauma-Related Disorders: Connecting the Body and the Mind. In S. Telles & N. Singh (Eds.), *Research-Based Perspectives on the Psychophysiology of Yoga* (pp. 218–240). Hershey, PA: IGI Global. doi:10.4018/978-1-5225-2788-6.ch013

Paholpak, P., Obler, L., & Lavretsky, H. (2018). Yoga for Seniors: Mechanisms of Response to Yoga Therapy in Older Adults. In S. Telles & N. Singh (Eds.), *Research-Based Perspectives on the Psychophysiology of Yoga* (pp. 151–174). Hershey, PA: IGI Global. doi:10.4018/978-1-5225-2788-6.ch009

Passi, S. J. (2017). Functional Foods and Cardiac Health. In H. Shekhar, Z. Howlader, & Y. Kabir (Eds.), *Exploring the Nutrition and Health Benefits of Functional Foods* (pp. 16–41). Hershey, PA: IGI Global. doi:10.4018/978-1-5225-0591-4.ch002

Patel, J. N., & Villadolid, J. (2017). Cancer Drug Delivery: Pharmacogenetics, Biomarkers, and Targeted Therapies. In R. Keservani, A. Sharma, & R. Kesharwani (Eds.), *Recent Advances in Drug Delivery Technology* (pp. 52–95). Hershey, PA: IGI Global. doi:10.4018/978-1-5225-0754-3.ch003

Peine, K. J., Chen, N., Bachelder, E. M., & Ainslie, K. M. (2017). Drug Delivery Strategies for Tolerogenic Therapy for Autoimmune Diseases in an Antigen-Specific Manner. In R. Keservani, A. Sharma, & R. Kesharwani (Eds.), *Recent Advances in Drug Delivery Technology* (pp. 23–51). Hershey, PA: IGI Global. doi:10.4018/978-1-5225-0754-3.ch002

Poonia, A. (2017). Antimicrobial Edible Films and Coatings for Fruits and Vegetables. In H. Shekhar, Z. Howlader, & Y. Kabir (Eds.), *Exploring the Nutrition and Health Benefits of Functional Foods* (pp. 301–319). Hershey, PA: IGI Global. doi:10.4018/978-1-5225-0591-4.ch014

Prakash, D., & Gupta, C. (2017). Phytopharmaceutical Applications of Nutraceutical and Functional Foods. In R. Keservani, A. Sharma, & R. Kesharwani (Eds.), *Recent Advances in Drug Delivery Technology* (pp. 263–285). Hershey, PA: IGI Global. doi:10.4018/978-1-5225-0754-3.ch009

Punetha, H., Kumar, S., Mudila, H., & Prakash, O. (2018). Brassica Meal as Source of Health Protecting Neuraceutical and Its Antioxidative Properties. In A. Verma, K. Srivastava, S. Singh, & H. Singh (Eds.), *Nutraceuticals and Innovative Food Products for Healthy Living and Preventive Care* (pp. 108–131). Hershey, PA: IGI Global. doi:10.4018/978-1-5225-2970-5.ch005

Santaella, D. F., Afonso, R. F., & Kozasa, E. H. (2018). Neurobiology of Yoga Practice. In S. Telles & N. Singh (Eds.), *Research-Based Perspectives on the Psychophysiology of Yoga* (pp. 52–66). Hershey, PA: IGI Global. doi:10.4018/978-1-5225-2788-6.ch004

Sen, S., & Chakraborty, R. (2017). Food in Health Preservation and Promotion: A Special Focus on the Interplay between Oxidative Stress and Pro-Oxidant/Antioxidant. In H. Shekhar, Z. Howlader, & Y. Kabir (Eds.), *Exploring the Nutrition and Health Benefits of Functional Foods* (pp. 265–300). Hershey, PA: IGI Global. doi:10.4018/978-1-5225-0591-4.ch013

Sidhu, J. S., & Zafar, T. A. (2017). Functional Foods of the Indian Subcontinent. In H. Shekhar, Z. Howlader, & Y. Kabir (Eds.), *Exploring the Nutrition and Health Benefits of Functional Foods* (pp. 347–375). Hershey, PA: IGI Global. doi:10.4018/978-1-5225-0591-4.ch016

Singh, P., Singh, S., & Kesharwani, R. K. (2017). Resealed Erythrocytes as Drug Carriers and Its Therapeutic Applications. In R. Keservani, A. Sharma, & R. Kesharwani (Eds.), *Recent Advances in Drug Delivery Technology* (pp. 340–366). Hershey, PA: IGI Global. doi:10.4018/978-1-5225-0754-3.ch012

Singh, U. P. (2018). Psychophysiological Effects of Yoga for Adults With Occupational Stress: Yoga in the Workplace. In S. Telles & N. Singh (Eds.), *Research-Based Perspectives on the Psychophysiology of Yoga* (pp. 359–382). Hershey, PA: IGI Global. doi:10.4018/978-1-5225-2788-6.ch019

Tangkiatkumjai, M. (2018). An Overview of Publications of Complementary and Alternative Medicine Research. In M. Tangkiatkumjai, A. Casarin, L. Chen, & D. Walker (Eds.), *Complementary and Alternative Medicine and Kidney Health* (pp. 43–59). Hershey, PA: IGI Global. doi:10.4018/978-1-5225-2882-1.ch003

Tangkiatkumjai, M., & Casarin, A. (2018). Integrative Medicine and Prospective Research on CAM. In M. Tangkiatkumjai, A. Casarin, L. Chen, & D. Walker (Eds.), *Complementary and Alternative Medicine and Kidney Health* (pp. 272–301). Hershey, PA: IGI Global. doi:10.4018/978-1-5225-2882-1.ch010

Tangkiatkumjai, M., & Kreepala, C. (2018). General Approach to Evaluating Beneficial and Adverse Effects of CAM Use in Kidney Diseases. In M. Tangkiatkumjai, A. Casarin, L. Chen, & D. Walker (Eds.), *Complementary and Alternative Medicine and Kidney Health* (pp. 60–99). Hershey, PA: IGI Global. doi:10.4018/978-1-5225-2882-1.ch004

Tangkiatkumjai, M., Kreepala, C., & Chen, L. (2018). Efficacy and Safety of CAM in Kidney Diseases. In M. Tangkiatkumjai, A. Casarin, L. Chen, & D. Walker (Eds.), *Complementary and Alternative Medicine and Kidney Health* (pp. 156–200). Hershey, PA: IGI Global. doi:10.4018/978-1-5225-2882-1.ch007

Tangkiatkumjai, M., Winit-Watjana, W., & Chen, L. (2018). How to Search and Critique Scientific Evidence for Decision-Making. In M. Tangkiatkumjai, A. Casarin, L. Chen, & D. Walker (Eds.), *Complementary and Alternative Medicine and Kidney Health* (pp. 100–123). Hershey, PA: IGI Global. doi:10.4018/978-1-5225-2882-1.ch005

Telles, S., & Sharma, S. K. (2018). Management of Obesity With Yoga: A Review. In S. Telles & N. Singh (Eds.), *Research-Based Perspectives on the Psychophysiology of Yoga* (pp. 185–202). Hershey, PA: IGI Global. doi:10.4018/978-1-5225-2788-6.ch011

Telles, S., & Singh, N. (2018). The Psychophysiology of Yoga Regulated Breathing (Pranayamas). In S. Telles & N. Singh (Eds.), *Research-Based Perspectives on the Psychophysiology of Yoga* (pp. 17–34). Hershey, PA: IGI Global. doi:10.4018/978-1-5225-2788-6.ch002

Thakur, K., Zhang, J. G., Wei, Z., Kumar, N., Tomar, S. K., & Pophaly, S. D. (2018). Cross Talk Between Functional Foods and Gut Health. In A. Verma, K. Srivastava, S. Singh, & H. Singh (Eds.), *Nutraceuticals and Innovative Food Products for Healthy Living and Preventive Care* (pp. 195–216). Hershey, PA: IGI Global. doi:10.4018/978-1-5225-2970-5.ch009

Travis, F. T. (2018). Long-Term Changes in Experienced Yoga Practitioners: Growth of Higher States of Consciousness. In S. Telles & N. Singh (Eds.), *Research-Based Perspectives on the Psychophysiology of Yoga* (pp. 35–51). Hershey, PA: IGI Global. doi:10.4018/978-1-5225-2788-6.ch003

Udupa, K., & Sathyaprabha, T. N. (2018). Influence of Yoga on the Autonomic Nervous System. In S. Telles & N. Singh (Eds.), *Research-Based Perspectives on the Psychophysiology of Yoga* (pp. 67–85). Hershey, PA: IGI Global. doi:10.4018/978-1-5225-2788-6.ch005

Uvanesh, K., Nayak, S. K., Sagiri, S. S., Banerjee, I., Ray, S. S., & Pal, K. (2018). Effect of Non-Ionic Hydrophilic and Hydrophobic Surfactants on the Properties on the Stearate Oleogels: A Comparative Study. In A. Verma, K. Srivastava, S. Singh, & H. Singh (Eds.), *Nutraceuticals and Innovative Food Products for Healthy Living and Preventive Care* (pp. 260–279). Hershey, PA: IGI Global. doi:10.4018/978-1-5225-2970-5.ch012

Verma, A. K., Singh, A., & Negi, M. S. (2018). Nutriproteomics: An Advance Methodology of Nutrichemical Analysis. In A. Verma, K. Srivastava, S. Singh, & H. Singh (Eds.), *Nutraceuticals and Innovative Food Products for Healthy Living and Preventive Care* (pp. 1–23). Hershey, PA: IGI Global. doi:10.4018/978-1-5225-2970-5.ch001

Vlasova, M., & Smirin, B. V. (2017). Personalized Approach in Nanomedicine: Understanding Adverse Effects and Their Risk Assessment. In R. Keservani, A. Sharma, & R. Kesharwani (Eds.), *Recent Advances in Drug Delivery Technology* (pp. 1–21). Hershey, PA: IGI Global. doi:10.4018/978-1-5225-0754-3.ch001

Vorkapic, C. F. (2018). Yoga for Children. In S. Telles & N. Singh (Eds.), *Research-Based Perspectives on the Psychophysiology of Yoga* (pp. 104–120). Hershey, PA: IGI Global. doi:10.4018/978-1-5225-2788-6.ch007

Walker, D., & Tangkiatkumjai, M. (2018). CAM Use From Western and Asian Perspectives: Overview of Different Cultural Beliefs of CAM Medicine and Prevalence of Use. In M. Tangkiatkumjai, A. Casarin, L. Chen, & D. Walker (Eds.), *Complementary and Alternative Medicine and Kidney Health* (pp. 24–42). Hershey, PA: IGI Global. doi:10.4018/978-1-5225-2882-1.ch002

Wani, K. A., Manzoor, J., Anjum, J., Bashir, M., & Mamta. (2018). Pesticides in Vegetables: Their Impact on Nutritional Quality and Human Health. In A. Verma, K. Srivastava, S. Singh, & H. Singh (Eds.), *Nutraceuticals and Innovative Food Products for Healthy Living and Preventive Care* (pp. 132-157). Hershey, PA: IGI Global. doi:10.4018/978-1-5225-2970-5.ch006

Wilson, M., & Shaw, M. R. (2017). Participant Perspectives on Benefits and Challenges of Engaging in an Online Pain Self-Management Program. *International Journal of Healthcare Information Systems and Informatics, 12*(4), 52–67. doi:10.4018/IJHISI.2017100104

Yadav, D., Pandey, V., Srivastava, S., & Tripathi, Y. B. (2017). New Herbal Approaches for the Treatment of Diabetic Kidney Diseases and Its Therapeutic Implications. In R. Keservani, A. Sharma, & R. Kesharwani (Eds.), *Recent Advances in Drug Delivery Technology* (pp. 368–406). Hershey, PA: IGI Global. doi:10.4018/978-1-5225-0754-3.ch013

Yagil, R. (2017). Cosmeceuticals: Camel and Other Milk – Natural Skin Maintenance. In R. Keservani, A. Sharma, & R. Kesharwani (Eds.), *Recent Advances in Drug Delivery Technology* (pp. 309–338). Hershey, PA: IGI Global. doi:10.4018/978-1-5225-0754-3.ch011

Index

G

H

I

J

M

N

O

P

Q

R

www.ingramcontent.com/pod-product-compliance
Lightning Source LLC
LaVergne TN
LVHW080606300926
849162LV00005B/1061